Forensic Learning Series

Domestic Violence
and Nonfatal
Strangulation Assessment

for Health Care Providers and First Responders

Forensic Learning Series

STM **Learning,** Inc.

Leading Publisher of Scientific, Technical, and Medical Educational Resources

Saint Louis

www.stmlearning.com

Domestic Violence
and Nonfatal
Strangulation Assessment

for Health Care Providers and First Responders

Forensic Learning Series

Diana K. Faugno, MSN, RN, CPN, SANE-A, SANE-P, FAAFS, DF-IAFN, DF-AFN
Forensic Nurse
Founding Board Director
End Violence Against Women International
Past President
Academy of Forensic Nursing

Valerie Sievers, MSN, RN, CNS, SANE-A, SANE-P, DF-AFN
Forensic Clinical Nurse Specialist
Forensic Healthcare Consultant
MedLaw Consultants, LLC

Michelle Shores, MSN, RN, MBA-HC, CEN, SANE-A, SANE-P
Director
Forensic Health Services
Palomar Health

Bill Smock, MD
Police Surgeon
Louisville Metro Police Department
Louisville, Kentucky
Medical Director
The Training Institute on Strangulation Prevention
San Diego, California

Patricia M. Speck, DNSc, CRNP, FNP-BC, DF-IAFN, FAAFS, DF-AFN, FAAN
Professor and Coordinator of Advanced Forensic Nursing
Department of Family, Community, & Health Systems
The University of Alabama at Birmingham School of Nursing

STM **Learning,** Inc.

Leading Publisher of Scientific, Technical, and Medical Educational Resources
Saint Louis
www.stmlearning.com

Publishers: Glenn E. Whaley and Marianne V. Whaley
Graphic Design Director: Glenn E. Whaley
Acquisitions Editor: Glenn E. Whaley
Associate Editor: Marika Betker
Book Design/Page Layout: Jennifer M. Jones and Glenn E. Whaley
Print/Production Coordinator: Jennifer M. Jones and Glenn E. Whaley
Cover Design: Jennifer M. Jones and Glenn E. Whaley
Color Prepress Specialist: Kevin Tucker
Developmental Editor: Marika Betker
Copy Editor: Marika Betker
Proofreader: Samantha Koester

Printed in the United States of America.

Publisher:
STM Learning, Inc.
Saint Louis, Missouri 63033
Phone: (314) 434-2424
http://www.stmlearning.com orders@stmlearning.com

Library of Congress Cataloging-in-Publication Data

Names: Faugno, Diana K., 1950- author. | Sievers, Valerie, author. | Shores, Michelle, author. | Smock, William S., author. | Speck, Patricia M., 1948- author.
Title: Domestic violence and nonfatal strangulation assessment for health care providers and first responders / Diana Faugno, Valerie Sievers, Michelle Shores, William Smock, Patricia M. Speck.
Other titles: SANE/SAFE forensic learning series.
Description: St. Louis, MO : STM Learning, Inc., [2020] | Series: Forensic learning series | Includes bibliographical references.
Identifiers: LCCN 2020004507 (print) | LCCN 2020004508 (ebook) | ISBN 9781936590834 (paperback) | ISBN 9781936590841 (epub)
Subjects: MESH: Domestic Violence | Asphyxia--diagnosis | Asphyxia--pathology | Forensic Medicine | Problems and Exercises | Case Reports
Classification: LCC RA1071 (print) | LCC RA1071 (ebook) | NLM W 618.2 | DDC 617.1/8--dc23
LC record available at https://lccn.loc.gov/2020004507
LC ebook record available at https://lccn.loc.gov/2020004508

Contributors

Kathryn L. Bell, MS, RN, SANE-A, SANE-P, DF-AFN
Forensic Nursing Administrator
Tulsa Police Department

Lynn Crosby, BSN, RN, SANE
liveSAFE Resources

Christine Foote-Lucero, MSN, RN, CEN, SANE-A, SANE-P
Forensic Program Manager
University of Colorado Hospital

Karen Marcus, RN, BS, SANE-A
Forensic Nurse
Forensic Health Services
Palomar Health

Sarah Marin, FNP-C, MSN, SANE-A, SANE-P
Forensic Nurse Practitioner
SART/Child Abuse
Forensic Nurses of SoCal, Inc.

Keri Sandy, RN, SANE-A
Forensic RN
Palomar Health Forensic Services

Angelia Trujillo, DNP, MS, RN, WHNP-BC, DF-AFN
Associate Professor of Nursing
University of Alaska Anchorage

Our Mission

To become the world leader in publishing and information services on child abuse, maltreatment, diseases, and domestic violence. We seek to heighten awareness of these issues and provide relevant information to professionals and consumers.

Foreword

As a forensic nurse with more than 17 years of experience working with victims of violence across the lifespan, I am pleased to have been given the opportunity to write the foreword to *Domestic Violence and Nonfatal Strangulation Assessment for Health Care Providers and First Responders*, part of the Forensic Learning Series. I have had the opportunity to work with the editors and many of the contributors to this text over the years, and I consider them colleagues and mentors working to improve the response to victims of violence.

The *Manual Nonfatal Strangulation Assessment* was published January 2017 as a part of STM Learning's Forensic Learning Series because the editors realized the need for training related to nonfatal strangulation assessment and care. Now, 3 years later, the editors and contributors to this text have updated the training manual for nonfatal strangulation to encompass domestic violence, male victim strangulation, and cases among the young and the old. There are a wide range of specialties that need a working knowledge of domestic violence and strangulation, including, but not limited to, nursing, medicine, emergency medical services, law enforcement, and legal system agencies. This text is designed to serve as:

— A companion resource to the other titles in the Forensic Learning Series

— An educational resource for forensic nurses seeking to prepare for specialty certification

— A valuable resource for the generalist

— An adjunct resource for nonmedical team disciplines

— An interdisciplinary text recognizing the common knowledge and unique skills of the multidisciplinary team

The editors and contributors bring decades of combined experience to the issue of strangulation assault, its impact on the human body, and the emotional impact to the victim whether they are male or female, young or old. The text relies on the use of standardized language, case studies, and case photographs to support the learning needs of health care providers responding to victims of domestic violence and strangulation. Unique case histories represent the myriad types of violence that impact men and women across the lifespan and the role that strangulation plays in the power and control sought by perpetrators of interpersonal violence. Chapters provide anatomic resources and activities for learning, and they demonstrate best practices for evidence collection, injury care, treatment, and follow-up examination options to serve victims of violence from the initial first responder to physicians/providers, hospitalists, and forensic examiners.

Recognition of strangulation injury and its sequelae has come a long way from a few short years ago when strangulation was considered "just choking," to today, when nonfatal manual strangulation is now recognized as a felony and life-threatening crime. These changes were due much in part to the work of the editors and contributors herein. It is my expectation that this book will provide an effective educational and reference tool for health professionals caring for victims of strangulation.

Angelia Trujillo, DNP, MS, RN, WHNP-BC, DF-AFN
Associate Professor of Nursing
University of Alaska Anchorage

Foreword

"Tell me and I forget, teach me and I may remember, involve me and I learn."

— Benjamin Franklin

It took the murders of 2 San Diego teenagers in 1995 to understand the seriousness and lethality of nonfatal strangulation. Before Casondra Steward and Tamara Smith were killed by their ex-partners, they were "choked." Both of them called the police for help, but neither case was prosecuted because of a lack of sufficient evidence to prove an assault had occurred. As former prosecutors, we should have known more and done more. Back then, we called them "choking" cases, and most choking cases were handled as misdemeanors or simply not prosecuted at all. It was the rare case where strangulation was charged and prosecuted as a felony. We were trained to look for external signs of injury, and many prosecutors believed you needed a cooperative victim to prove a choking case, including testifying about her injuries. But choking victims often said they were fine and rarely requested paramedics or sought medical attention. They often would not remember the details of the assault. This seemed like it made the case even weaker. The usually said they were "fine" or "okay," and it caused us to think they were fine too. But we were wrong.

The deaths of Casondra and Tamara triggered profound changes in San Diego. After their deaths, we needed answers. The San Diego City Attorney's Office immediately launched one of the first and largest studies of nonfatal strangulation cases by conducting a careful analysis of 300 cases submitted for prosecution by the San Diego Police Department. The results of that study proved that most victims of strangulation did not present with visible injuries; however, there were subtle, identifiable signs and symptoms that could be documented by well-trained professionals. With the support of adequate laws, protocols, and leadership, the cases could be handled much more effectively.

Today, it is understood unequivocally that strangulation is one of the most lethal forms of domestic violence. Victims may have no visible injuries, but because of underlying brain damage or other internal injuries caused by the lack of oxygen during the strangulation assault, they may sustain serious internal injuries. They may die days or weeks after the attack because of a stroke, suffer a traumatic brain injury, or experience other long-term physical and mental health consequences. Nonfatal strangulation and suffocation assaults are also more prevalent than we realized years ago, with prevalence rates between 68% to 80% for high-risk domestic violence victims.

When a victim is strangled, she is at the edge of a homicide. Strangulation is one of the most accurate predictors for the subsequent homicide of victims of domestic violence. One study showed that the odds of becoming an attempted homicide victim increased by about seven fold for women who had been strangled by their partner. Women who are strangled multiple times are at even higher risk.

Strangulation has also been linked to officer-involved critical incidents, officers killed in the line of duty in intentional homicides, and mass murders. The research clearly shows the need for all professionals to improve their screening and documentation of strangulation cases. When working with a strangled victim, advocates, detectives, nurses, and prosecutors must all make good use of risk assessment tools, encourage medical treatment, create personalized safety plans, and offer long-term follow-up. Today, we know far more about strangulation than we knew in 1995.

It is now our responsibility to do something about it. We cannot continue to hear the words "He choked me," and treat this assault like we would a slap or a punch. The difference between life and death in most strangulation assaults is only a matter of seconds. We have an opportunity to stop stranglers before they kill, but we must seize that opportunity.

We must learn to more effectively investigate and prosecute near-fatal and nonfatal strangulation assaults as felony offenses even with little or no external visible injury. We must pursue these complicated cases even without victim participation or testimony whenever possible. We must work in Family Justice Centers and multidisciplinary teams to effectively hold offenders accountable and provide the victim the medical advocacy and support survivors need. Every time we hold a strangler accountable, we reduce the likelihood of a homicide, and we send a message to men who strangle and suffocate women: We see you, and we will not let you commit life-threatening and often brain-damaging assaults with impunity.

Thankfully, 25 years later, San Diego has figured it out and is leading the way in felony strangulation prosecutions with a 96% conviction rate thanks to a county-wide protocol that includes strong on-scene and follow-up investigation; domestic violence and strangulation medical assessments by forensic nurses; expert testimony; and specially trained dispatchers, paramedics, prosecutors, and probation officers.

The authors of the *Domestic Violence and Nonfatal Strangulation Assessment,* Diana Faugno, Valerie Sievers, Michelle Shores, Patricia Speck, and William Smock, are some of the leading experts in the field of nonfatal strangulation. They all serve as advisors, mentors, faculty, and friends of our internationally recognized Training Institute on Strangulation Prevention, which we officially launched in 2011.

There is a growing body of peer-reviewed articles published in medical, social science, and legal journals about all aspects of nonfatal strangulation cases, including signs and symptoms, internal injuries, and delayed or long-term consequences. Education and training for professionals who deal with strangulation patients has dramatically improved. Advancements in the field now allow for more accurate evaluations of findings, or lack of findings, in strangulation patients.

Domestic Violence and Nonfatal Strangulation Assessment for Health Care Providers and First Responders is one of those valuable tools available to all disciplines. This workbook will allow both new and experienced practitioners the opportunity to build skills in identification, documentation, assessment, and treatment of strangulation assaults. We strongly recommend this material as a valuable addition to every basic training curriculum and to every professional handling nonfatal strangulation cases, but especially to medical and emergency medical services professionals. Had this workbook been available back in 1995, we are confident both Casondra and Tamara would be alive today because police officers and prosecutors would have known how to investigate and prosecute these cases, victims would have been adequately assessed and treated by medical professionals, and offenders would have been held accountable for their crimes.

Thank you, Diana, Valerie, Michelle, Patricia, and Bill for creating this powerful, effective tool for the field. It will be a lifesaver and a hope-giver.

Gael Strack, Esq.
CEO & Co-Founder
Training Institute on Strangulation Prevention
A Project of Alliance for HOPE International

Casey Gwinn, Esq.
President & Co-Founder
Training Institute on Strangulation Prevention
A Project of Alliance for HOPE International

Preface

In the last 35 years, the published literature has evolved to address violence against women with a variety of titles and terms including: battered wives, battered women syndrome, domestic violence, and perhaps the more widely used reference, intimate partner violence. According to the Centers for Disease Control and Prevention,[1] the overall definition for intimate partner violence includes physical violence, sexual violence, stalking, and psychological aggression (including coercive tactics) by a current or former intimate partner (ie, spouse, boyfriend/girlfriend, dating partner, or ongoing sexual partner). Physical violence is defined as the intentional use of physical force with the potential for causing death, disability, injury, or harm. Physical violence includes, but is not limited to scratching, pushing, shoving, throwing, grabbing, biting, ***choking***, shaking, hair-pulling, slapping, punching, hitting, burning, use of a weapon (gun, knife, or other object), and use of restraints or one's body, size, or strength against another person.[1]

Currently, intimate partner violence is widely recognized as a public health issue. In the past 17 years, recognition of nonfatal strangulation within the context of intimate partner violence has garnered a lot of attention, largely in response to a seminal study that has helped to shape law enforcement responses, health care practice, legislation, and research. The study of 300 victims of nonfatal strangulation conducted in San Diego identified that most victims reporting strangulation lacked physical, observable injuries; 50% of the victims had no visible injuries, and 35% of the victims had injuries too minor to photograph. Additionally, many of these victims did not present or were not referred to an emergency department for evaluation.[2] The impact of early studies has increased awareness that nonfatal strangulation is more serious than has previously been considered and may have been the impetus for legislation and developing best practices for clinical evaluation and treatment recommendations.[3]

While much of the published literature on nonfatal strangulation has identified that women of child-bearing age are most often the victims of this form of trauma, other vulnerable populations cannot be overlooked by health care and law enforcement professionals, including children and the elderly. Professionals providing a response to these vulnerable groups should also consider that these patients may have been injured by forms of smothering or suffocation.

In 44 states and the District of Columbia, health care professionals are obligated to report elder abuse to adult protective services.[4] Elder abuse is defined as an intentional act, or failure to act, by a caregiver or another person in a relationship involving an expectation of trust that causes or creates a risk of harm to an older adult. (An older adult is defined as someone age 60 or older.) Forms of elder abuse are recognized to include physical abuse, sexual abuse or abusive sexual contact, emotional or psychological abuse, neglect, and financial abuse or exploitation.[5]

The incidence of strangulation and subtle nature of associated symptoms and injury are not easily distinguished if health care professionals, law enforcement, and pre-hospital personnel are not exposed to education and training about identification, screen-

1. *Breiding MJ, Basile KC, Smith SG, Black MC, Mahendra RR. Intimate Partner Violence Surveillance: Uniform Definitions and Recommended Data Elements, Version 2.0. Atlanta, GA: National Center for Injury Prevention and Control, Centers for Disease Control and Prevention; 2015.*
2. *Strack GB, McClane, GE, Hawley, D. A review of 300 attempted strangulation cases part I: criminal legal issues.* J Emerg Med. *2001;21(3):303-309.*
3. *McClane, GE, Strack, GB, Hawley, D. A review of 300 attempted strangulation cases part II: clinical evaluation of the surviving victim.* J Emerg Med. *2001;21(3):311-315.*
4. *Daly JM, Jogerst GJ. Statute definitions of elder abuse.* J Elder Abuse Negl. *2003;13(4):39-57.*
5. *Hall, JE, Karch, DL, Crosby, AE. Elder Abuse Surveillance: Uniform Definitions and Recommended Core Data Elements for Use in Elder Abuse Surveillance, Version 1.0. Atlanta (GA): National Center for Injury Prevention and Control, Centers for Disease Control and Prevention, 2016.*

ing, assessment, and treatment. In addition, forensic nurses have a pivotal role in not only evaluating patients seen after strangulation, but providing in depth evidentiary examinations and accurate medical-forensic documentation. A variety of case studies, best practice recommendations, and tools to support evaluation and documentation are reviewed in the following chapters.

Diana K. Faugno, MSN, RN, CPN, SANE-A, SANE-P, FAAFS, DF-IAFN, DF-AFN
Valerie Sievers, MSN, RN, CNS, SANE-A, SANE-P, DF-AFN
Michelle Shores, MSN, RN, MBA-HC, CEN, SANE-A, SANE-P
Bill Smock, MD
Patricia M. Speck, DNSc, CRNP, FNP-BC, DF-IAFN, FAAFS, DF-AFN, FAAN

Reviews

Domestic Violence and Nonfatal Strangulation Assessment *is a valuable tool to educate first responders, SAFE/SANE nurses, and medical providers on how to assess, document, and treat victims of nonfatal strangulation. It starts by standardizing basic definitions and moves on to discuss the anatomy, signs and symptoms, and injuries seen in victims of strangulation. Information on the various imaging modalities and what each specific technique visualizes is provided. The multiple case studies, along with the resources in the appendices and the recommended readings, serve to standardize our documentation. This book provides invaluable, evidence-based information to both novice providers and experienced providers alike.*

Rosalyn Berkowitz, BSN, RN, FNE A/P
Forensic Nurse Examiner
SAFE and Domestic Violence Program
Greater Baltimore Medical Center
Towson, Maryland

Strangulation victims most often do not have signs or symptoms of strangulation. The Domestic Violence and Nonfatal Strangulation Assessment *is very important to implement in every health care provider's practice. This guide does a great job presenting case studies from everyday practice and gives you the knowledge you will need to assess the strangulation victim while using the best evidence-based practices and tools. Photos are used to discuss the anatomic location of common injuries and proper documentation of those injuries. Safety and proper discharge planning are essential in these patients and are discussed in the guide with great resource recommendations for the victims. Overall, this an excellent guide from a very knowledgeable group of expert authors.*

Natalie Calow, MSN, RN, CEN
Forensic Nurse
IUH Methodist Hospital
Indianapolis, Indiana

The case studies used in this comprehensive guide can be extremely helpful for newer forensic nurses or for those working in rural areas that may not have seen the volume of forensic examinations a busier metropolitan area has. The pictures and activities at the end of each chapter will help prepare these nurses for the injuries they might see during a strangulation examination.

Kristin Hall, BSN, RN, CEN
Clinical Director
Family Justice Center SANE

The Domestic Violence and Nonfatal Strangulation Assessment for Health Care Providers and First Responders *will be a tremendous asset for those that encounter a victim of strangulation. Often, first responders may not be trained on the signs and symptoms of a strangulation assault and may overlook some important information and assessments. The use of case studies and imaging in this guidebook will assist first responders and health care providers in recognizing some of the physical signs that may be present, but also the verbal identifiers the victim may report. This guide will provide a quick and easily accessible reference to understand the uniqueness of this form of violence and provide the necessary steps to provide the best practice initial care and compassion these individuals will need upon first contact with health care or law enforcement.*

Lori Combs, BS, RN, LNC
Forensic Nurse Expert/Forensic Consultant
Critical Analysis Consulting RN
Fort Myers/Cape Coral, Florida

Domestic Violence and Nonfatal Strangulation Assessment for Health Care Providers and First Responders *is a collection of case studies that presents relevant discussions and activities to enhance the user's knowledge base surrounding nonfatal strangulation. Leaders in the field have compiled pertinent case studies, including photographs, which promote discussion of the challenges surrounding nonfatal strangulation cases and provide best practice recommendations for these cases. We keep this workbook in our "library." It is used as a teaching aid and reference for SANEs.*

Each case study provides an anatomic skill review that reinforces areas of interest or concern when caring for victims of nonfatal strangulation. An injury identification activity for each case study provides visual cues for photodocumentation and can bolster the provider's documentation skills by incorporating key descriptive words to use when describing findings. Case studies also provide activities to enhance the user's assessment and evidence collection skills. Activities are designed to encourage the user to outline appropriate care and referrals for each patient.

Jennifer Knowlton, RN, SANE-A
Chief Executive Officer
Chesapeake Forensic Specialists
Chesapeake, Virginia

This workbook lays the foundation of fundamental concepts necessary for evidence-based clinical and medical-forensic assessment and care of the strangulation patient. It addresses key information that underlies the background and dynamics of domestic violence and applies it toward a holistic care approach. Each case study looks at the unique medical and psychosocial implications. A literature-based discussion is provided, which drives clinical decision making, safety planning, and mental and behavioral health guidance. Health care providers can rely on this resource to enhance their care plans to meet the comprehensive set of needs of the strangulation patient.

Amber O'Malley, MSN, RN, SANE-A, SANE-P
Forensic Nurse Examiner
NWA Forensic Nurses
Bentonville, Arkansas

The Domestic Violence and Nonfatal Strangulation Assessment *is an outstanding guide for those who provide care to victims of domestic and intimate partner violence affected by strangulation. This workbook is all-encompassing and addresses the physical, mental, emotional, social, and legal challenges victims and providers experience when providing care to those impacted by violence. It highlights evidence-based practice screening tools, diagnostic testing, assessment pearls, evidence collection, and resources, enhancing a provider's ability to deliver safe, quality, comprehensive medical-forensic treatment and care. This workbook is not only a must-read for forensic nurses, but for all health care providers.*

Jennifer Barrett, MSN, RN, CNS, SANE-A, SANE-P
Sexual Assault Nurse Examiner,
Forensic Clinical Nurse Specialist
Denver Health Medical Center
Denver, Colorado

Contents in Brief

Contents in Detail

Domestic Violence
and Nonfatal
Strangulation Assessment

for Health Care Providers and First Responders

Forensic Learning Series

STM **Learning,** Inc.

Leading Publisher of Scientific, Technical, and Medical Educational Resources
Saint Louis
www.stmlearning.com

Section I

Definitions and Anatomic Review

Objectives

After reviewing the information presented in this section, the participant will be able to:

1. *Identify anatomic structures of the neck.*
2. *Define strangulation and the language associated with strangulation.*
3. *Describe the possible signs and symptoms experienced during and after strangulation.*
4. *Recognize the different presentations of complications occurring after strangulation.*
5. *Critically analyze recommended treatment pathways for the patient who experiences strangulation.*

Instructions

An anatomic diagram of the neck helps the participant correctly identify anatomic landmarks. Participants, refer to the anatomic diagram using definitions that follow for documentation of normal anatomy, identifying and describing injury, and noting other conditions or findings throughout *Domestic Violence and Nonfatal Strangulation Assessment.*

Additionally, the authors encourage participants to review the sections on presenting and developing symptoms, the potential for lethality, and recommended assessments and treatment as a supplement to the exercises in *Domestic Violence and Nonfatal Strangulation Assessment.* With the structured learning presented in this publication, students will familiarize themselves with signs and symptoms of strangulation and current treatment recommendations available to better identify and respond to cases of strangulation and properly document visible physical injuries.

Strangulation Language and Definitions

— ***Abrasion (scratches and scrapes):*** Superficial injuries to the skin that are limited to the epidermis and superficial dermis. Abrasions are normally caused by rubbing, sliding, or compressive forces against the skin.[1] A variety of traumatic abrasions may result from strangulation:

— ***Chin abrasion:*** Incurred when, in an effort to protect the neck, the victim instinctively lowers the head and creates a compression sliding of the chin against whatever is applying external pressure to the neck.

— ***Impression mark abrasion:*** Occurs when fingernails abrade the skin leaving a curvilinear (ie, semicircular) mark(s).

— ***Ligature mark abrasions:*** Typically horizontal abrasions left on the neck that follow a predictable pattern. Distinguishable from suicidal hanging marks because the suicidal suspension ligature mark rises diagonally toward the ear. However, if pressure is applied with a ligature at an upward angle, the mark may be indistinguishable from suicidal hanging marks.

— ***Scratch mark abrasion:*** Long, superficial abrasions that may be as wide or narrow as the fingernail itself. Scratch marks may be caused by the assailant or may be a defensive wound caused by the victim trying to remove the hand(s) or object applying pressure to their neck.

- *Alternative light source (ALS light):* A valuable tool that helps detect the presence of potential forensic evidence (eg, urine, sweat, semen, saliva, vaginal secretions, fibers) and other substances (eg, lotion, oils, powders) that would otherwise remain invisible to the naked eye. The area fluoresces, or glows, allowing samples to be collected; however, the collector cannot confirm the origin of the substance or fiber at the time of collection.[2,3]
- *Anoxia:* The absence of oxygen. During strangulation the brain suffers an anoxic injury when the blood supply is completely obstructed.
- *Anoxic seizure:* Tonic-clonic seizure activity lasting 2 to 8 seconds; results from an anoxic insult to the brain.[4]
- *Asphyxia:* A general term which indicating the body is deprived of oxygen. Causes of asphyxia are divided into 4 primary categories: suffocation, strangulation, mechanical asphyxia, and drowning.[5,6]
- *Bruise or contusion:* An area of hemorrhage of soft tissue caused by the rupture of blood vessels from blunt trauma. Contusions may be present in skin and internal organs. Some contusions express a pattern. A ***patterned injury*** is one which has a distinct pattern that may reproduce the characteristic of the object that caused the injury. The pattern may be caused by the impact of a weapon or other object on the body or by contact of the body with a pattered surface. Deep bruising is typically not visible externally. However, in physical injury, pain over an area without visible hemorrhage is presumed to be bruised/contused. Estimation of the age of contusions based on its color is imprecise and not supported by forensic science evidence.[5] However, there is staging of bruising and injury associated with healing stages—hemostasis, inflammation, proliferation, maturation—where bruise staging is possible during microscopic evaluation at autopsy.
  - *Chin bruise:* Occurs when, in an effort to protect the neck, the victim instinctively lowers the head causing the chin to press against the hands of the assailant, and the small vessels are torn and leak to form a bruise.
  - *Clustering bruises:* Usually located on the sides of the neck and on the jawline. May extend onto the chin and collar bones. Consistent with fingers in a hand-grasp strangulation.
  - *Fingertip bruises:* Circular, oval-shaped bruises consistent with the assailant's grasp.
  - *Single bruise on neck:* Most frequently caused by the assailant's thumb. Because the thumb generates more pressure than any other finger, this bruise is found more often than fingertip bruises in a hand-grasp strangulation.
- *Buccal swabs:* Cotton swabs used to collect cheek cells for DNA samples from the inside of the mouth.[2]
- *Choking:* Blockage of respiratory passage(s) with a foreign body. Choking results from materials such as food or other objects obstructing the airway and preventing the exchange of oxygen and carbon dioxide.
- *Computed tomographic angiography or angiogram (CTA):* CTA is used to evaluate the arterial vessels. CTA is the gold standard for the evaluation of the carotid and vertebral arteries for a strangulation-induced dissection. CTA is sensitive for bony, cartilaginous, and soft tissue trauma as well as vascular injuries (**Appendix** 7).
- *Computed tomography (CT):* CT is an imaging technique which is fast and provides a detailed view of the internal organs and structures. CT imaging will identify injuries to neck structures (bones and cartilage); however it fails to evaluate injuries to the vasculature of the neck. A CT is not recommended to determine if there are injuries to the carotid or vertebral arteries (**Appendix** 7).

— ***Deoxyribonucleic acid (DNA):*** A valuable piece of biologic forensic evidence. DNA can be transferred between the assailant and the victim during an assault. Swabbing of the victim's neck, the suspect's injuries, and other locations is an important component of a strangulation examination.

— ***Dysphonia:*** Involves difficulty in speaking because of a physical disorder of the mouth, tongue, throat, or vocal cords.[9,10] Spastic dysphonia is a condition of the voice box or larynx, causing the voice to "break." It is a lifelong condition thought to begin after an upper respiratory infection, injury to the larynx, voice overuse, or stress.[11,12]

— ***Dyspnea:*** Shortness of breath or difficulty breathing.[9,13]

— ***ENT:*** Acronym for "ears, nose, and throat."[14]

— ***Examiner:*** The term refers to a health care provider conducting a medical forensic examination after trauma. Titles for the role are determined by license, education, and job description in the institution or organization. The term "examiner" has roots in English law and Scotland Yard and is not used by most state licensing boards or educational institutions. For the purposes of this document, the term "examiner" is used for the health care provider. Additional terms used in this document include the "medical forensic provider," the "sexual assault forensic examiner" (SAFE), the "sexual assault examiner" (SAE), the "forensic nurse," and the "forensic nurse examiner" (FNE). Many communities refer to the SAE by more specific acronyms and have justification in the specific license, practitioner role, or achievement of specialized education and clinical experiences.[15]

— ***Forensic nurse:*** A registered nurse or advanced practice nurse who has received specific education and training. Forensic nurses provide specialized care for patients who are experiencing acute and long-term health consequences associated with victimization or violence and have unmet evidentiary needs related to being victimized. Forensic nurses also provide consultation and testimony for civil and criminal proceedings. Forensic nursing care is not separate and distinct from other forms of medical care. It is integrated into the overall care needs of individual patients.

— ***Hypoxia:*** The deficiency of sufficient oxygen in the blood, tissues, or cells to maintain normal physiological function.

— ***Magnetic resonance with angiography (MRA):*** MRA is used to evaluate the carotid and vertebral arteries for a possible dissection after strangulation. MRA is equally as sensitive as CTA for arterial dissection and does not involve ionizing radiation (**Appendix** 7).

— ***Magnetic resonance imaging (MRI):*** MRI is a technique that uses a magnetic field and radio waves to create detailed images of the organs and tissues within the body. An MRI machine also produces 3D images that can be viewed from many different angles.[16]

— ***Odynophagia:*** Pain when swallowing.[9]

— ***OLDCARTS:*** Acronym (Onset, Location, Duration, Character, Aggravating/relieving, Radiation, Timing, Severity) used by health care providers when completing a comprehensive symptom history in the great subjective history provided by the patient.

— ***Petechial hemorrhages:*** Small, pinhead-sized hemorrhages caused by increased venous pressure in the capillary bed. Capillaries may be singular or multiple in appearance and may occur in any part of the body. The development of petechial hemorrhages in strangulation requires venous obstruction without obstruction of arterial flow. May be found under the eyelids (conjunctive), around the eyes, scalp, or anywhere on the face and neck in and above the area of constriction. Petechial hemorrhages can also result from nontraumatic causes, including forceful vomiting, coughing, childbirth, infection, and bleeding disorders.[5]

— ***Positional asphyxia (postural asphyxia):*** A form of asphyxia occurring when the position of a person's body or external pressure prevents the person from breathing adequately.[17] External pressure on the chest, neck, or abdomen restricts respiration and the exchange of oxygen and carbon dioxide resulting in hypoxia and elevated levels of carbon dioxide.

— ***Pulse oximetry:*** A device that measures the oxygen saturation of arterial blood in a subject. A sensor is usually attached to a finger, toe, or ear to determine the percentage of oxyhemoglobin in the blood pulsating through a network of capillaries.[18]

— ***Sexual assault forensic examiner (SAFE):*** Advanced practice providers, including nurse practitioners, physician assistants, and physicians with specialized education in the forensic aspects of health care for sexual assault patients.[1,15]

— ***Sexual assault nurse examiner (SANE):*** A registered nurse who has specialized education in the forensic aspects of health care for sexual assault patients.[1,15]

— ***Sexual assault response or resource team (SART):*** Coalitions of agencies that serve sexual assault victims. Core membership for SARTs typically includes victim advocates, law enforcement officers, medical forensic providers, forensic scientists, and prosecutors. Multidisciplinary SARTs work together to formalize interagency guidelines that prioritize victims' needs, hold offenders accountable, and promote public safety.[19,20]

— ***Strangulation:*** A form of asphyxiation characterized by closure of the air passage and/or blood vessels of the neck from the application of external pressure to the neck.

— ***Subconjunctival hemorrhage:*** Capillary rupture and bleeding into the white portion of the eye (ie, sclera).

— ***Suffocation:*** Obstruction or restriction of breathing by external mechanical forces. Suffocation does not require blunt force.[9]

— ***Swelling (edema) of the neck:*** Notable puffiness or tight appearance of the neck caused by tissue trauma, bleeding, or subcutaneous emphysema; may also be slight visible puffiness with more significant swelling inside, compromising the airway. Patient may complain of feeling tightness or fullness in the neck. Examiner may see jewelry impressions on the neck.

— ***Victim advocate:*** Someone who provides immediate crisis intervention, confidential emotional support, and information and advocacy to victims and their loved ones. The advocate is part of a coordinated response team and facilitates medical and legal services while providing trauma-informed, victim-centered care.

Methods of Strangulation

— ***Complete hanging:*** Suspension from a ligature around the neck holding the full body weight.

— ***Incomplete hanging:*** Suspension from a ligature around the neck holding partial body weight (ie, the feet, legs, pelvis, or torso is in contact with the ground).

— ***Ligature strangulation:*** Strangulation without suspension using some form of flexible linear object (eg, cord-like item).

— ***Manual strangulation:*** Strangulation using the hands, fingers, arms, or legs.

Mechanisms of Strangulation

— ***Compression of the laryngopharynx, larynx, or trachea:*** Inhibits inhalation and exhalation causing hypoxia and eventually anoxia.

— ***Compression over the carotid artery ganglion:*** May stimulate the carotid sinus reflex; produces bradycardia and hypotension; however, it does not cause cardiac arrest.[21,22]

— ***Sustained compression of the carotid arteries:*** Prevents 80% to 85% of oxygenated blood flow to the brain, which leads to cerebral anoxia and unconsciousness within 10 seconds.

— ***Sustained compression of the carotid and vertebral arteries:*** Prevents 100% of oxygenated blood flow to the brain. Without any arterial inflow to the head, no petechial hemorrhages develop, leading to "pale strangulation" or "pale hanging."

— ***Sustained compression of the jugular veins:*** Prevents outflow of venous blood from the brain. Leads to a gradual backup of venous blood into the face and brain causing "venous congestion" and eventually petechial hemorrhages. However, the jugular vein and the carotid artery are anatomically side-by-side, and the difference between the collapse of the jugular vein and the carotid artery is only 7 pounds of pressure.

Anatomy of the Neck

To best understand the clinical features associated with strangulation, one must understand the basic anatomy and functions of the neck (**Figure 1**). The neck is comprised of subcutaneous fat, muscle, cartilage, bone, vessels, nerves, lymph nodes, and salivary glands. The underlying neck structures that are especially vulnerable to the intentional external pressure from strangulation are located in the anterior and anterolateral neck. These structures include the hyoid bone, larynx, trachea, jugular veins, and carotid arteries. The vertebral arteries are located on the side of the neck (**Figure 2-a** and **b**). To grasp the importance of these structures, it is important to understand the role of the individual structure in the cardiovascular and respiratory system.

Life-sustaining oxygenation depends on the combination of air and blood flow. Respiration starts with the free movement of oxygenated air through the upper air passages (ie, the nose and mouth). Then, the air *must flow freely* through the larynx, to the trachea, and finally, to the lungs. Oxygenation occurs when the lungs shift oxygen from inhaled air into the blood. Then, the cardiovascular system pumps oxygenated blood through the heart and up into the carotid and vertebral arteries of the neck for oxygenation of the brain. At the brain's cellular level, blood exchanges oxygen for CO_2 gas, which is then transported down the neck's jugular veins to the lungs for exhalation. Other liquid and solid waste products travel through the circulatory system and are excreted by the kidneys and gastrointestinal track.

Vital Neck Structures

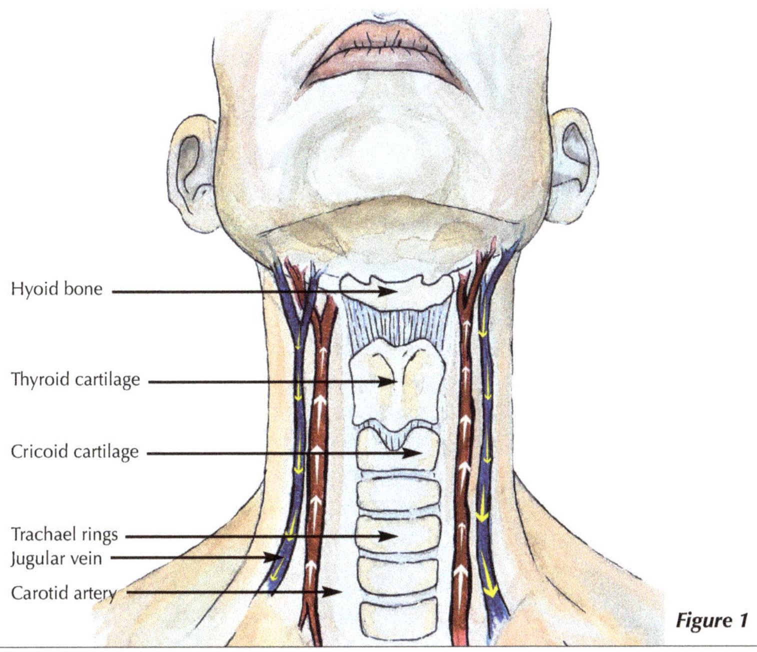

Figure 1

Figure 1. *Vital neck structures. (Illustration courtesy Yesenia Aceves and the Training Institute on Strangulation Prevention.)*

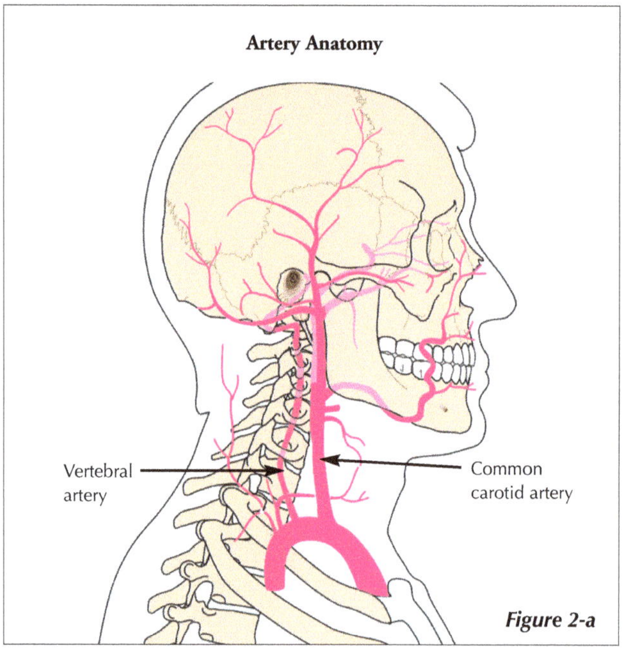

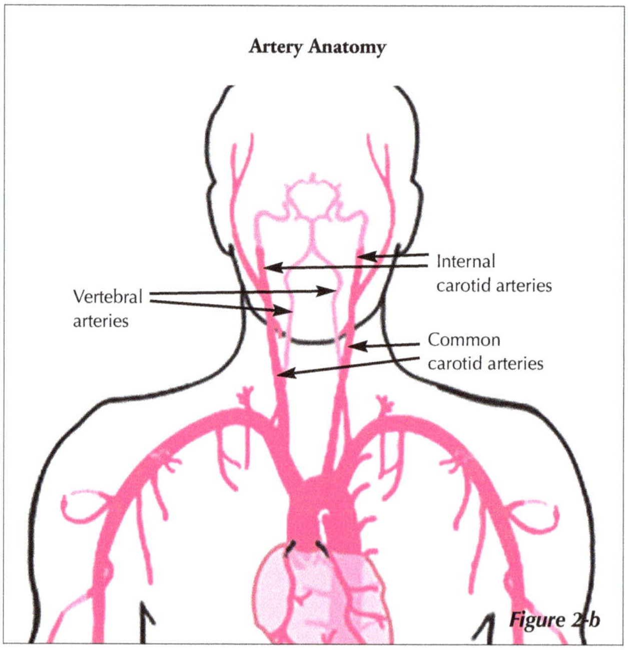

Figure 2-a and b. *Carotid and vertebral arteries.*

Cessation of oxygenated blood flow to the brain cells leads to anoxia. Hypoxia (eg, decreased oxygen levels) results from strangulation when pressure to the neck compromises air flow. Anoxia and hypoxia from compressive force on the arteries and air passages of the neck is the most common cause of death in strangulation. Based on videotapes of hanging death, the last breath occurs between 62 and 157 seconds.[6,23] Injuries to neck structures may also lead to compromised air and blood flow. Pressure to the neck can result in hyoid bone or laryngeal fractures, carotid or vertebral artery dissections, intrinsic neck muscle bleeding, cervical spine ligament tears, nerve injury, and cervical spine fractures. Injury-associated bleeding, swelling, and/or functional disability in maintaining a patent airway interferes with oxygenation leading to hypoxia. The following is a more detailed explanation of underlying neck structures, including their location, function, and susceptibility to compressive forces of strangulation.

Carotid Arteries

The carotid arteries originate from the aortic arch at the top of the heart and are located on the left and right side of the neck. Protected by neck muscles, the carotid arteries lie slightly deeper and medial to the jugular veins. The carotid arteries carry approximately 80% of the oxygenated, nutrient-rich blood from the heart to the head and brain. Pressure inside the carotid arteries exerts the force required not only to deliver oxygenated blood but to diffuse oxygen throughout the brain tissues.

It takes approximately 11 pounds of pressure to occlude the carotid arteries and compromise oxygenated blood flow to the brain. Sustained pressure causes unconsciousness within 10 seconds as a result of immediate cessation of oxygenated blood flow. Immediate relief of pressure allows consciousness to return in approximately 10 seconds. Death occurs within 1 to 2.5 minutes of constant pressure on the arteries.[23] A tear, called a dissection, can occur to the internal lining of the carotid arteries. The body's response to a dissection is to form a blood clot around the tear and begin the hemostasis phase of healing. Blood clots can completely occlude the artery or can break off, travel to the brain, and compromise blood flow and oxygenation, resulting in neurologic compromise and stroke. The clot may not break off until days, weeks, or months after injury, and the strangulation victim remains asymptomatic until the moment of the stroke.[24] A screening CTA is required to rule out the presence of a carotid artery dissection (**Appendix 7**).

Vertebral Arteries

The vertebral arteries originate from the subclavian arteries and are the primary blood supply to the upper spinal cord, brainstem, cerebellum, and the posterior circulation of the brain. They carry 15% to 20% of the brain's blood supply. When the carotid arteries are occluded but the vertebral arteries remain patent, the vertebral arterial blood flow is primarily responsible for the development of petechial hemorrhages on the integument skin and mucous membrane surfaces of the face and the oto-oral-pharyngeal areas. There are 2 mechanisms for occluded vertebral arteries. First, if pressure is applied just above the collarbone to occlude the subclavian arteries[4,25] or second, if lateral neck pressure is applied from a thin ligature or with hands in a choke hold, 100% of arterial blood flow to the brain can be blocked.[26] Compression of both the carotid and vertebral arteries will result in a "pale strangulation" or a "pale hanging" because petechiae will not develop. A screening CTA is required to rule out the presence of a vertebral artery dissection (**Appendix** 7).

Carotid Artery Ganglion

The carotid artery ganglion, also called the carotid body, is a cluster of cells located at the bifurcation of the carotid artery. An important neurologic sensor, the carotid body is primarily stimulated by oxygen and is highly sensitive to carbon dioxide. The carotid body's main function is to trigger nerve impulses, relaying important information to the central nervous system. Although it requires a specific area of compression with strangulation, sustained stimulation of the carotid body for 3 to 4 minutes could activate the carotid sinus reflex, resulting in bradycardia and hypotension. However, death does not occur from carotid sinus stimulation.[21,22]

Hyoid Bone

The hyoid bone is a horseshoe-shaped bone located at the base of the mandible and above the larynx (**Figure 3**). It is free-floating (ie, not connected to any other bone in the body). The hyoid bone's main function is to support a wide range of tongue, pharyngeal, and laryngeal movements, including swallowing. A fracture of the hyoid bone may lead to difficulty swallowing (ie, dysphagia), painful swallowing (ie, odynophagia), and pain on neck rotation. Effective swallowing is important to maintain uncompromised air flow during respiration. Therefore, the impact of a hyoid bone fracture on swallowing, as well as the potential for associated bleeding and/or swelling, may compromise airway patency. Hyoid bone fracture is reported with a frequency of 17% to 71% in fatal strangulation[27] and occurs during manual strangulation, ligature strangulation, and in hangings. Hyoid bone fracture is infrequently recognized in nonfatal strangulation.[28]

Figure 3. *The hyoid bone. The greater horns (cornu) are the most common location for fractures.*

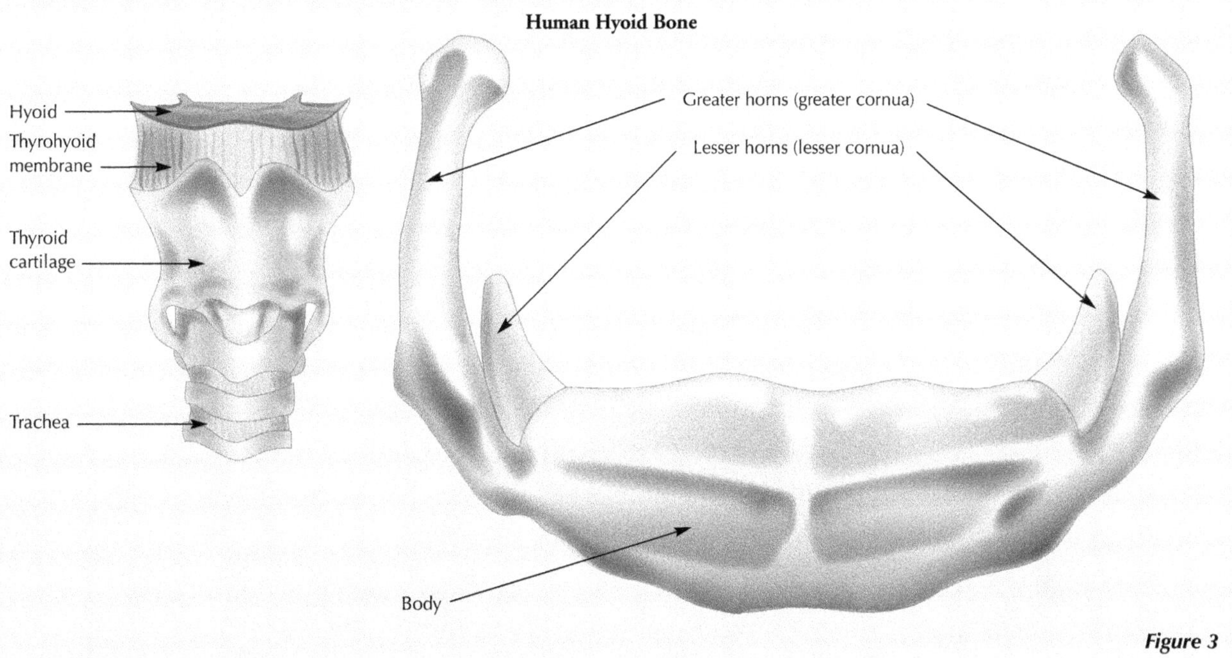

Figure 3

Jugular Veins

The jugular veins are vessels located on the left and right side of the anterior neck and are more external and lateral to the carotid arteries. The jugular veins return the majority of CO_2 gases in deoxygenated blood from the brain and head back to the heart and lungs where the CO_2 gases are exhaled as waste.

It takes approximately 4.4 pounds of pressure to occlude the jugular veins. This occlusion causes venous outflow obstruction, resulting in deoxygenated blood backing up into vessels of the head and brain. This build-up of deoxygenated blood is known as stagnant hypoxia. If venous outflow is obstructed without carotid artery occlusion, the veins above the level of constriction begin to dilate in order to accommodate the incoming blood that cannot exit the neck. This obstructive process causes the veins to engorge, resulting in increased internal venous pressure. When pressure is sustained for approximately 20 to 30 seconds without complete arterial (carotid and vertebral) occlusion, the dilated vessels rupture, causing pinpoint hemorrhages known as petechiae. Petechiae may occur anywhere above the level of constriction, including the brain, scalp, skin, conjunctiva of the eyes, soft palate of the mouth, and the external ear canal.

Larynx

The larynx (ie, voice box) is a tubular structure of cartilage between the superior hyoid bone and inferior trachea. The larynx serves 2 important functions: first, it is part of the respiratory tract, allowing inhaled air to pass while simultaneously keeping food and liquid from obstructing the airway; second, the larynx is the area with vocal cords and subsequently functions to produce sound and vocalizations. The larynx contains the following structures, which are important to swallowing and vocalization.

— ***Cricoid cartilage:*** A ring-shaped structure providing the transition from larynx to trachea. Provides an attachment point for the cartilage, ligaments, and muscles involved in sound production and the opening and shutting of the airway.

— ***Epiglottis:*** An elastic, spoon-shaped flap extending from the posterior tongue to the anterior border of the thyroid cartilage. During swallowing, the epiglottis folds over to cover the opening of the larynx (ie, glottis) to block any food or fluid from entering the airway.

— ***Thyrohyoid membrane:*** A fibrous, elastic membrane connecting thyroid cartilage to the hyoid bone by a mucosa bursa that aids the upward movement of the larynx in swallowing.

— ***Thyroid cartilage:*** A semicircular structure positioned on the anterior larynx. Consists of a fusion of 2 cartilage plates. The external point of fusion is the laryngeal prominence (ie, Adam's apple) and is more pronounced in men. The thyroid cartilage supports and protects the upper larynx and anchors the anterior portion of the vocal cords.

— ***Vocal cords:*** Situated in the mucous membrane on each side of the larynx opening. As exhaled air moves through the larynx, the vocal cords vibrate and produce sound.

The compressive forces of strangulation may lead to occlusion, fractures, and hemorrhages of the larynx's cartilaginous framework. It takes approximately 22 pounds of force for airway occlusion at the level of the thyrohyoid membrane, 31.5 pounds of force to fracture the thyroid cartilage, and 41 pounds of force to fracture the cricoid. Laryngeal fractures often allow air to escape into the soft tissues of the neck, producing subcutaneous emphysema (ie, subcutaneous crepitation), which can result in potential airway compromise that can develop into acute asphyxia, and eventually, death. Subsequent hemorrhages and swelling may also play a role in airway compromise as a result of these injuries. If these fractures or hemorrhages go untreated or unrecognized, the victim may survive initially, but over hours, or even days, the victim may develop life-threatening airway complications, leading to a delayed death. Vocal cord injury that leads to swelling or hematoma formation may result in temporary or long-term vocal dysfunction that includes a hoarse voice (ie, dysphonia) or the inability to produce a voice (ie, aphonia).

Trachea

The trachea is a hollow tube located along the body's midline that connects the larynx to the 2 main bronchi of the lungs. Incomplete, highly elastic, C-shaped cartilage rings are located anteriorly along the tracheal wall. The trachea's primary function is to allow air flow to and from the lungs. It takes approximately 33 pounds of pressure to completely occlude the trachea. Tracheal occlusion inhibits the inhalation of oxygen and the exhalation of carbon dioxide, resulting in multisystem hypoxia and acidosis. The force of the strangulation pressure may also fracture the trachea, causing subcutaneous emphysema and subsequent airway compromise.

Anatomy of the Ear

When documenting injuries on a patient after strangulation, it is important to inspect and photograph both sides of the ears (**Figure 4**). Initial injury, unless it involves dermal capillary injury, may not be visible but over time may surface, allowing for reassessment and documentation.

— ***Triangular fossa:*** A shallow depression in the anterior part of the top of the ear's auricle between the 2 crura into which the antihelix divides.

— ***Scaphoid fossa:*** A shallow oval depression that is situated above the pterygoid fossa on the pterygoid process of the sphenoid bone and that provides attachment for the origin of the tensor veli palatini muscle.

— ***Helix:*** The outer rim of the ear that extends from the superior insertion of the ear on the scalp (root) to the termination of the cartilage at the earlobe. The helix can be divided into 3 approximate parts: the ascending helix, which extends vertically from the root; the superior helix, which begins at the top of the ascend-

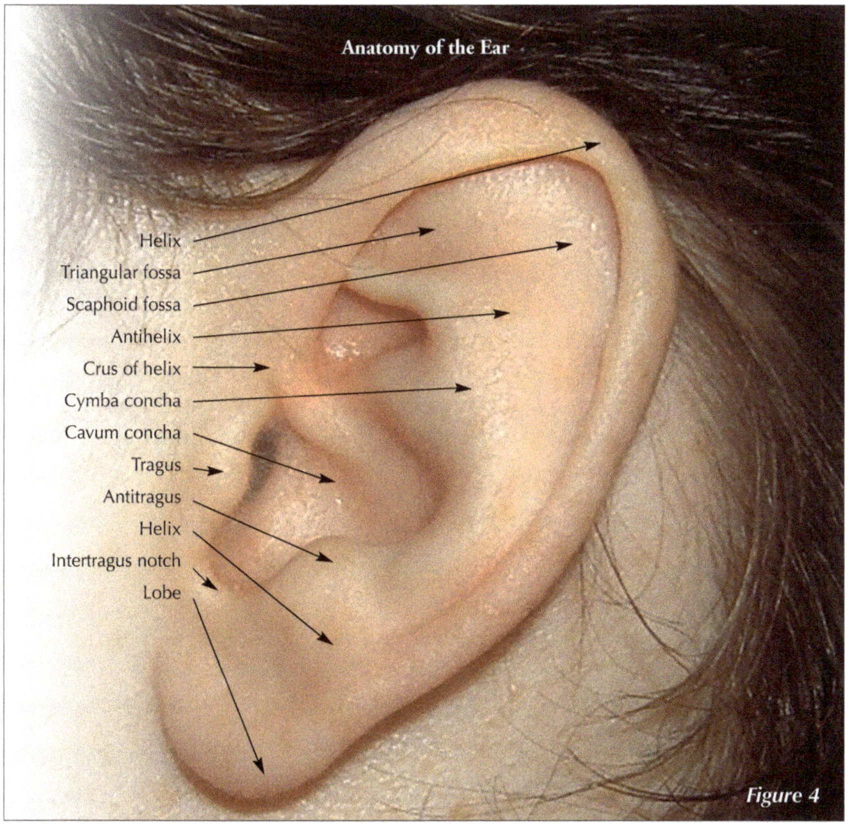

Figure 4. Anatomy of the ear.

ing portion, extends horizontally, and curves posteriorly to the site of Darwin tubercle; and the descending helix (sometimes called posterior), which begins inferior to Darwin tubercle and extends to the superior border of the earlobe. The lower portion of the posterior part is often noncartilaginous. The border of the helix usually forms a rolled rim, but the helix is highly variable in shape.

— ***Crus of helix:*** The continuation of the anteroinferior ascending helix, which extends in a posteroinferior direction into the cavity of the concha above the external auditory meatus. The average crus helix extends about one-half to two-thirds the distance across the concha.

— ***Antihelix:*** A Y-shaped curved cartilaginous ridge arising from the antitragus and separating the concha, triangular fossa, and scapha. The antihelix represents a folding of the conchal cartilage, and it usually has similar prominence to a well-developed helix. The stem (the part below the bifurcation) of the normal antihelix is gently curved and branches about two-thirds of the way along its course to form the broad fold of the superior (posterior) antihelical crus and the more sharply folded inferior (anterior) crus. The inferior and superior crura of the antihelix can vary both in volume and degree of folding.

— ***Tragus:*** A posterior, slightly inferior, protrusion of skin-covered cartilage, anterior to the auditory meatus. The inferoposterior margin of the tragus forms the anterior wall of the incisura.

— ***Intertragic notch:*** The space that separates the tragus from the antitragus in the outer ear.

— ***Antitragus:*** The anterosuperior cartilaginous protrusion lying between the incisura and the origin of the antihelix. The anterosuperior margin of the antitragus forms the posterior wall of the incisura.

— ***Concha:*** The fossa bounded by the tragus, incisura, antitragus, antihelix, inferior crus of the antihelix, and root of the helix, into which opens the external auditory canal. It is usually bisected by the crus helix into the cymba superiorly and cavum inferiorly.

— ***Cavum concha:*** The inferior portion of the cavity of the auricle of the ear. It leads to the external acoustic meatus.

— ***Cymba concha:*** The narrowest end of the concha.

— ***Lobe:*** The soft, fleshy lower part of the external ear.

Strangulation-Related Injuries and Conditions

The learner may find reviewing the following definitions useful in completing the activities within this book. Terminology for indicators of direction when documenting findings in a medical forensic examination include anterior (nearer the front), posterior (nearer the back), inferior (nearer the bottom), superior (nearer the top), medial (to the middle), lateral (to the side), proximal (nearer the center of the body), and distal (away from the center of the body) (**Figure 5**).

Signs and Symptoms of Strangulation

— ***Breathing changes:*** Difficulty breathing (dyspnea), hyperventilation, inability to breathe (apnea)

— ***Evidence of hypoxia/anoxia and near-unconsciousness:*** Changes in vision (eg, tunnel vision, blurred, "curtain closing in," spots, flashes of light), changes in hearing (eg, hearing loss, ringing), loss of control over body (eg, weakness, limpness)

— ***Evidence of anoxia and unconsciousness:*** Loss of memory, unexplained injuries, brain damage, involuntary urination or defecation

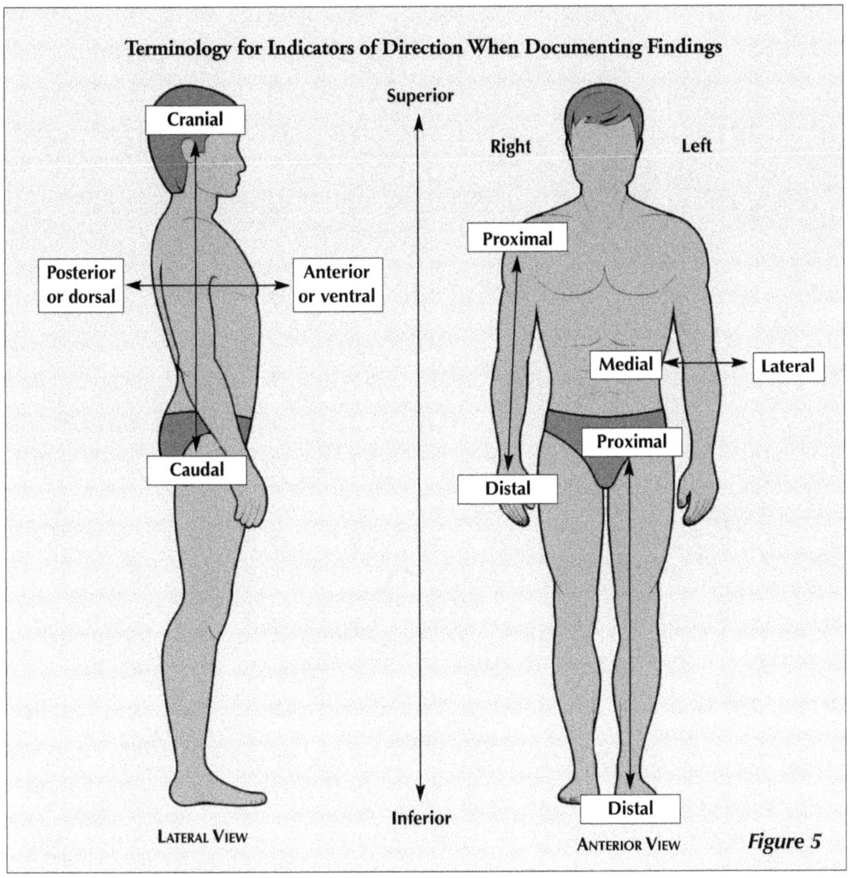

Figure 5. *Terminology for indicators of direction when documenting findings.*

— ***Mental status changes:*** Restlessness/combativeness, seizure activity, frank psychosis/amnesia

— ***Swallowing changes (larynx/hyoid bone injury):*** Difficult, but not painful, swallowing (dysphagia); painful swallowing (odynophagia); drooling

— ***Symptomatic voice changes:*** Hoarse or raspy voice (dysphonia), complete loss of voice (aphonia)

Lethality of Strangulation

Lethality refers to capacity to cause death. Therefore, lethality of strangulation refers to one's chances of dying as a result of strangulation.[29]

Lethality as a Result of External Pressure

— ***Anoxia:*** In cases of strangulation, the absence of oxygen depriving the brain of oxygenated blood. Characterized by tachycardia, hypertension, dizziness, mental confusion, and unconsciousness.

— ***Neck swelling:*** May present as soft tissue trauma/inflammation, internal bleeding (carotid dissection), laryngeal injury (subcutaneous emphysema). May progress slowly.

— ***Pneumonitis:*** Inflammation of the lung, resulting from inhaled emesis where the gastric juices begin to digest lung tissue.

— ***Post-anoxic encephalopathy:*** Decrease in blood flow to the brain by which some brain cells die immediately while others survive for days. Surviving brain cells eventually succumb to the cerebral anoxia. Surviving patients may incur lifelong brain damage and neurologic deficits. May be fatal: "brain death," persistent vegetative coma, cerebral edema (ie, brain swelling), and herniation of the brain. The hippocampus (part of the limbic system) is the most sensitive part of the brain to anoxia and is the first area to experience damage with anoxia.

— ***Pulmonary edema:*** Accumulation of extravascular fluid in lung tissues and alveoli. Caused by excessive negative respiratory pressures resulting from victim's attempts to breathe while external neck pressure impedes the airway.

Lethality of Interpersonal Violence with Nonfatal Strangulation: Risk for Homicide*

— Nonfatal strangulation has been reported in 45% of attempted homicides.

— Nonfatal strangulation has been reported in 43% of completed homicides.

— With nonfatal strangulation, odds of attempted homicide increase sixfold.

— With nonfatal strangulation, odds of completed homicide increase sevenfold.

Tests and Treatment

— ***CT of the neck:*** Sensitive for bony, cartilaginous, and soft tissue injuries. Also identifies edema, hemorrhage, and subcutaneous emphysema. However, CT without angiography does not evaluate the carotid or vertebral arteries for vascular damage.

— ***CTA of the neck:*** Very sensitive test for the detection of vascular injuries in the carotid and vertebral arteries. CTA is also sensitive for the detection of bony and cartilaginous injuries. The CTA is the gold standard for the emergent radiologic evaluation of nonfatal or near-fatal strangulation patients (**Appendix** 7).

— ***Discharge planning:*** Considered safe if patient experienced no loss of consciousness, presents with no or minimal soft tissue neck injury, and no objective/subjective neurologic findings. Encourage the patient to stay with someone, or have someone stay with them, for the 24 hours after discharge to help monitor for any increase in symptoms. Patients with significant trauma can be safely discharged if the CTA is negative for injury or dissection.

— ***Fiberoptic laryngoscopy:*** Visually evaluates the soft tissues of the oropharynx; however, this approach does not offer evaluation of deep soft tissue injuries.

— ***MRI and MRA:*** MRI and MRA are used to produce 2- or 3-dimensional images of the structures inside your body, including your blood vessels. Both an MRI and MRA are noninvasive and painless diagnostic tools used to view tissues, bones, or organs inside the body. An MRI creates detailed images of organs and tissues. An MRA focuses more on the blood vessels than the tissue surrounding it. Usually, the MRA is done in conjunction with the MRI. MRAs evolved from MRIs to give doctors the ability to look at blood vessels more thoroughly.

— ***Plain radiographs:*** Images that identify bone and laryngotracheal injuries. Plain radiographs are not recommended for emergent evaluation of the vasculature in nonfatal strangulation (**Appendix** 7).

References

1. Faugno DF, Speck PM, Spencer MJ, Giardino AP, eds. Sexual Assault Quick Reference: For Health Care, Social Service, and Law Enforcement Professionals. 2nd ed. Saint Louis, MO: STM Learning, Inc; 2016.
2. Ditton M, Gray L. The ABC's - Anatomy, "Bunk" and the Courtroom of Sexual Assault. Fort Wayne, IN: Socratic Parenting, LLC; 2015.
3. Pollitt EN, Anderson JC, Scafide KN, Holbrook D, D'Silva G, Sheridan DJ. Alternate light source findings of common topical products. *J Forensic Nurs.* 2016;11(3)97-103.
4. Herman Kabat. Acute arrest of cerebral circulation in man. *Arch Neurol.* 1943;50(5):510-528.

**Data from Glass N, Laughon K, Campbell J, et al. Non-fatal strangulation is an important risk factor for homicide in women.* J Emerg Med. *2008;35(3):329-335.*

5. Matusz EC, Schaffer JT, Bachmeier BA, et al. Evaluation of nonfatal strangulation in alert adults. *Ann Emerg Med.* 2019;S0196-0644(19)30594-3.

6. Sauvageau A, Boghossian E. Classification of asphyxia: the need for standardization. *J Forensic Sci.* 2010;55(5):1259-1267.

7. Stark P. Principles of computed tomography of the chest. UpToDate Web site. http://www.uptodate.com/contents/principles-of-computed-tomography-of-the-chest?source=preview&search=CAT+Scan&language=en-US&anchor=H1&selectedTitle=1~150#H1. Updated April 22, 2019. Accessed December 4, 2019.

8. Raby BA. Basic principles of genetic disease. UpToDate Web site. http://www.uptodate.com/contents/basic-principles-of-genetic-disease?-source=machineLearning&search=DNA&selectedTitle=1~150&section-Rank=1&anchor=H5203404#H5203404. Updated May 31, 2019. Accessed December 4, 2019.

9. Training Institute on Strangulation Prevention, California District Attorneys Association. The Investigation and Prosecution of Strangulation Cases. San Diego, CA: California District Attorneys Association, California Emergency Management Agency; 2013.

10. Schwartz SR, Cohen SM, Dailey SH, et al. Clinical practice guideline: hoarseness (dysphonia). *Otolaryngol Head Neck Surge.* 2009;141(3 suppl 2):S1-S31.

11. Spasmodic dysphonia. Johns Hopkins Medicine Web site. https://www.hopkinsmedicine.org/health/conditions-and-diseases/spasmodic-dysphonia. Accessed May 28, 2020.

12. Spasmodic dysphonia. National Institute on Deafness and Other Communication Disorders Web site. https://www.nidcd.nih.gov/health/spasmodic-dysphonia. Updated March 6, 2017. Accessed May 28, 2020.

13. Bass JB Jr. Dyspnea. In: Walker HK, Hall WD, Hurst JW, eds. Clinical Methods: The History, Physical, and Laboratory Examinations. 3rd ed. Boston, MA: Butterworths; 1990. National Center for Biotechnology Web site. https://www.ncbi.nlm.nih.gov/books/NBK357/. Accessed December 4, 2019.

14. What's an ENT? American Academy of Otolaryngology - Head and Neck Surgery Web site. https://www.enthealth.org/whats-an-ent/. Accessed December 4, 2019.

15. US Department of Justice, Office on Violence Against Women. A National Protocol for Sexual Assault Medical Forensic Examinations: Adults/Adolescents. 2nd ed. Washington, DC: US Department of Justice, Office on Violence Against Women; 2013. National Criminal Justice Reference Service Web site. https://www.ncjrs.gov/pdffiles1/ovw/241903.pdf. Accessed December 4, 2019.

16. MRI. Mayo Clinic Web site. http://www.mayoclinic.org/tests-procedures/mri/home/ovc-20235698. Accessed December 4, 2019.

17. Parkes J, Thake D, Price M. Effect of seated restraint and body size on lung function. *Med Sci Law.* 2011;51(3):177-181.

18. Pulse oximetry. Johns Hopkins Medicine Web site. http://www.hopkinsmedicine.org/healthlibrary/test_procedures/pulmonary/oximetry_92,p07754/. Accessed December 4, 2019.

19. National Sexual Violence Resource Center. Sexual Assault Response Team Development: A Guide for Victim Service Providers. Enola, PA: National Sexual Violence Resource Center; 2011.

20. Introduction to the SANE Program Development and Operation Guide. Office for Victims of Crime Training and Technical Assistance Center Web site. https://www.ovcttac.gov/saneguide/introduction/. Accessed December 4, 2019.

21. Ungar A, Rivasi G, Rafanelli M, et al. Safety and tolerability of Tilt Testing and Carotid Sinus Massage in the octogenarians. *Age Ageing*. 2016;45(2):242-248.

22. Doberentz E, Schyma C, Madea B. Histological examination of the carotid bifurcation in case of violence against the neck. *Forensic Sci Int*. 2012;216(1-3):135-140.

23. Sauvageau A, Laharpe R, King D, et al. Agonal sequences in 14 filmed hangings with comments on the role of the type of suspension, ischemic habituation, and ethanol intoxication on the timing of agonal responses. *Am J Forensic Med Pathol*. 2011;32(2):104-107.

24. Chokyu I, Tsumoto T, Miyamoto T, Yamaga H, Terada T, Itakura T. Traumatic bilateral common carotid artery dissection due to strangulation. A case report. *Interv Neuroradiol*. 2006;12(2):149-154.

25. Rossen R, Kabat H, Anderson JP. Acute arrest of cerebral circulation in man. *Arch Neurol Psychiatry*. 1943;50(5):510-528.

26. Smith BA, Clayton EW, Robertson D. Experimental arrest of cerebral blood flow in human subjects: the red wing studies revisited. *Perspect Biol Med*. 2011;54(2):121-131.

27. Fineron PW, Turnbull JA, Busuttil A. Fracture of the hyoid bone in survivors of attempted manual strangulation. *J Clin Forensic Med*. 1995;2(4):195-197.

28. Iacovou E, Nayar M, Fleming J, Lew-Gor S. A pain in the neck: a rare case of isolated hyoid bone trauma. *J Surg Case Rep*. 2011;2011(7):3.

29. Sorenson SB, Joshi M, Sivitz E. A systematic review of the epidemiology of nonfatal strangulation, a human rights and health concern. *Am J Public Health*. 2014;104(11):e54-e61.

Section II

Case Studies

Objectives

After completing the exercises presented in this chapter, the student will be able to:

1. *Correctly identify the anatomy of strangulation patients.*
2. *Identify and document injuries based on an analysis of case photographs.*
3. *List at least 3 items of evidence that should be collected.*
4. *Discuss treatment and discharge instructions.*

Key Terms

— ***Carotid artery:*** Arteries supplying oxygenated blood from the heart to the brain.

— ***Choking:*** Blocking of a respiratory passage by constriction of the neck, obstruction in the trachea, or swelling of the larynx.

— ***Hanging:*** Suspension from a cord or cord-like object wound around the neck.

— ***Jugular vein:*** Veins transporting deoxygenated blood from the brain back to the heart.

— ***Lethality of strangulation:*** Odds of death as a result of strangulation.

— ***Ligature strangulation:*** Strangulation without suspension using a cord-like object.

— ***Manual strangulation:*** Strangulation using the hands, fingers, or other extremities.

— ***Petechial hemorrhage:*** Subcutaneous hemorrhages presenting as small purple or red spots on the skin. Characteristic of asphyxia by external force.

— ***Strangulation:*** Asphyxia characterized by closure of the air passage or vessels of the neck as a result of external pressure.

— ***Suffocation:*** External prevention of respiration via occlusion of nose and mouth with an object.

Introduction

The following cases represent a compilation of many different patients and are not intended to represent an individual case. Any similarity is purely coincidental. The photographs are from individual cases, but the patient's faces have been obscured for the purposes of this publication.

The *Domestic Violence and Nonfatal Strangulation Assessment* assists first responders, nurses and physicians, nurse practitioners, physician assistants, emergency room health care providers, attorneys, and law enforcement personnel in the assessment and documentation of strangulation cases.

First responders and health care providers evaluating patients who have been strangled often face challenges related to lack of education, knowledge, experience, and competence. The reasons include limited contact with this particular patient population, lack of access to experts who provide ongoing evaluation and peer review, and increasing demands from employers to manage all patients effectually. To maintain and improve highly specialized skills necessary for the evaluation of patients who have been strangled, this workbook improves provider's understanding about the assessment, documentation, and treatment of strangulation, thereby improving competency and allowing for improved quality of care for strangulation patients.

Chapter 1

32-Year-Old Female Strangulation Patient with Hyoid Bone Fracture and Suicidal Ideation

Case History

Janice, a 32-year-old, arrives at a Family Justice Center approximately 2 hours after being strangled by her ex-boyfriend, Jason. She was going to walk to meet her dad, and when she went outside, Jason was there. He walked up to her, and after they argued for a bit, he grabbed her by the throat with 1 hand. He stopped when he thought someone might be watching. She reports that he said he is "tired of me hurting him and tired of my disrespect." Jason wanted her to go inside, but she feared for her life because she knew if they were out of view of the public, he would hurt her badly. Janice states that Jason had previously beaten her, hit her on the head, strangled her, and threatened to burn her house down with her inside it. When she refused to go inside with him, he pulled her into the house. This time, he did not continue to physically assault her, but he threatened to. Janice's dad began calling, but Jason would not let her answer the phone. When the phone kept ringing, he finally left. Janice spoke to her dad and he brought her to the Family Justice Center where she was initially triaged, and because of the history of strangulation, she was immediately taken to the nurse.

During examination, Janice discloses the nature of the strangulation and says that her neck hurts. There is an area of abrasion on the right side of her neck. She states the right side of her jaw and the middle of her jaw on the bone are very tender. She states she had trouble breathing during the incident and had some visual changes. She also describes pain when she rotates her neck, trouble swallowing (dysphagia), and painful swallowing (odynophagia). She complains of pain and pulls away when the examiner palpates the area under the jaw. The tissue is crepitus as well. Her first set vital signs show that her blood pressure is 167/97, pulse is 81, and pulse oximeter is 97%. She states the assaults have been going on for the past 1½ years. Lately, the assaults have been happening every week. She has a Danger Assessment score of 28/37. During the conversation about the Danger Assessment, Janice discloses that she has attempted suicide in the past and currently felt it would be better if she were dead. The HELPS Brain Injury Screening Tool was scored (**Appendix 5**). She answered affirmatively to 14 of the 20 questions. Once the forensic medical examination, including safety planning, is complete, the patient is referred to the emergency department (ED). She leaves the center with her dad for further evaluation and treatment for strangulation, traumatic brain injury, and suicidal ideation.

Janice reports the strangulation and suicidal ideation to the ED physician. She denies any specific plan to harm herself but feels she is "a bother and burden to my family." She tells the physician that she was sexually assaulted by Jason over a week ago, and she is worried about sexually transmitted infections (STIs). She is assigned a "sitter" while in the ED. She has no pertinent medical history other than the long-term physical, sexual, and emotional abuse. Computed tomography angiography (CTA) is negative for any vascular abnormalities. CT of soft tissue shows nondisplaced hyoid fracture on the right. An emergent psychiatric evaluation is implemented, and the physician determines Janice is not a threat to herself, so it is safe to discharge her. She is empirically treated for STIs. She is discharged in stable condition and is told to follow-up with a gynecologist; ear, nose, and throat specialist; and a behavioral health professional.

Case Discussion

Studies are being done to better understand the overall epidemiology of strangulation, and more are needed to better understand the magnitude, risk, and consequences of strangulation.[1] Only then can policies, protocols, and clinical interventions be developed. Nonfatal strangulation is a common circumstance and presents significant health risks within a violent intimate partner relationship.[2] Studies have shown consistently high incidents of strangulation events in domestic violence situations, from 60% to 89%.[2-4] Reporting the incident immediately or soon after the incident is uncommon. Strack et al[5] reported that 5% of their sample reported within 48 hours and that the report was usually associated with concerning symptoms. It is common for symptoms that should be cause for concern (eg, loss of consciousness, loss of bladder control, pain in throat or neck, hoarseness, trouble swallowing) to be minimized by the patient.[6]

Contrary to what one might think, visible injury is not common in cases of strangulation. One study found only 15% of injuries were of the quality to photograph.[5] Injuries are a result of blunt force trauma inflicted by either the victim while trying to remove the constriction from around their neck or from whatever is causing the strangulation. Skin injuries, when present, in the form of bruises or scratches (contusions or abrasions) on the neck may be faint circular bruises, curved or linear scratches, or petechiae.[4,8-10] One or 2 hands from the front are the most common approaches to the victim's neck.[1,11] Internal injury with accompanying symptoms are common and can be deadly days, weeks, or years after the incident. Potential for brain injury and memory loss should be considered during assessment.[6,7]

The hyoid bone is a horseshoe-shaped bone that is located at the base of the mandible and above the larynx.[12] It supports the tongue and assists in swallowing, speaking, and movement of the tongue. It is the only bone in the body not articulated to any other bone.[12] It is protected by the mandible and the cervical spine.[12] Mature hyoid bones comprise a central body to which a pair each of greater and lesser horns are attached. These horns are joined to the body by cartilaginous joints and later in life by bony fusion.[8] Ossification begins at birth, and care must be taken to avoid confusing a fracture with delayed ossification.[8] While hyoid bone fracture is rare because it is protected by the mandible, most hyoid bone injuries are caused by strangulation.[13]

Hyoid bone fractures in nonfatal strangulation are also not frequently recognized.[8,14] Therefore, the true rate of hyoid bone fracture in nonfatal strangulation is unknown.[10] Rates of hyoid bone fracture in fatal cases range from 13% to 71%.[9] Studies have shown that hyoid bone fractures are more common in the older population (older than 50) as a result of more calcification of the bone than found in the younger population.[8] When fracture occurs in the younger population, it could support a history of a vigorous attack with significant use of force. Hyoid bone fractures rarely cause life-threatening findings. However, pharyngeal and supraglottic edema can occur, leading to life-threatening situations.[11,14]

Hyoid fracture should be suspected in every case of anterior neck pain associated with soft tissue findings.[14] Hyoid bone fracture is one possible cause of painful or compromised swallowing after strangulation.[9] De Boos[9] states that these fractures result from pressure above the larynx and may be asymptomatic at rest but tender on palpation and when swallowing.

In addition to the strangulation and physical assault, Janice disclosed that she was sexually assaulted. Sexual assault is a common form of intimate partner violence (IPV). Prevalence studies show that 17% to 25% of women and 1% to 3% of men will be sexually assaulted in their lifetime.[15] Sexual violence affects millions of people each year in the United States. Sexual assaults are often not reported, so the true prevalence is unknown. Victims may be ashamed, embarrassed, or afraid to tell the police, friends, or family about the violence. Victims may also not report because they have been threatened with further harm if they tell anyone, or they do not think that anyone will help them.

Sexual abuse of an intimate partner is common and takes on many forms. It can range from birth control sabotage to rape to human trafficking. The violence and trauma associated with the fact that the offender is someone the victim loves is oftentimes much worse than what is seen in acquaintance and stranger assaults. There may be a certain threshold that leads a victim to report. Once that threshold is reached, they may seek help.[16] For some victims, the escalation of violence to include strangulation is that threshold. The co-occurrence of sexual violence and IPV is often identified in the medical forensic examination. The situation is more complicated than the statistics show. The two may appear separate, but they are tightly intertwined.[17]

Lethality in IPV can be either at the hands of the perpetrator or the victim. A history of strangulation substantially increases a woman's risk of homicide.[18,19] Persons who experience IPV have a 7 times higher incidence of suicidal ideation than those who have not.[20] Nearly 1 in 5 adult female victims of IPV have threatened or attempted suicide during their lifetime.[20] Sexual assault also leads to significant forms of psychopathology, including suicidal ideation. One study indicated that 23% to 44% of victims of sexual assault experience suicidal ideation, and 2% to 19% attempt suicide.[15] Life-threatening ingestion and overdoses of medications can complicate the assessment of strangulation.[21] When the combination of strangulation and suicidal ideation or attempt exist, a thorough psychiatric evaluation is necessary and may necessitate admission to the hospital under suicide precautions.

Eighty-three percent of those who die by suicide saw a health care provider in the year before their death.[22] Assessment tools provide useful information about suicide risk but do not predict the likelihood of a completed suicide. A study by Cochran,[17] although small, indicated that 31% of sexual assault victims were at high risk of suicide after experiencing the sexual assault. The Emergency Nurses Association provides a thorough evidence-based review of various assessment tools and resources in their Clinical Practice Guideline: Suicide Risk Assessment.[23]

Clinical judgment is needed to determine what actions should be taken to keep the patient safe. The key to determining the actual level of risk will be in the examiner's ability to communicate effectively in an environment where the patient feels safe to share truthfully their thoughts regarding their suicidal ideation. These conversations for assessment will include the means a person would use to die (ie, gun, hanging, pills) and their intent. Are they thinking about it or have they taken action toward it (ie, bought a gun, stockpiled pills)? Finally, what is their plan (ie, the details of how, when, and where a person will commit suicide)? Questions about suicide and suicide attempts are asked as part of the Danger Assessment. One question is aimed at the offender and the other, although it does not count as part of the score, is about the patient's personal experience with suicidal thoughts and actions. In Janice's situation, after discussing with the psychiatrists, it was felt that she was safe to discharge home with information on access to and referrals for follow-up psychiatric treatment.

As part of the forensic medical examination, the forensic nurse assessed Janice's safety. The nurse completed a Danger Assessment and took a history. The Danger Assessment should be a routine component in the assessment of an IPV patient. The original Danger Assessment was a 20-question instrument designed to assess the likelihood of lethality or near lethality occurring.[24] The most current Danger Assessment can accurately identify the majority of women that are at risk of homicide. Women often underestimate the potential for homicide. A study by Campbell et al[24] showed that only 46% of women killed by their partners assessed their partner as capable of killing them according to family members. Having a discussion with the patient about the findings of these types of studies is often eye-opening. Once the health care provider has their attention, the specific components identified can be used in safety-planning activities.

For more acute settings such as the ED, the DA-5 may be the most appropriate Danger Assessment tool.[25,26] The difference between the original Danger Assessment and the DA-5, other than the number of questions, is that the DA-5 was developed for a quick assessment of homicide or near homicide risk among IPV survivors. It gives the nurse a clearer picture of the immediate risks for death, making it easier for them to understand the need for immediate referral for safety planning and further services. Therefore, it is extremely important that a protocol be established so it is clear what the next step in the care of this patient will be once they leave the hospital setting.

References

1. Sorenson SB, Joshi M, Sivitz E. A systematic review of the epidemiology of nonfatal strangulation, a human rights and health concern. *Am J Public Health.* 2014;104(11):e54-e61.
2. Messing JT, Patch M, Wilson JS, Kelen GD, Campbell J. Differentiating among attempted, completed, and multiple nonfatal strangulation in women experiencing intimate partner violence. *Womens Health Issues.* 2018;28(1):104-111.
3. Wilbur L, Higley M, Hatfield J, et al. Survey results of women who have been strangled while in an abusive relationship. *J Emerg Med.* 2001;21(3):297-302.
4. Faugno D, Waszak D, Strack GB, Brooks MA, Gwinn CG. Strangulation forensic examination: best practice for health care providers. *Adv Emerg Nurs J.* 2013;35(4):314-327.
5. Strack GB, McClane GE, Hawley D. A review of 300 attempted strangulation cases. Part 1: criminal legal issues. *J Emerg Med.* 2001;21(3):303-309.
6. Patch M, Anderson JC, Campbell JC. Injuries of women surviving intimate partner strangulation and subsequent emergency health care seeking: an integrative evidence review. *J Emerg Nurs.* 2018;44(4):384-393.
7. Strack GB, Gwinn C, Hawley D, Green W, Smock B, Riviello R. Why didn't someone tell me? Health consequences of strangulation assaults for survivors. *Domestic Violence Report.* 2014;19(6):87-90.
8. Fineron PW, Turnbull JA, Busuttil A. Fracture of the hyoid bone in survivors of attempted manual strangulation. *J Clin Forensic Med.*1995;2(4):195-197.
9. De Boos, J. Review article: non-fatal strangulation: hidden injuries, hidden risks. *Emerg Med Australas.* 2019;31(3):302-308.
10. Plattner T, Bolliger S, Zollinger U. Forensic assessment of survived strangulation. *Forensic Sci Int.* 2005;153(2-3):202-207.
11. Line WS Jr, Stanley RB Jr, Choi JH. Strangulation: a full spectrum of blunt neck trauma. *Ann Otol Rhinol Laryngol.* 1985;94(6 pt 1):542-546.
12. Iacovou E, Nayar M, Fleming J, Lew-Gor S. A pain in the neck: a rare case of isolated hyoid bone trauma. *J Surg Case Rep.* 2011;2011(7):3.
13. Kuo LC, Lin HL, Chen CW, Lee WC. Traumatic hyoid bone fracture in patient wearing a helmet: a case report. *Am J Emerg Med.* 2008;26(2):251.e1-e2.

14. Angoules AG, Boutsikari EC. Traumatic hyoid bone fractures: rare but potentially life threatening injuries. *Emerg Med.* 2013;3(1):e128.

15. Dworkin ER, Menon SV, Bystrynski J, Allen NE. Sexual assault victimization and psychopathology: a review and meta-analysis. *Clin Psychol Rev.* 2017;56:65-81.

16. Mitchell C, Anglin D. *Intimate Partner Violence: A Health-Based Perspective.* New York, NY: Oxford University Press; 2009.

17. Cochran CB. An evidence-based approach to suicide risk assessment after sexual assault. *J Forensic Nurs.* 2019;15(2):84-92.

18. Thomas KA, Joshi M, Sorenson SB. "Do you know what it feels like to drown?": Strangulation as coercive control in intimate relationships. *Psychol Women Q.* 2014;38(1):124-137.

19. Glass N, Laughon K, Campbell J, et al. Non-fatal strangulation is an important risk factor for homicide of women. *J Emerg Med.* 2008;35(3):329-335.

20. Cavanaugh CE, Messing JT, Del-Colle M, O'Sullivan C, Campbell JC. Prevalence and correlates of suicidal behavior among adult female victims of intimate partner violence. *Suicide Life Threat Behav.* 2011;41(4):372-383.

21. Dunn RJ, Lopez RA. *Strangulation Injuries.* Treasure Island, FL: StatPearls Publishing; 2019.

22. Ahmedani BK, Simon GE, Stewart C, et al. Health care contacts in the year before suicide death. *J Gen Intern Med.* 2014;29(6):870-877.

23. Zaleski ME, Johnson ML, Valdez AM, et al; 2017 ENA Clinical Practice Guideline Committee. Clinical practice guideline: suicide risk assessment. *J Emerg Nurs.* 2018;44(5):505.e1-505.e33.

24. Campbell JC, Webster DW, Glass N. The danger assessment: validation of a lethality risk assessment instrument for intimate partner femicide. *J Interpers Violence.* 2009;24(4):653-674.

25. Snider C, Webster D, O'Sullivan CS, Campbell J. Intimate partner violence: development of a brief risk assessment for the emergency department. *Acad Emerg Med.* 2009;16(11):1208-1216.

26. Campbell R, Dworkin ER, Cabral G. An ecological model of the impact of sexual assault on women's mental health. *Trauma Violence Abuse.* 2009;10(3):225-246.

27. Messing JT, Campbell JC, Snider C. Validation and adaptation of the danger assessment-5: a brief intimate partner violence risk assessment. *J Adv Nurs.* 2017;73(12):3220-3230.

Anatomic Skills 1-1

Refer to **Figure 1-1**. Using the letters that correspond to the structure in the photograph, label the anatomic locations.

A.____

B.____

C.____

D. ____

E.____

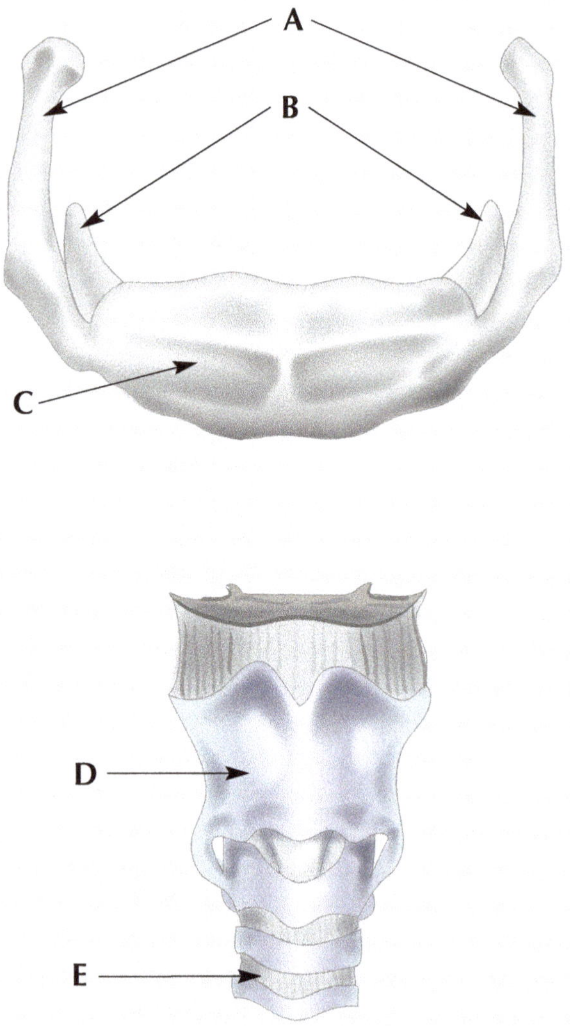

Figure 1-1

Activities

Activity 1-1. Injury Identification

Refer to **Figures 1-2** and **1-3**. Identify any injuries in respect to their anatomic location. Write objective descriptions when documenting findings.

F. ____

G. ____

H. ____

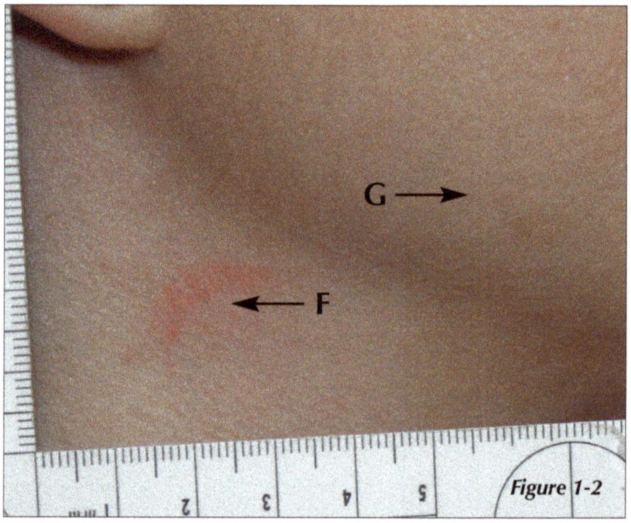

Figure 1-2

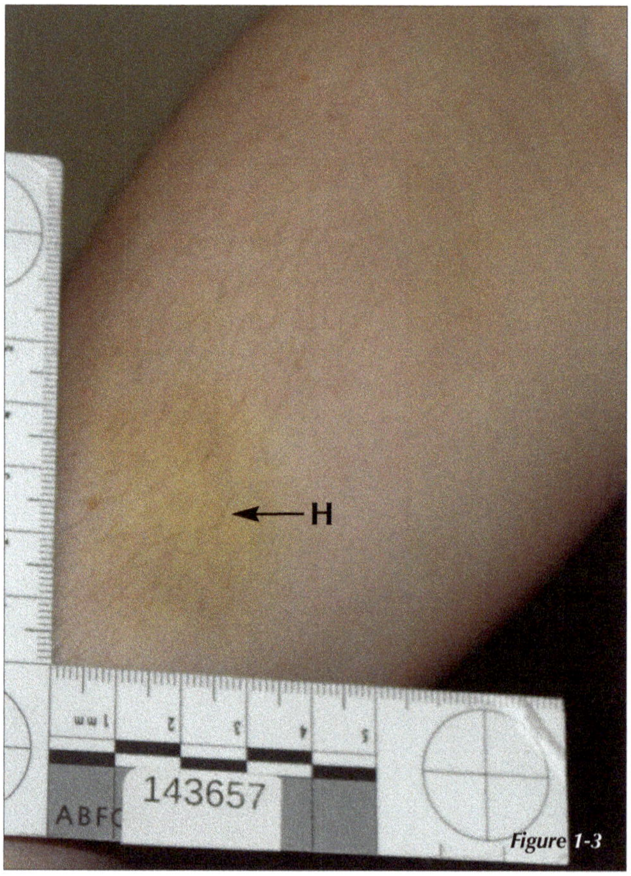

Figure 1-3

Activity 1-2. Assessment

List 3 additional questions that the forensic nurse asks regarding the physical findings (eg, symptom Onset, Location/radiation, Duration, Character, Aggravating factors, Relieving factors, Timing, and Severity [OLDCARTS]; demonstration of method of injury [if known]; level of consciousness).

Activity 1-3. Physical Assessment

Remember that injury is progressive throughout the healing phases. Because of the nature of neck and brain injury (eg, closed/open spaces with continued bleeding), there is potential for diminished function throughout the assessment. Therefore, assessment for potential serious sequelae is continuous in all patients, and when decline in function is recognized, an immediate referral to an advanced practice nurse, physician, or physician assistant is urgent and necessary. List 3 to 6 additional procedures you should consider.

Activity 1-4. Evidence Collection

The nurse has the patient demonstrate on a mannequin how the offender's hands were placed on her neck (**Figure 1-4**). List 3 to 6 other photos that should be added to what you have also observed. What evidence would you collect given the patient's history? What findings would promote evidence collection even if the history is deficient?

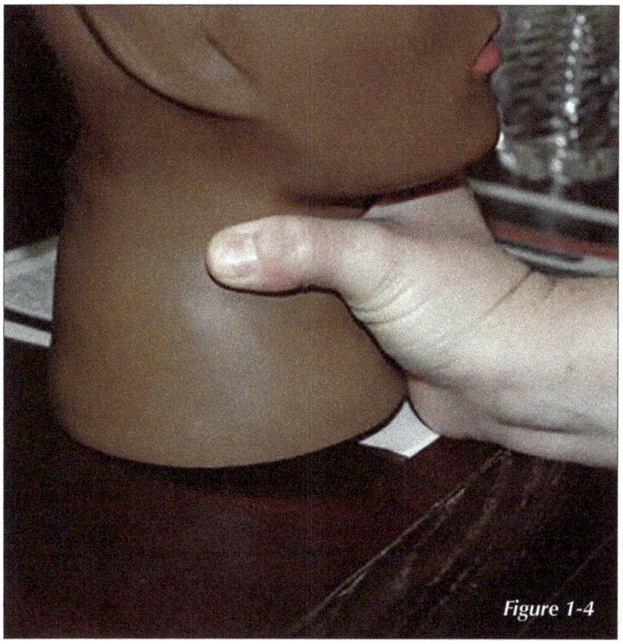

Figure 1-4

Activity 1-5. Treatment and Care

Based on the history and your findings, what treatment would you offer this patient? Would you report this case to the police?

Activity 1-6. Lethality Assessment

During care and as part of discharge planning, all patients who are suspected to be victims of domestic violence should be assessed for risk of immediate danger. List 4 indicators of escalating danger for a person who has experienced domestic violence. What questions should you ask a patient to assess his or her risk of immediate danger?

Chapter 2

21-Year-Old Male Patient Assaulted by an Acquaintance

Case History

Ralph is a 21-year-old man who met with another man from a dating website. They met in the backyard of a house that was closed for the summer. The suspect became very aggressive and wanted to have sex immediately. Ralph said no, and the suspect grabbed Ralph and "choked" him with his forearm. Ralph lost consciousness and woke to the suspect on top of him penetrating his anus. A security camera had recorded all activities in the backyard, and a police investigation discovered all of the events recorded, happening as described by Ralph.

Ralph states, "I tried to move, but his forearm went on my neck again, and that's the last thing I remember. When I woke up, he was still on top of me. He choked me again, and I passed out. I woke up again, and I didn't move. He was still on top of me, and his penis was in my anus. I just let him finish. Then I got up, pulled my pants up, ran with my cell phone, and called 911. Paramedics brought me to the hospital. I can barely talk now."

Case Discussion

Myths, stereotypes, and unfounded beliefs about male sexuality—and in particular, male homosexuality—are widespread in legal and medical communities, as well as among agencies providing services to sexual assault victims. Men and boys who have been sexually assaulted or abused have many of the same feelings and reactions as other survivors of sexual assault, but they may also face additional challenges because of social attitudes and stereotypes about men and masculinity. Because of this, sexual assaults with male victims are underreported.[1,2] There is also a lack of appropriate services for male victims. Male victims of stranger assaults are more likely to experience assaults involving deadly weapons[3] and physical violence.[4]

Some common experiences shared by men who have been sexually assaulted include anxiety, depression, posttraumatic stress disorder, flashbacks, and eating disorders; feeling on-edge, being unable to relax, and having difficulty sleeping; and withdrawal from relationships and friendships and an increased sense of isolation. After a sexual assault, many men also have concerns or questions about sexual orientation, have feelings of being "less of a man," feel a sense of shame from not being able to stop the assault, and worry about disclosing for fear of judgement or disbelief.[5] When a man reports sexual assault to a heath care provider, it is important to listen, validate the patient's feelings, express concern, and provide appropriate treatment and resources.

Approximately 26% of gay men and 37% of bisexual men experience rape, physical violence, or stalking by an intimate partner, compared with 29% of heterosexual men.[4] This vulnerable population has increased risk and problems after sexual assault and violence.

In this case, strangulation was also involved. The guidelines for strangulation assessment should be followed to ensure a complete analysis of injury. Another concern for

Ralph is bias and discrimination by health care professionals, a major deterrent for gay men to seek health care. Sexual orientation determines who a person is attracted to, whether it is a man, a woman, both, or a combination of gender characteristics.[6] Ralph never told his parents nor his health care provider that he is gay. Young gay men without social acceptance are at risk for suicide. Social support is necessary for gay men to express their fears and concerns before revealing their sexual orientation.

Another potential risk is exposure to human immunodeficiency virus (HIV). Ralph was tested and provided postexposure prophylaxis (PEP). Instructions to follow up with his health care provider addressed some of Ralph's concerns about disclosure. A good rule of thumb is to routinely test men who have sex with men for HIV, assess HIV-negative patients for risk behaviors, and prescribe preexposure prophylaxis (PrEP) as needed.[7] Knowledgeable health care providers have a critical role in addressing all HIV prevention and intervention efforts for patients like Ralph.

In this case, after 2 years, the accused pled to an agreement that included incarceration, and Ralph did not have to testify in the courtroom.

Community-specific resources include the following:

— LGBT National Help Center Online Chat[8]

— The Human Rights Campaign[9]

As a caring society of professionals, health care providers should recognize the barriers faced by sexually nonconforming persons when choosing whether to speak out about a sexual assault. When men do choose to come forward, it is important that male survivors, like all survivors, are believed and supported by those around them and allowed to make trauma-informed, evidence-based decisions about what are necessary actions to take.[10]

References

1. Info & stats for journalists: statistics about sexual violence. National Sexual Violence Resource Center Web site. https://www.nsvrc.org/sites/default/files/2015-01/publications_nsvrc_factsheet_media-packet_statistics-about-sexual-violence_0.pdf. Accessed December 10, 2019.
2. Masho SW, Anderson L. Sexual assault in men: a population-based study of Virginia. *Violence Vict.* 2009;24(1):98-110.
3. Lipscomb GH, Muram D, Speck PM, Mercer BM. Male victims of sexual assault. *JAMA.* 1992;267(22):3064-3066.
4. Bullock CM, Beckson M. Male victims of sexual assault: phenomenology, psychology, physiology. *J Am Acad Psychiatry Law.* 2011;39(2):197-205.
5. Sexual assault of men and boys. Rape, Abuse, & Incest National Network Web site. https://www.rainn.org/articles/sexual-assault-men-and-boys. Accessed May 11, 2020.
6. Psychology Today. How many genders are there? Psychology Today Web site. https://www.psychologytoday.com/us/basics/gender. Accessed October 29, 2019.
7. Finlayson T, Cha S, Xia M, et al; National HIV Behavioral Surveillance Study Group. Changes in HIV preexposure prophylaxis awareness and use among men who have sex with men - 20 urban areas, 2014 and 2017. *MMWR Morb Mortal Wkly Rep.* 2019;68(27):597-603.
8. LGBT national online peer-support chat. LGBT National Help Center Web site. https://www.glbthotline.org/chat.html. Accessed October 29, 2019.
9. Sexual assault and the LGBTQ community. Human Rights Campaign Web site. https://www.hrc.org/resources/sexual-assault-and-the-lgbt-community. Accessed October 29, 2019.
10. Student Life Sexual Assault Prevention and Awareness Center. Male survivors of sexual assault. University of Michigan Web site. https://sapac.umich.edu/article/53. Accessed October 29, 2019.

Anatomic Skills 2-1

Refer to **Figures 2-1** through **2-3**. Using the letters that correspond to the structure in the photograph, label the anatomic locations.

A. ______________________________

B. ______________________________

C. ______________________________

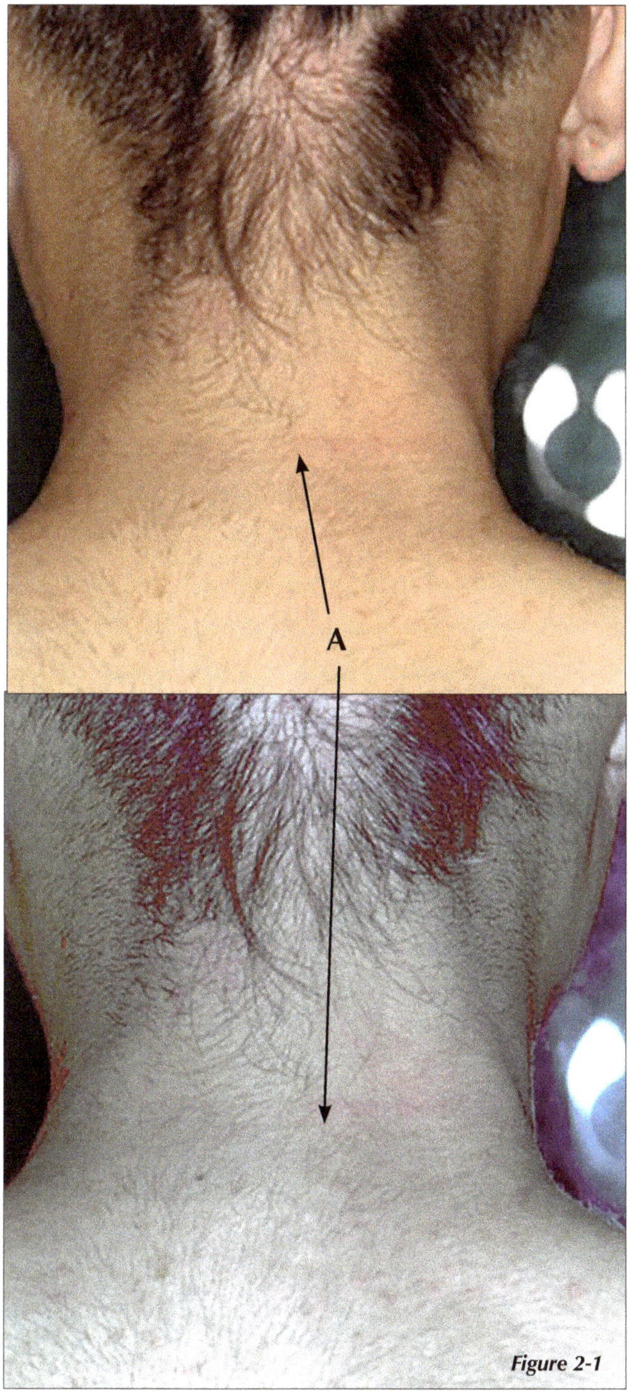

Figure 2-1

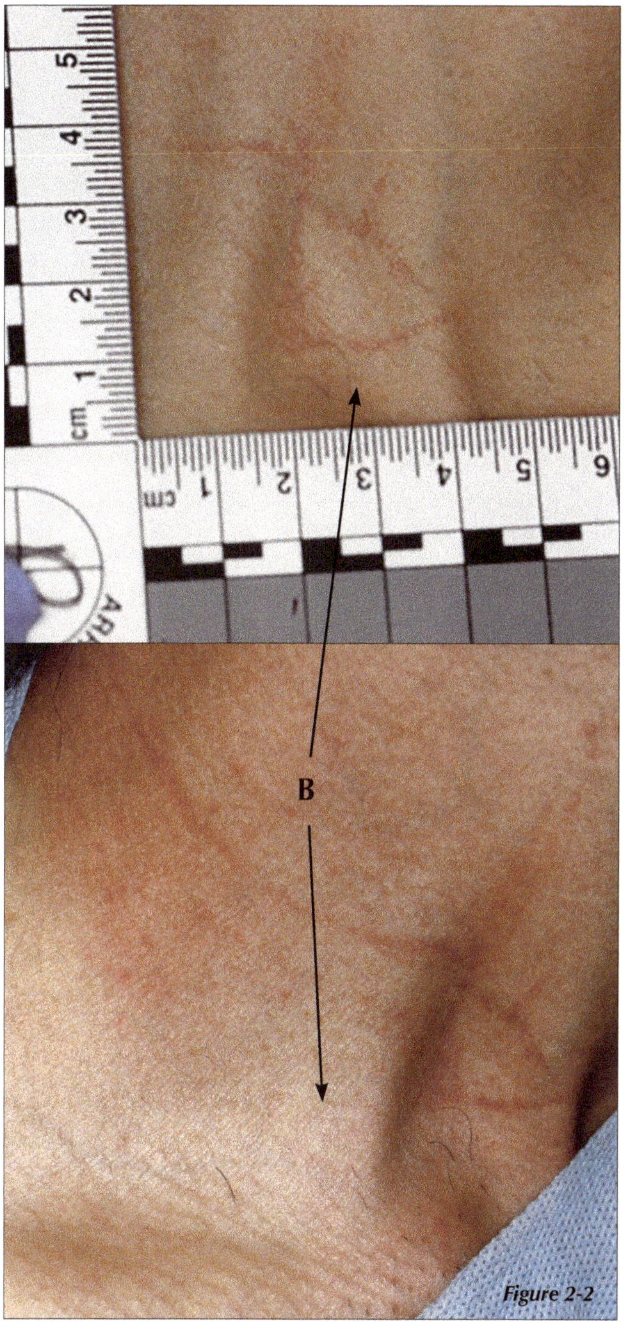

Figure 2-2

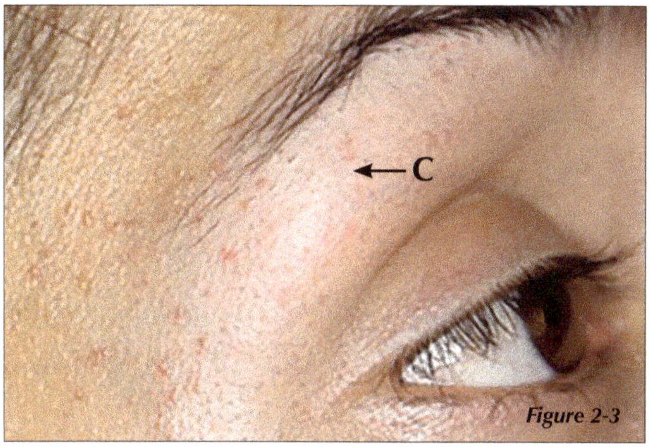

Figure 2-3

Activities

Activity 2-1. Injury Identification

Refer to **Figures 2-1** through **2-4**. Identify any injuries in respect to their anatomic location. Give objective descriptions when documenting findings.

A. ______________________________

B. ______________________________

C. ______________________________

D. ______________________________

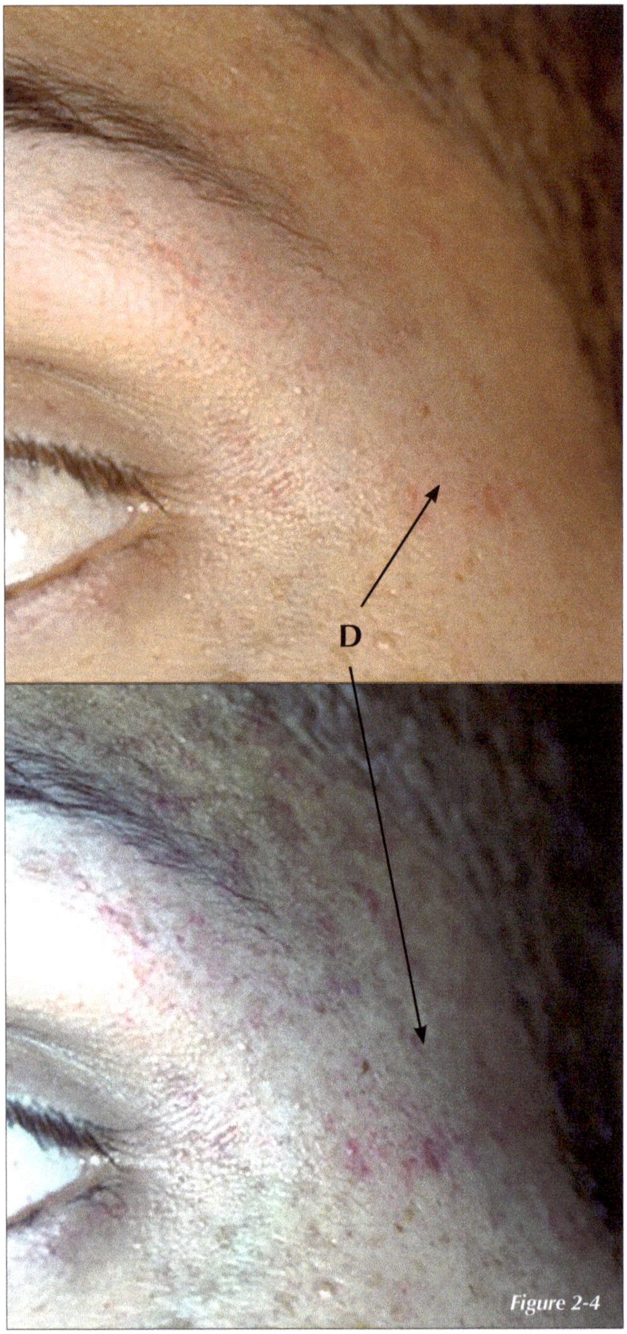

Figure 2-4

Activity 2-2. Assessment

List 3 additional questions that the forensic nurse should ask regarding the physical findings.

Activity 2-3. Physical Assessment

Remember that because of the potential for diminished function, assessment is continuous in all patients, and when diminished function is recognized, it requires immediate referral (eg, to an advanced practice nurse, physician, or physician assistant). List 3 to 6 additional physical assessment procedures you should consider.

Activity 2-4. Evidence Collection

Using the patient's history, what evidence would you collect?

Activity 2-5. Treatment and Care

Based on the history and your findings, what treatment would you offer this patient? Would you report this case to the police?

Chapter 3

66-Year-Old Female Patient Assaulted by Her Son

Case History

Mary is a 66-year-old woman who lives at home with her 69-year-old husband and 42-year-old son. She reports to the nurse that she was in the kitchen when her son came home and started to yell at her and hit her. She says he was mad "because he ran out of money again." The suspect grabbed the patient's neck from the front with one hand and threw her to the floor. "I don't remember falling down, but I remember feeling that his hand never came off my neck," Mary says. She remembers being on the ground on her back with the suspect leaning over her, and his left hand was still on her neck while he held a gun to her head with his right hand. "It was hard to remember exactly what he was saying, but he told me to give him money or he was gonna shoot me." The patient says her husband was in the bedroom but came into the kitchen when he heard the commotion. He started "a fight with our son," Mary says. She then describes that during the confrontation, the suspect physically assaulted his father with his fist and the gun. Mary says her son fled the residence through the front door when she called 911. Her husband was transported to the emergency department (ED), but she did not disclose her strangulation to law enforcement. Her injuries were not evaluated in the ED until the next day when they became visible to the nurses caring for her husband.

> ***Clinical Pearl:***
> *97% of strangulation victims are strangled manually with hands.*

Mary is examined by a forensic nurse in the ED 24 hours after the assault. She states, "I think he only choked me once, because he pushed me to the floor by my neck. He was squeezing so hard. When he pulled out the gun, he squeezed even harder." Mary states, "He deals drugs, and he is just not right. He doesn't know what he's doing! He never hurt us like this before. It was like he was crazy."

The forensic nurse continues to ask Mary questions about her symptoms after the physical assault and strangulation. Mary reports that she lost her hearing during the event. She says she could not hear what her husband was saying when he and their son were fighting. Mary says, "It seemed quiet during that time even though I could see them yelling at each other." She says, "I got my hearing back once I heard my husband yell after my son hit him. It felt like slow motion, then it all went really fast." Other symptoms Mary discloses are weakness and numbness in bilateral upper extremities, chest pain, sore throat, coughing, difficulty swallowing, raspy voice, and nausea. Mary is disoriented to time and place when asked simple questions about her demographics and living situation. She is unsure if she lost consciousness but does not actually remember falling to the floor (**Appendix 14**). The patient is admitted to the hospital for 24-hour observation.

During the physical assessment, the patient does not disclose physical blows. She does have bruising to the right side of the upper lip area and the lateral and inferior corpus of the tongue that she cannot explain. She is asked about possibly clenching her jaw or biting her own tongue during strangulation and she states she does not remember because "it happened so fast."

The patient is seen for a follow-up examination 4 days (96 hours) later. The bruising on her tongue is almost completely gone after 4 days. However, she has new emerging and visible bruising on her right mandible area that was not seen during the evaluation 24 hours after the assault. She states that, although she was discharged from the hospital after 1 day, she continues to have neck pain, headaches, and dizziness.

Case Discussion

Forensic nurses and other forensic providers should follow best practices and a structured protocol to guide the evaluation and to capture all visible and painful injury. The nurse did a complete head-to-toe assessment, examining 360 degrees around the head and neck of the patient, and used traumagrams (**Figure 3-1**) to designate signs of the detectable injury. Using a standardized examination process decreases and minimizes errors in documentation. An example of standard strangulation examination protocols for both adults and pediatrics are on the Secure Digital Forensic Imaging website.[1]

The forensic nurse found injury on the patient's tongue. Injury in this area is easily missed if it is not part of the provider's standard oral cavity examination. It is important to note that the forensic nurse scheduled a follow-up examination with the patient. The next evaluation found additional injuries on the patient that were not present at the time of the initial examination. If a follow-up examination is not possible, tell the patient to contact law enforcement if new injuries arise or to self-photograph injury progression.

In the initial history, the patient did not remember or disclose everything that happened to her during the attack. That is expected, and there are several reasons for this (eg, trauma to the head and subsequent brain injury, anoxic injury, some memories take time to fall into place after a traumatic experience). In this instance, the suspect grabbed the patient's neck with one hand and pushed her to the floor, all while clasping her throat. The patient does not remember falling, suggesting she experienced an anoxic injury.

Figure 3-1. *Traumagrams for documentation of detectable injury in nonfatal strangulation.*

Traumagrams for Documentation of Injury in Nonfatal Strangulation

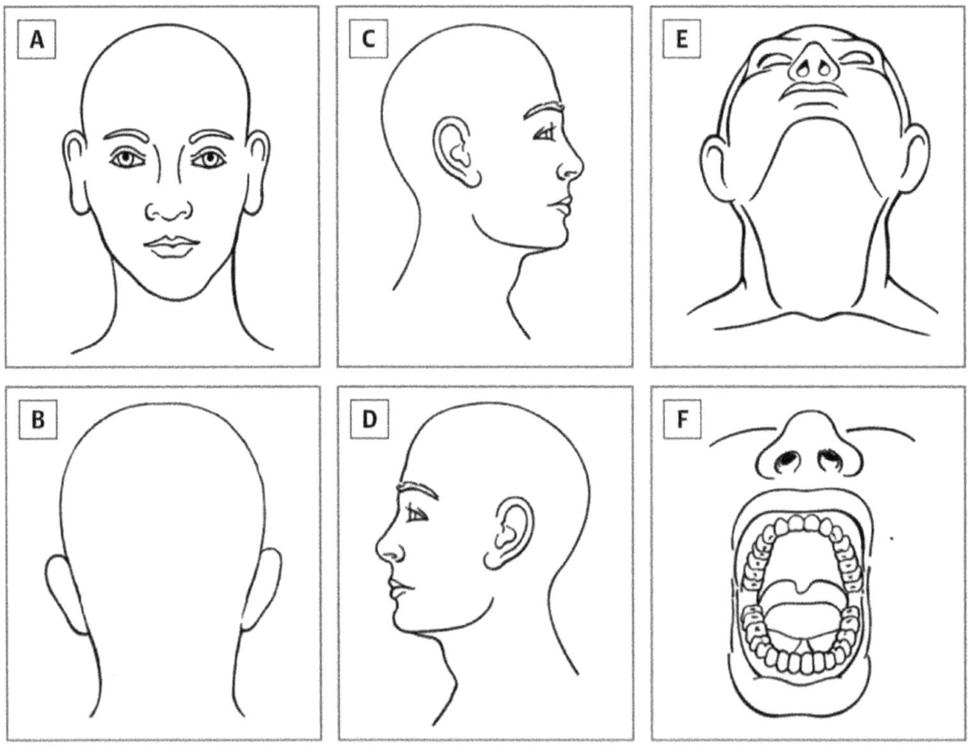

Figure 3-1

Safety planning is a significant consideration for this elderly couple. A social assessment looking to identify other family members in the area and community organizations that have services to support them would be very helpful. If their caregiver is their son, they may wonder if other family members will believe them or shun them, leaving them with nowhere to turn for assistance. A caregiver is mandated to cross-report to adult protective services. Often, elders are ashamed after facing violence and worry about losing their homes; therefore, they do not want to burden other family members, and as a result, they keep serious internal family troubles to themselves.[2]

There are coordinated community responses in place to assist victims of elder abuse, whether it is sexual abuse or other types of maltreatment. Depending on the community, maltreated elders receive an array of services to address their unique situation. Some may have had negative experiences with law enforcement and therefore decline to report.[3] It is important to remember that elders have the capacity to make informed decisions and have the right to decline any and all services offered by the coordinated response community.

Estimates indicate that 1 million elderly people are victims of domestic violence every year, and 40% of cases occur when adult children victimize their parents. Maltreatment of elderly persons is a growing problem because of the intimate nature of parent-child relationships. Researchers believe that elder parent abuse is one of the most underreported forms of violence.[4]

The National Center for Elder Abuse[5] provides the latest information regarding research, training, best practices, news, and resources on elder maltreatment (eg, abuse, neglect, financial exploitation) to professionals and the public. There are also a wide variety of tools available to help screen for elder abuse.[6]

In this case, the patient and her husband are victims of elder maltreatment, including emotional and physical abuse. The Centers for Disease Control and Prevention[7] defines elder abuse as an "intentional act, or failure to act, by a caregiver or another person in a relationship involving an expectation of trust that causes or creates a risk of harm to an older adult." An older adult is someone age 60 years or older. Physical elder abuse is the intentional use of physical force that results in acute or chronic illness, body injury, physical pain, functional impairment, distress, or death. Physical abuse may include, but is not limited to, violent acts such as striking (with or without an object or weapon), hitting, beating, scratching, biting, strangling, suffocating, pushing, shoving, shaking, slapping, kicking, stomping, pinching, and burning. Emotional or psychological abuse is verbal or nonverbal behavior that results in the infliction of anguish, mental pain, fear, or distress (eg, holding a gun to a person's head).[7]

The power of controlling a victim's next breath makes strangulation a tactic frequently used by abusers. In manual strangulation, it can take fewer than 10 seconds for a person to lose consciousness, and death may occur in under 5 minutes.[8]

The identification rate of intimate partner violence in health care settings is high.[9,10] Strangulation Medical Guidelines advise the medical care after strangulation. Often, communities do not have an understanding of the treatment or documentation of strangulation. Community-based education on strangulation is necessary to create standardization in care. One standard is mandatory reporting laws, which require certain groups, including health care providers, to tell designated authorities about reasonable suspicions of elder abuse.[11]

References

1. Pediatric non-fatal strangulation photodocumentation protocol. Secure Digital Forensic Imaging Web site. http://www.sdfi.com/eCommerce/sdfi-pediatric-non-fatal-strangulation-protocol. Accessed August 28, 2019.

2. Lin MC, Giles H. The dark side of family communication: a communication model of elder abuse and neglect. *Int Psychogeriatr.* 2013;25(8):1275-1290.

3. Posick C. Victimization and reporting to the police: the role of negative emotionality. *Psychol Violence.* 2014;4(2):210-223.

4. Springer A. Elderly abuse: why they don't report it. Gloucester Times Web site. https://www.gloucestertimes.com/news/lifestyles/elderly-abuse-why-they-don-t-report-it/article_0c43c405-63a4-543f-b46c-f07ebbb3f7ac.html. Published April 26, 2013. Accessed September 5, 2019.

5. National Center on Elder Abuse Web site. https://ncea.acl.gov/. Accessed September 5, 2019.

6. Ries NM, Mansfield E. Elder abuse: the role of general practitioners in community-based screening and multidisciplinary action. *Aust J Gen Pract.* 2018;47(4):235-238.

7. Violence prevention: elder abuse definitions. Centers for Disease Control and Prevention Web site. https://www.cdc.gov/violenceprevention/elderabuse/definitions.html. Updated May 28, 2019. Accessed August 28, 2019.

8. Strack GB, McClane G. How to improve your investigation and prosecution of strangulation cases. National Center on Domestic and Sexual Violence Web site. http://www.ncdsv.org/images/strangulation_article.pdf. Updated May 1999. Accessed June 4, 2020.

9. Messing JT, Patch M, Wilson JS, Kelen GD, Campbell J. Differentiating among attempted, completed, and multiple nonfatal strangulation in women experiencing intimate partner violence. *Womens Health Issues.* 2018;28(1):104-111.

10. Yon Y, Ramiro-Gonzalez M, Mikton CR, Huber M, Sethi D. The prevalence of elder abuse in institutional settings: a systematic review and meta-analysis. *Eur J Public Health.* 2019;29(1):58-67.

11. State elder abuse statues. The United States Department of Justice Web site. https://www.justice.gov/elderjustice/elder-justice-statutes-0. Accessed September 5, 2019.

Anatomic Skills

Anatomic Skills 3-1

Refer to **Figure 3-2**. Using the letters that correspond to the structures in the photograph, label the anatomic locations.

Arrow A. ____________________

Arrow B. ____________________

Arrow C. ____________________

Arrow D. ____________________

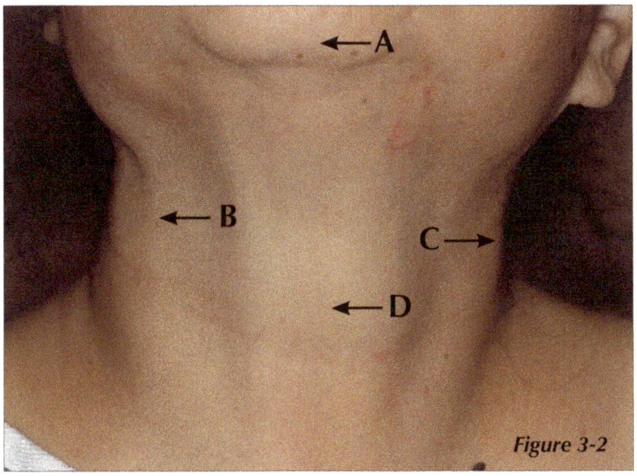

Figure 3-2

Anatomic Skills 3-2

Refer to **Figure 3-3**. Using the letters that correspond to the structures in the photograph, label the anatomic locations.

Arrow E. ____________________

Arrow F. ____________________

Arrow G. ____________________

Arrow H. ____________________

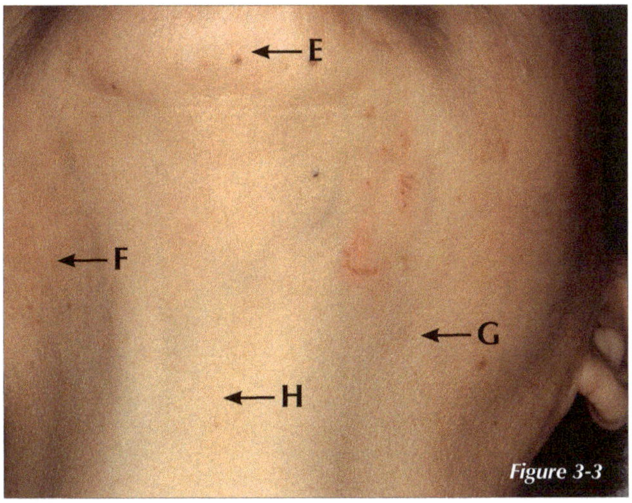

Figure 3-3

Activities

Activity 3-1. Injury Identification

Refer to **Figures 3-4** through **3-8**. Identify any injuries in respect to their anatomic location. Write objective descriptions when documenting findings.

Arrow I. ____________________

Arrow J. ____________________

Arrow K. ____________________

Arrow L. ____________________

Arrow M. ____________________

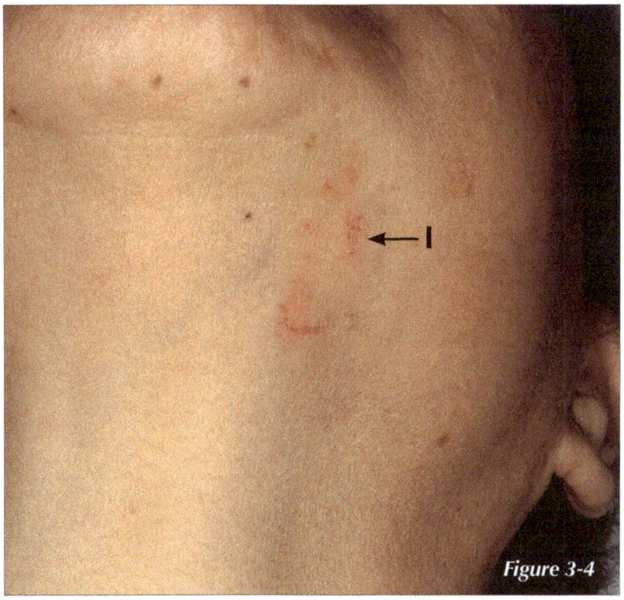

Figure 3-4

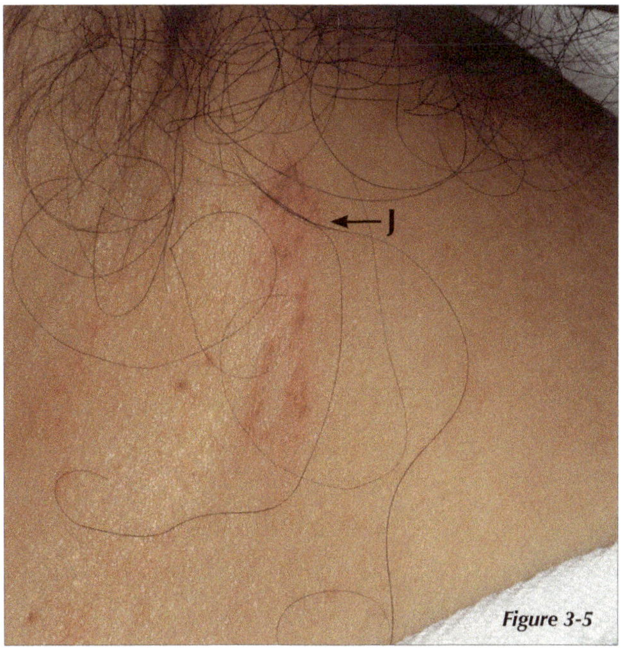

Figure 3-5

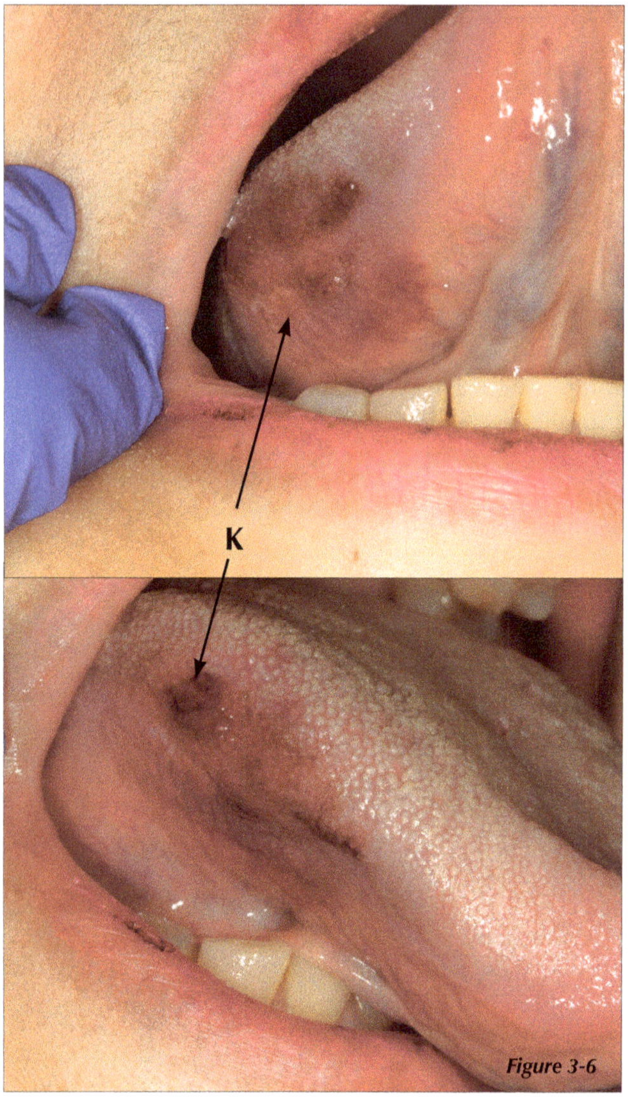

Figure 3-6

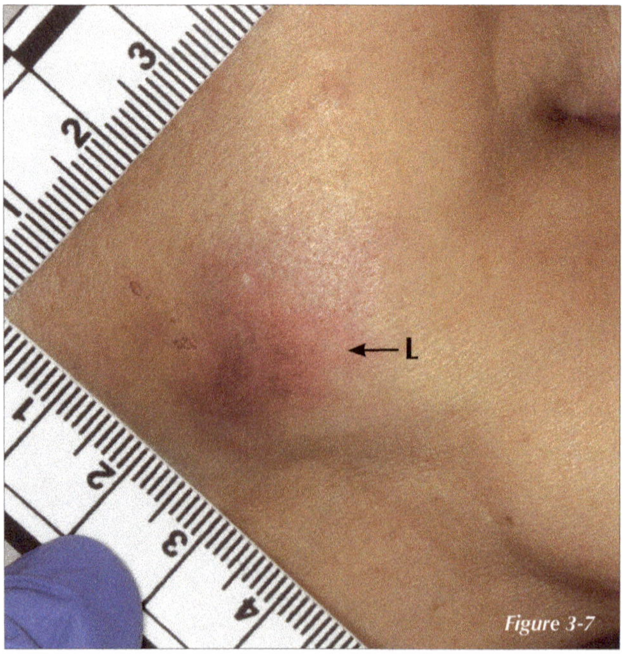

Figure 3-7

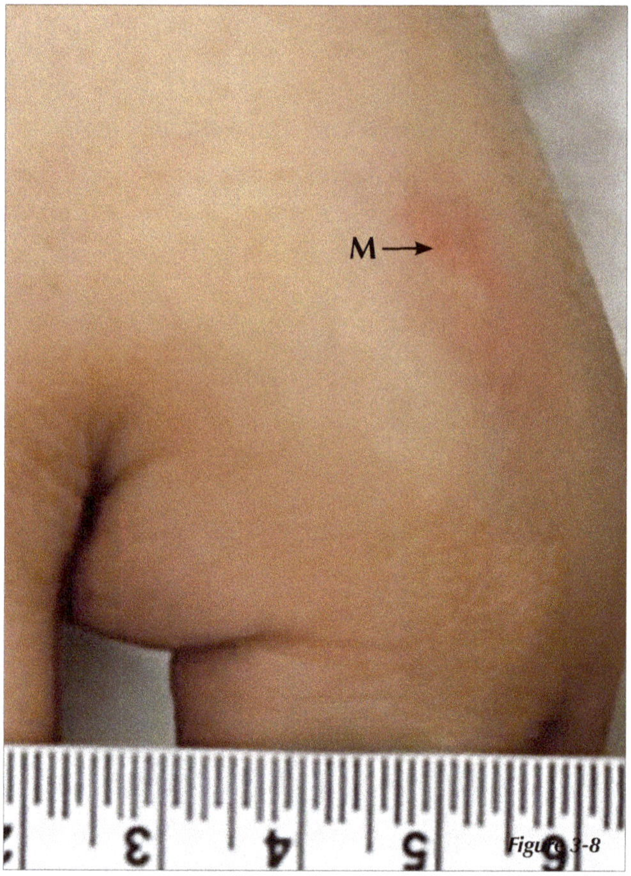

Figure 3-8

ACTIVITY 3-2. ASSESSMENT

List 3 additional questions that the forensic nurse in SANE care asks regarding the physical findings (eg, symptom Onset, Location/radiation, Duration, Character, Aggravating factors, Timing and Severity [OLDCARTS]; demonstration of method of injury [if known]; level of consciousness).

Activity 3-3. Physical Assessment

Remember that injury is progressive throughout the healing phases. Because of the nature of neck and brain injury (eg, closed/open spaces with continued bleeding), there is potential for diminished function throughout the assessment. Therefore, assessment for potential serious sequelae is continuous in all patients, and when decline in function is recognized, an immediate referral to an advanced practice nurse, physician, or physician assistant is urgent and necessary. List 3 to 6 additional physical assessment procedures you should consider.

Activity 3-4. Evidence Collection

What evidence would you collect given the patient's history? What findings would promote evidence collection even if history is deficient?

Activity 3-5. Treatment and Care

Based on the history and your findings, what treatment would you offer this patient? Would you report this case to the police or adult protective services or both?

Activity 3-6. Lethality Assessment

During care and as part of discharge planning, all patients who are suspected to be victims of domestic violence should be assessed for risk of immediate danger. List 4 indicators of escalating danger in a person who has experienced domestic violence. What questions should you ask a patient to assess his or her risk of immediate danger?

Chapter 4

17-Year-Old Female Patient Assaulted by a Nonintimate Acquaintance Stalker

Case History

Linda is a 17-year-old girl with a history of foster care and no family ties. She had been in foster care since age 6 when her parents died in an accident. She aged out of foster care, and she and her 1-year-old daughter currently live with friends. Linda usually works the evening shift with her friend José, when there are only a few employees scattered throughout the building. José had been asking Linda to go out with him, and she told him she was not interested in "that kind of relationship."

She says that José sexually assaulted her when they were together at work. She states, "He got really angry after looking at my Facebook account. He told me he was going to hit me for every guy he saw on my page. He repeatedly hit and slapped me on the left side of my face, back, thighs, and tummy. He tied my hands up with his tie and just punched and kicked my body all over. He had me in a choke hold when he dragged me into the copy room." She reports being "crumpled on the floor" and "crying" asking for help. She says, "No one came," and "that's where he forced me to have sex with him." Someone from the office called 911.

> ***Clinical Pearl:***
> *35% of strangulation victims are strangled as well as sexually assaulted/abused, and 9% of victims are also pregnant.*

Emergency medical responders arrived with law enforcement, and after a rapid triage process, attached her to a backboard, applied a neck brace, and inserted an intravenous (IV) line. Her clothing was cut off and bagged, and Linda was bleeding from the genital area. They transported Linda to the emergency department where the trauma team was waiting. Police remained on the scene. Linda was crying and sobbing through her oxygen mask. She does not have health insurance and states, "I don't have any money and now I won't have a job because of this. What do you want me to do?" The forensic nurse is called and responds to the hospital to see Linda. After Linda is stabilized, the forensic examination is started with Linda's consent. An advocate is present for the examination. The patient examination is conducted 6 hours after the assault. Linda tells the nurse that José had sex with her. The nurse confirms "sex" was penile-vaginal penetration.

Case Discussion

A full battery of laboratory testing and imaging is completed, reflecting the assault history, and the patient is released to the forensic nurse for the medical forensic evaluation. Often, when gathering the history of an assault, the forensic nurse may not suspect strangulation, and therefore, will not ask about it. It is recommended that communication with the patient includes common, understandable vocabulary. Even if the health care provider uses the word ***choking***, the patient may not see that as strangulation. The recommendation from San Diego County Forensic Nurses is to ask, "Did anything touch your neck or mouth?" Using open-ended, descriptive language often triggers the patient's need to divulge a history of strangulation.[1] In this case, the patient does disclose strangulation in the form of a "choke hold" and being dragged. If not evaluated during the acute workup following triage, the recommendation for testing is computed tomographic (CT) angiogram of the carotid/vertebral arteries (the gold standard for evaluation of vessels and bony/cartilaginous structures, although it is less sensitive for soft tissue trauma) or CT of the neck with contrast (less sensitive than CT angiogram for vessels but good for bony/cartilaginous structures). In addition, CT angiography combines a CT scan with the injection of dye through an IV line that starts in the arm or hand. The contrast dye technique creates detailed images of the blood vessels in the head and neck, discovering minor dissections. It is important that the nurse does not rub the carotid artery or palpate this area in a nonfatal strangulation case, because that pressure could dislodge a clot. The poststrangulation evaluation information will need to be given to the patient in order to receive consent authorization for this type of examination. The goals of this procedure also need to be explained to the patient, which are to evaluate the vertebral and carotid arteries as well as the soft tissue neck structure and head injury.

When presented with the information about further evaluation, Linda stated she was worried because she does not have insurance. Linda also stated she did not have anywhere for her or her child to go or any friends who would help her now. She also said that she was very scared. The social worker or case manager is notified to discuss her minor status. Without a job and housing, the court should collaborate with Linda to create a safety plan to protect her. Because Linda's assault will be filed as a crime, victim witness services may be helpful. She may qualify for federal or state assistance as well. The social worker assists Linda through the hospital process before discharge. When discharged, the community advocate helps Linda with the child protective services' (CPS) safety plan and court's protection order and helps her find support from someone who can stay with her and monitor her for a few days.[2,3] The advocate notifies a local shelter that could provide long-term services to assist Linda, and she is taken to the shelter after discharge. Follow-up with a medical provider was arranged and approved by CPS with a local clinic. CPS also brought her child to the shelter.

In summary, Linda's case is complex, requiring a number of government, non-governmental, and volunteer organizations' collaborative efforts to support Linda throughout her recovery.

References

1. County of San Diego Health and Human Services Agency. Intimate partner violence in San Diego County. San Diego County Web site. https://www.sandiegocounty.gov/content/dam/sdc/hhsa/programs/phs/cahan/communications_documents/02-12-19.pdf. Published February 12, 2019. Accessed December 4, 2019.

2. Crawford-Jakubiak JE, Alderman EM, Leventhal JM; Committee on Child Abuse and Neglect, Committee on Adolescence. Care of the adolescent after an acute sexual assault. *Pediatrics*. 2017;139(3):e20164243.

3. Mollen CJ, Goyal M, Lavelle J, Scribano P. Evaluation and treatment of the adolescent sexual assault patient. *Adolesc Med State Art Rev*. 2015;26(3):647-657.

Anatomic Skills 4-1

Refer to **Figure 4-1**. Using the letters that correspond to the structures in the photograph, label the anatomic locations.

Arrow A: ______________________________

Arrow B: ______________________________

Arrow C: ______________________________

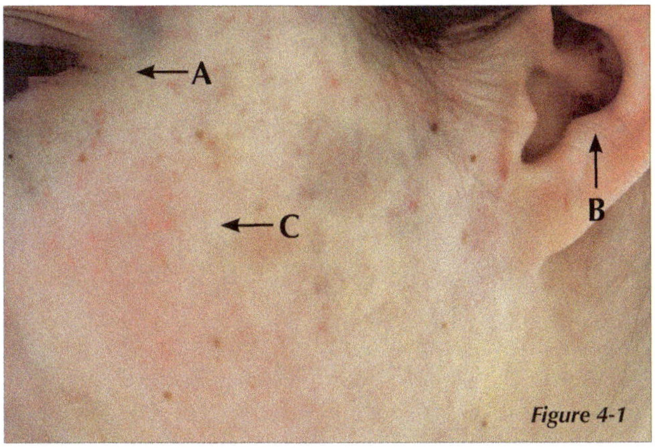

Figure 4-1

Activities

Activity 4-1. Injury Identification

Refer to **Figures 4-2** and **4-3**. Identify any injuries in respect to their anatomic location. Write objective descriptions when documenting findings.

Arrow D. ______________________________

Arrow E. ______________________________

Arrow F. ______________________________

Arrow G. ______________________________

Arrow H. ______________________________

Arrow I. ______________________________

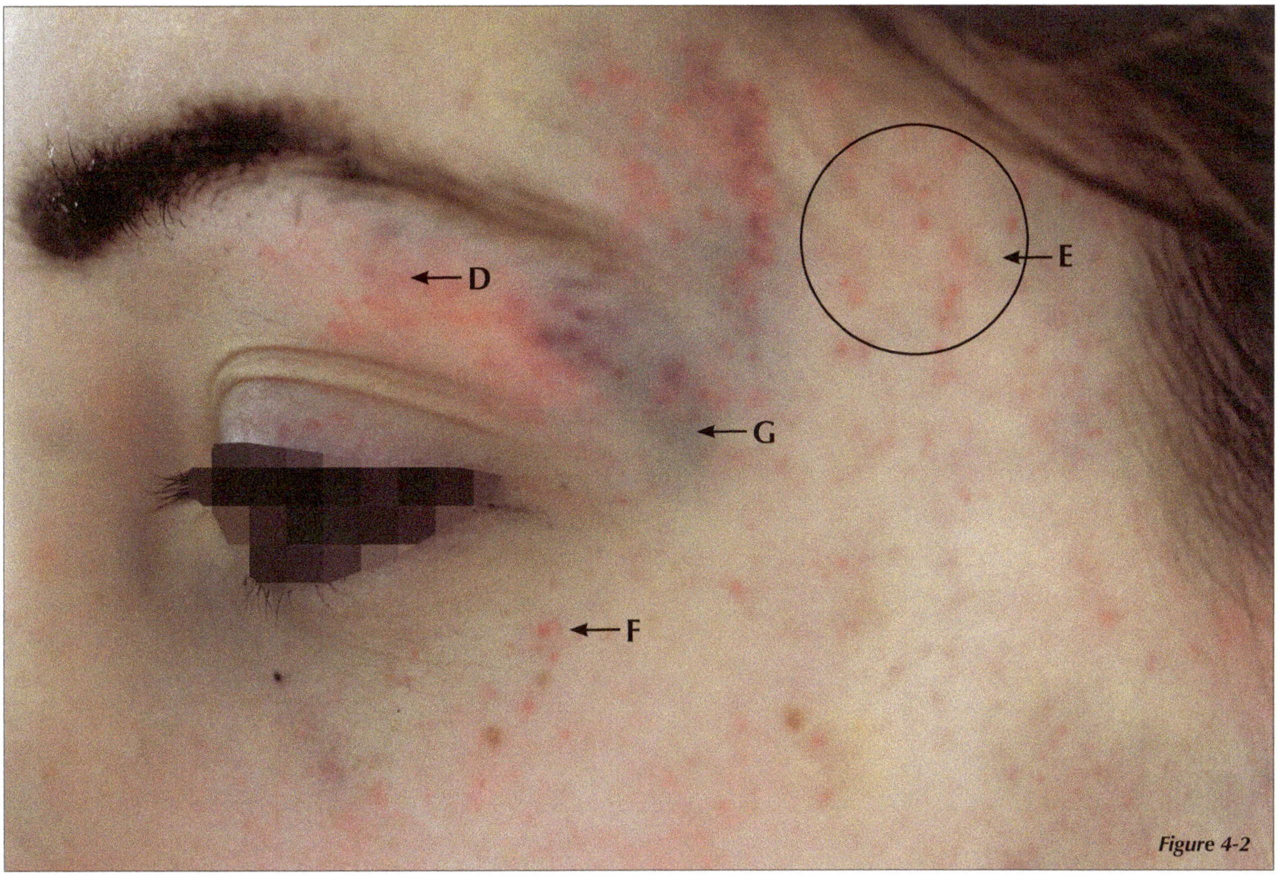

Figure 4-2

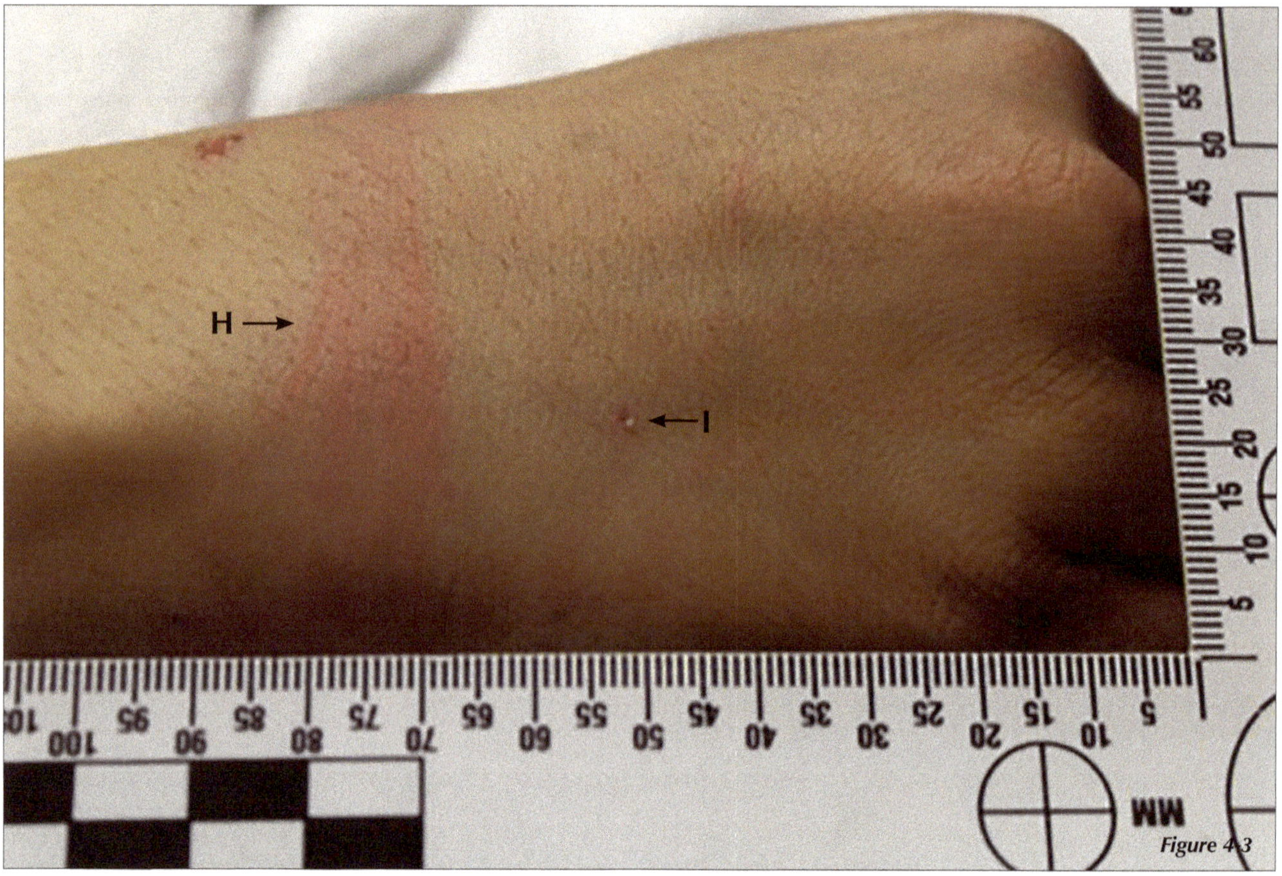

ACTIVITY 4-2. ASSESSMENT

List 3 additional questions that the forensic nurse in SANE care asks regarding the physical findings (eg, symptom Onset, Location/radiation, Duration, Character, Aggravating factors, Timing and Severity [OLDCARTS]; demonstration of method of injury [if known]; level of consciousness).

ACTIVITY 4-3. PHYSICAL ASSESSMENT

Remember that injury is progressive throughout the healing phases. Because of the nature of neck and brain injury (eg, closed/open spaces with continued bleeding), there is potential for diminished function throughout the assessment. Therefore, assessment for potential serious sequelae is continuous in all patients, and when decline in function is recognized, an immediate referral to an advanced practice nurse, physician, or physician assistant is urgent and necessary. List 3 to 6 additional physical assessment procedures you should consider.

Activity 4-4. Evidence Collection

What evidence would you collect given the patient's history? What findings would promote evidence collection even if the history is deficient?

Activity 4-5. Treatment and Care

Based on the history and your findings, what treatment would you offer this patient? Would you report this case to the police or child protective services or both?

Additional Photos

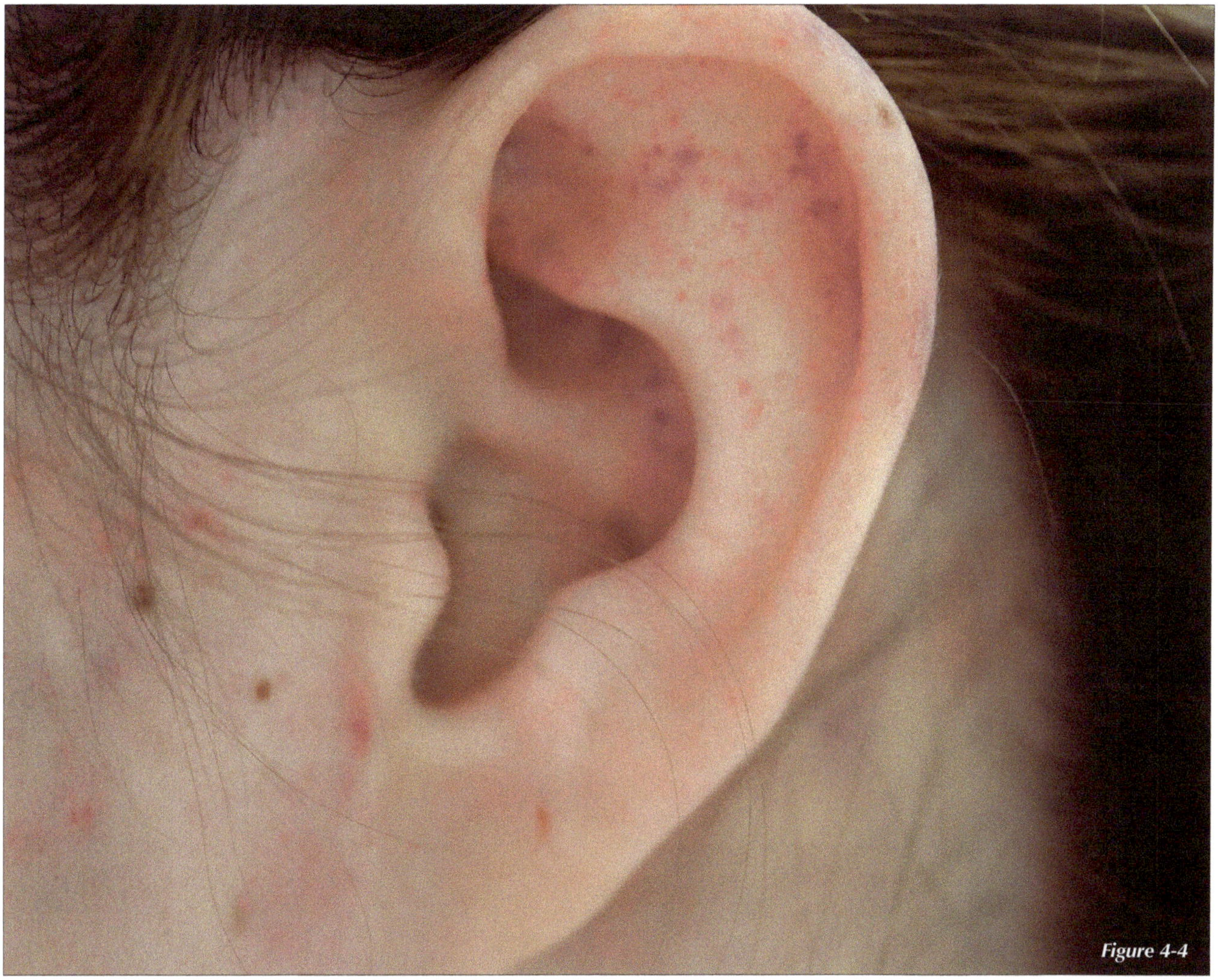

Figure 4-4

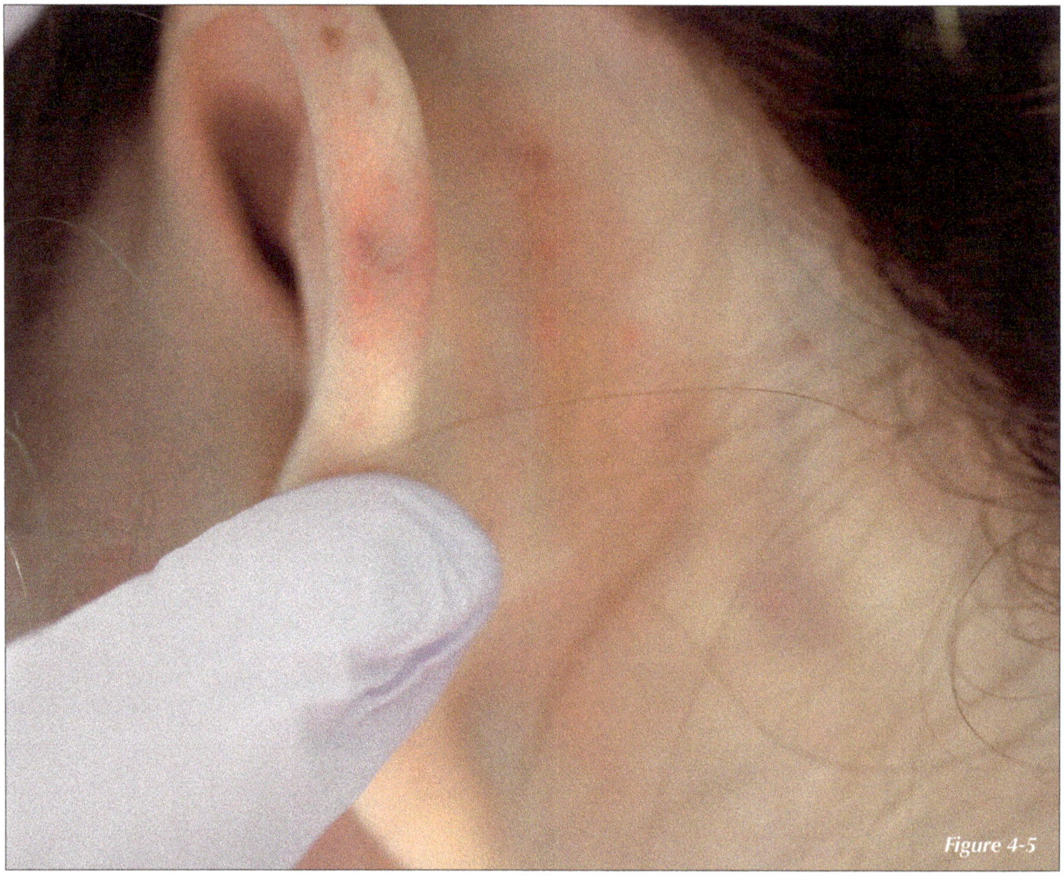

Figure 4-5

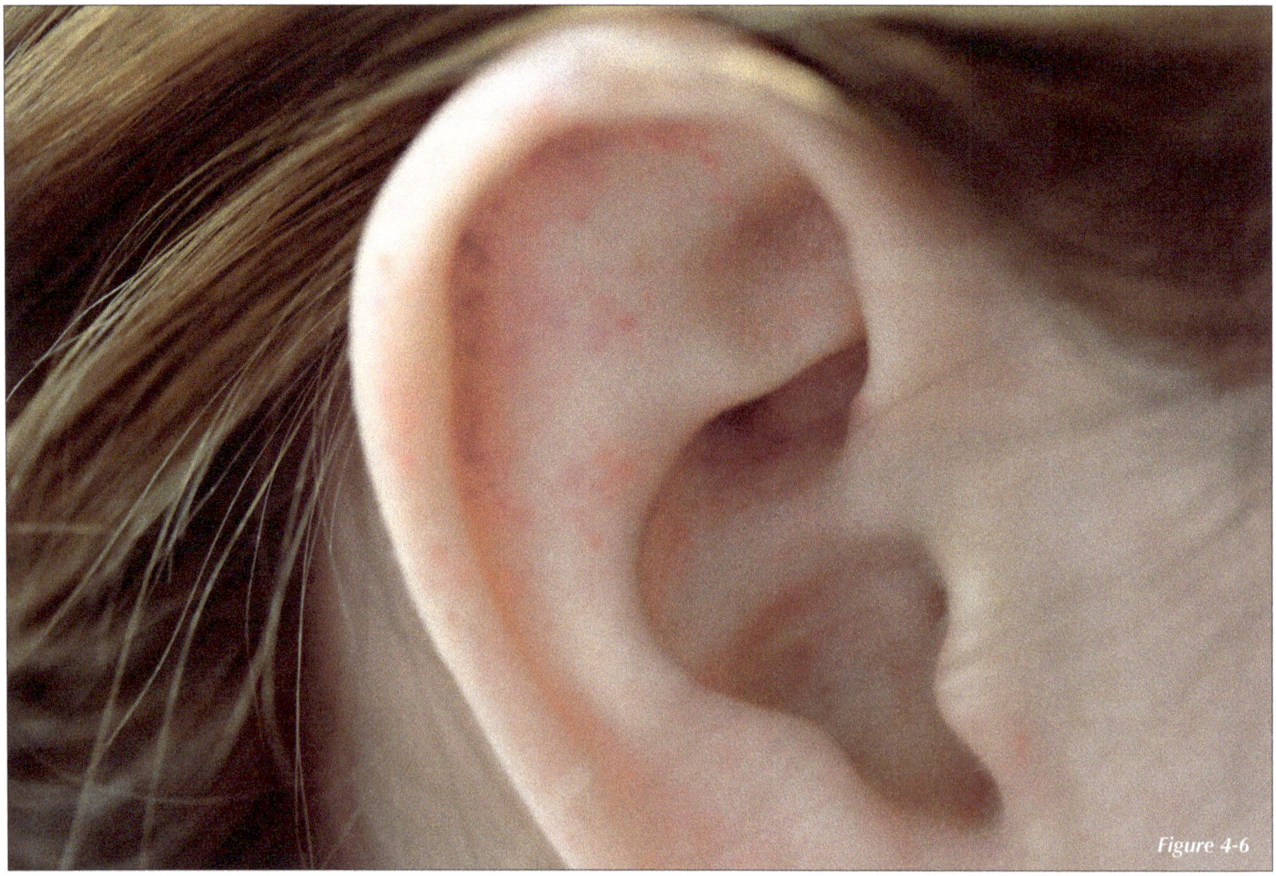

Figure 4-6

Chapter 5

26-Year-Old Female Patient Assaulted by a Former Intimate Partner

Case History

Maria is a 26-year-old woman who is a service maid at a resort hotel. She was in the shower getting ready for work when Tom, her estranged partner and the father of her son, entered the home through the kitchen window. Tom approached her in the shower, grabbed her by the neck, and pulled her out of the shower. At first, she did not recognize him. Once she realized it was her ex-partner, she protested loudly, "You shouldn't do this! Stop!" He squeezed down harder on her neck, and she could not yell anymore. Maria reports that Tom directed her to have sex with him, and she complied. Their son was sleeping upstairs, but he woke up. When Tom realized their child was coming down the stairs, he released Maria's neck and punched her in the mouth. Then Tom got off Maria, and she ran to the bathroom to finish dressing; she continued pleading for him to leave. Tom zipped his pants, and before leaving the home, threatened to kill Maria and their son if she told anyone about the assault.

Maria drove their son to Tom's mother's house so she could watch the child. Without disclosing the crime, Maria told Tom's mother that she was going to work. Instead of reporting for work, Maria called the police, who brought her to the hospital. She is cleared under the Emergency Medical Treatment and Labor Act and meets with the forensic nurse for a medical forensic examination. During the medical forensic history, Maria discloses the strangulation again. She also talks about how Tom verbally abuses her and uses her words against her.

> ***Clinical Pearl:***
> *Women who suffer one nonfatal strangulation by an intimate partner are 750% more likely to be killed with a gun by the same person.*

During examination, Maria says, "His hands are so large … and he only needs one hand on my neck to grab hold, and I can't breathe. He's done this so many times before… I give in because I know it will only get worse if I don't do what he wants." When asked how she explains the bruising on her face and neck, she says, "I usually tell the people I work with that they are suck marks. I don't discuss what happens to me when I am with him. I need the work." There are no other injuries noted on the head-to-toe domestic violence and nonfatal strangulation examination. Swabs are collected from the neck and fingernails, with reference DNA samples from Maria. All samples are submitted to the police department with the forensic report.

Case Discussion

Maria's case was difficult because she remained disengaged throughout the history and said she wanted to go back to work. Weighing her options, she verbalized to the forensic nurse that she was very worried about her job and who she could count on to take care of her child if the police report became public. When asked about her relationship with her son's grandmother, Maria said that the grandmother was their babysitter and often made excuses for Tom's behavior, accusing Maria of not being a good mother or partner. When asked if her son was safe with the grandmother, Maria assured the forensic nurse that the grandmother loved him and he loved her.

The child's presence during domestic violence is considered child endangerment, so all medical providers involved with this case are mandatory reporters of the crime. In some states, upon conviction, penalties for domestic violence are increased when it is substantiated that children were present during the event.

A number of factors in intimate partner violence are identified with an increased risk of morbidity and mortality, and victims often do not understand their increased risk. For example, when intimate partners are excessively jealous and constantly want to know the partner's location, they use rage as a weapon and are lethally dangerous. A jealous batterer often tries to control their partner's behavior and often projects that the partner is having affairs. These abusers often stalk their partners when they leave the relationship or move out of the house.[1] In this case, the abuser came in through an open window to gain access to his ex-partner. An abuser's history, such as Tom's, of using strangulation during an assault increases lethality risk with each subsequent assault.

After the physical assessment, the forensic nurse used the Danger Assessment with Maria to help her begin to process her risk of lethality. It was explained that her partner's increasing number of episodes of strangulation and rapes predict an increasing risk of death. Maria was given a calendar and asked to mark the approximate dates during the past year when she was beaten, raped, or strangled by Tom. She was instructed to write on each of those dates how bad the incident was according to the following scale[2]:

1. Slapping, pushing; no injuries and/or lasting pain
2. Punching, kicking; bruises, cuts, and/or lasting pain
3. "Beating up;" severe contusions, burns, broken bones
4. Threat to use weapon; head injury, internal injury, permanent injury
5. Use of weapon; wounds from weapon

During the medical forensic examination, the forensic nurse noted that Maria's demeanor was flat, and she played games on her phone. She never engaged with the calendar activity, even with support from the forensic nurse. She remained disengaged throughout the entire evaluation. The forensic nurse and health care provider discussed safety planning with Maria. She had no support present for the examination, and no advocate was available. The forensic nurse, providing patient-centered and trauma-informed care, supported Maria's decision to leave when she became impatient and asked if she could go to work, opening the door for her to seek services again. Maria did not take the calendar or the lethality scale with her when she left. She did not follow up with the agency or return for follow-up care.

Later, Maria called the district attorney's office and said, "everything's fine," and she would not cooperate with pressing charges against her child's father. A criminal case was not pursued, and the case was dropped. It is not uncommon for women in domestic violence situations to avoid all legal actions, including pressing charges. Research reveals that victims of domestic violence often provide a number of reasons for their choices, including a lack of money to afford leaving their abuser and fear of homelessness. Other reasons include individual religious beliefs and marriage vows. Often, the offender provides financial support and threatens withdrawal of support when arrested and in jail. Additionally, offenders will minimize the event (eg, "You're exaggerating what happened;" "It wasn't that bad;" "I wouldn't do that to you") (**Appendix 17**) and reinforce their love for the victim while promising that "it won't happen again."

During the examination, Maria also talked about some of the emotional abuse she experienced from Tom. She said Tom would tell her, "You're a rotten mother. You're a whore." This caused Maria to doubt that she was a good mother, and she verbalized fears that her son would be taken away from her. Reframing and twisting words or experiences is called gaslighting[3] and is a common method used to emotionally break down and abuse intimate partners. Gaslighting is a very effective form of emotional abuse, because once an abusive partner has broken down the victim's ability to trust their own perspective, the individual may be more vulnerable to the effects of abuse, making it more difficult to leave the abusive relationship. Gaslighting also increases isolation from family and friends.

References

1. Stop Violence Against Women. Lethality assessments. University of Minnesota Human Rights Library Web site. http://hrlibrary.umn.edu/svaw/domestic/link/lethality.htm. Accessed October 29, 2019.

2. Campbell JC. Danger assessment. National Center on Domestic and Sexual Violence Web site. http://www.ncdsv.org/images/DANGERASSESSMENT.pdf. Accessed October 29, 2019.

3. A deeper look into gaslighting. National Domestic Violence Hotline Web site. https://www.thehotline.org/2019/11/22/a-deeper-look-into-gaslighting/. Published November 22, 2019. Accessed January 2, 2020.

Anatomic Skills 5-1

Refer to **Figure 5-1**. Using the letters that correspond to the structure in the photograph, label the anatomic locations.

Arrow A. ____________________

Arrow B. ____________________

Arrow C. ____________________

Arrow D. ____________________

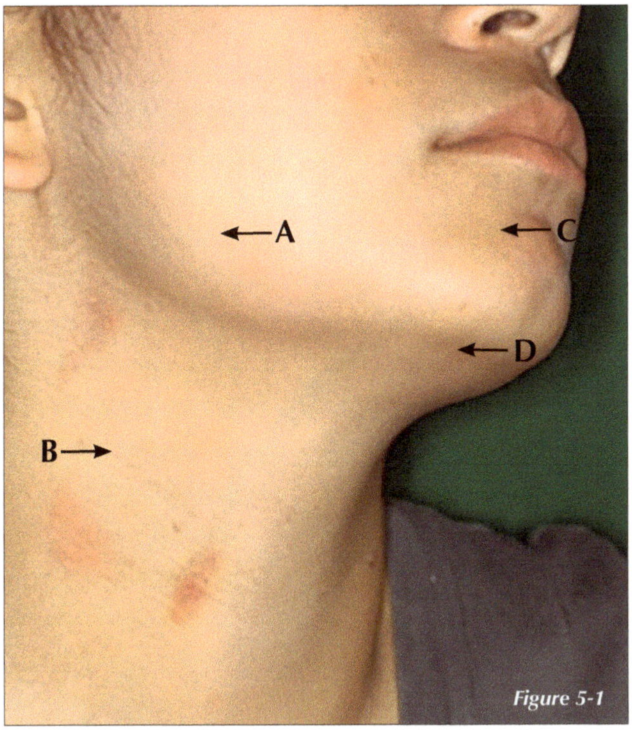

Figure 5-1

Activities

Activity 5-1. Injury Identification

Refer to **Figure 5-2**. Identify any injuries in respect to their anatomic location. Write objective descriptions when documenting findings.

Arrow E. ____________________

Arrow F. ____________________

Arrow G. ____________________

Arrow H. ____________________

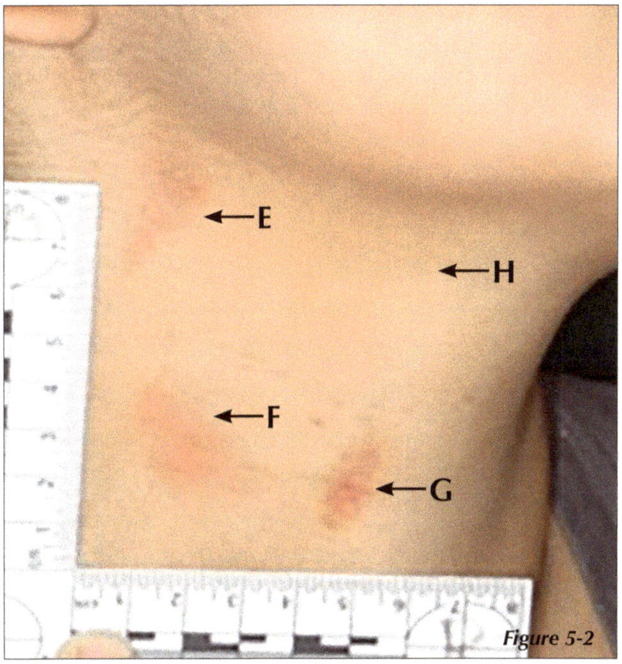

Figure 5-2

Activity 5-2. Assessment

List 3 additional questions that the forensic nurse in SANE care asks regarding the physical findings (eg, symptom Onset, Location/radiation, Duration, Character, Aggravating factors, Timing and Severity [OLDCARTS]; demonstration of method of injury [if known]; level of consciousness).

Activity 5-3. Physical Assessment

Remember that injury is progressive throughout the healing phases. Because of the nature of neck and brain injury (eg, closed/open spaces with continued bleeding), there is potential for diminished function throughout the assessment. Therefore, assessment for potential serious sequelae is continuous in all patients and, when decline in function is recognized, an immediate referral to an advanced practice nurse, physician, or physician assistant is urgent and necessary. In addition, if the patient is in need of emergent care, take note of existing injury at time of arrival because lifesaving measures will alter the body's appearance. List 3 to 6 additional physical assessment procedures you should consider.

Activity 5-4. Evidence Collection

What evidence would you collect given the patient's history? What findings would promote evidence collection even if the history is deficient?

Activity 5-5. Treatment and Care

Based on the history and your findings, what treatment would you offer this patient? Would you report this case to the police or child protective services or both?

Activity 5-6. Lethality Assessment

During care and as part of discharge planning, all patients who are suspected to be victims of domestic violence should be assessed for risk of immediate danger. List 4 indicators of escalating danger in a person who has experienced domestic violence. What questions should you ask a patient to assess his or her risk of immediate danger?

____

____

____

____

____

____

____

____

____

____

____

____

Additional Photos

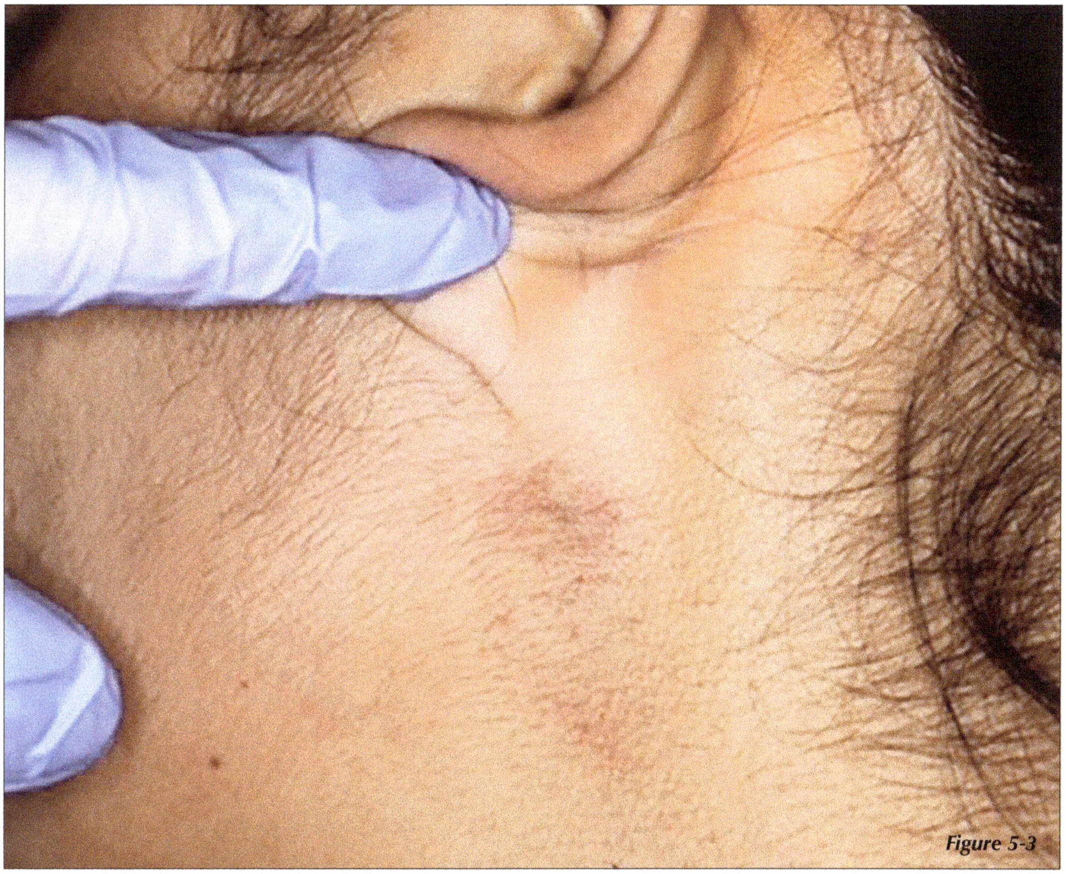

Figure 5-3

Additional Photos

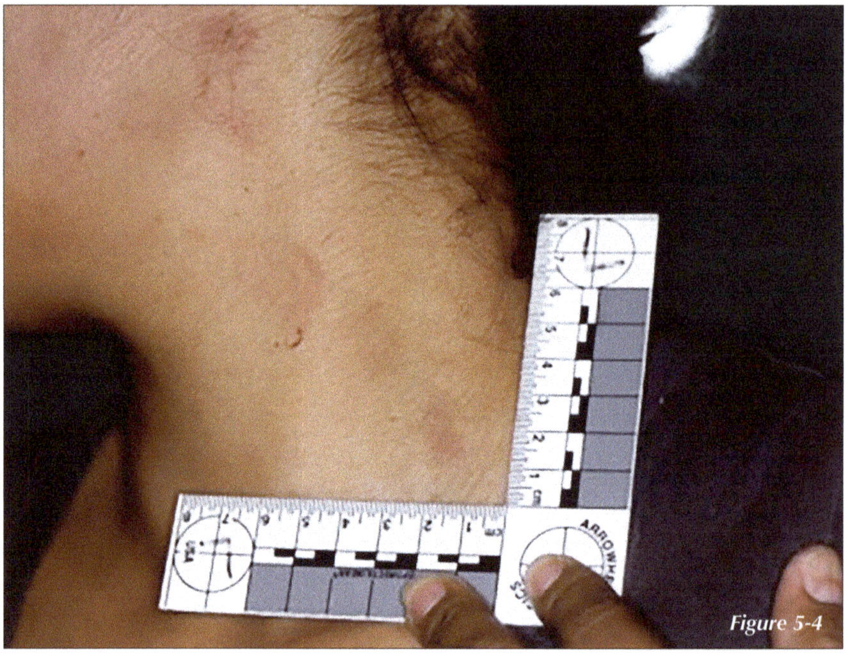

Figure 5-4

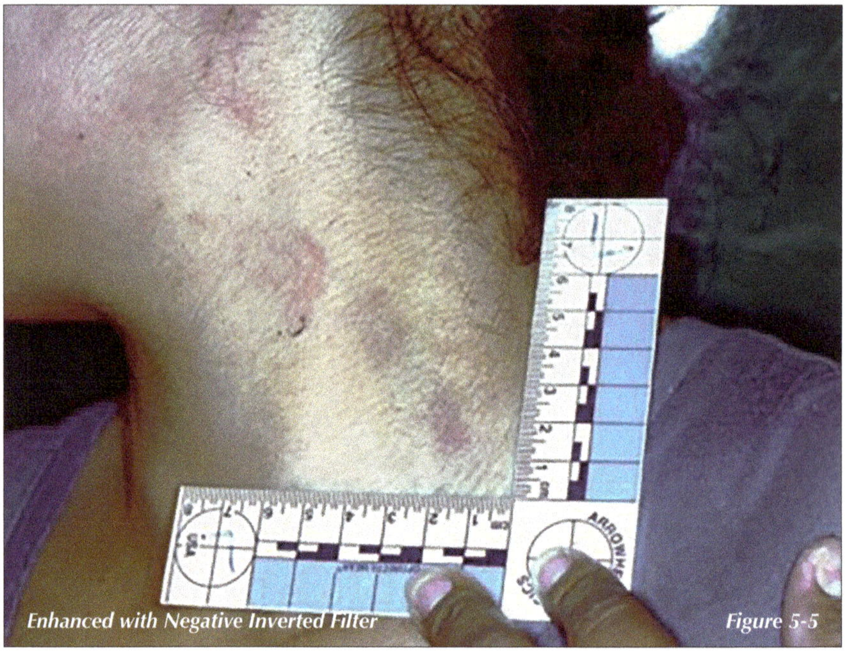

Enhanced with Negative Inverted Filter

Figure 5-5

Chapter 6

15-year-old Female Patient Assaulted by a Stranger

Case History

Latisha is a 15-year-old African immigrant who was walking home from a friend's house. She remembers being grabbed from behind and that a rope was put around her neck. The next thing she remembers is waking up naked and alone in an alley. She locates her clothes and walks to a store nearby. The shop owner calls the police and fire department. Emergency medical services bring Latisha to the emergency department for a medical forensic evaluation with the on-call forensic nurse. The police accompany her to the hospital and tell the forensic nurse about the circumstances of Latisha's experience. The officer tells the forensic nurse that Latisha was reported missing last night when she did not return home, and her mother was on the way to the hospital to support her daughter. Latisha expresses worry about how her mother will react. She states, "My mom gets angry and yells when I do not do what she wants." The advocate reassures Latisha that she will help both Latisha and her mother.

Even without a known history of sexual assault, Latisha agrees to a medical forensic examination that includes a total body inspection for injury, including inspection of her anogenital structures for possible sexual assault. On a scale of 1 to 10, Latisha says her neck pain is a 7 out of 10. She also says she has a sore throat and notes that her voice is hoarse, which is audible to the forensic nurse. The nurse also notices a large bruise on Latisha's left arm and a laceration on her forehead.

> ***Clinical Pearls:***
> *During a strangulation event, loss of consciousness can occur within 5 to 10 seconds, and death can occur within minutes.*

Case Discussion

Latisha lost consciousness quickly. Because Latisha is 15 years old, consider an interview with a trained forensic interviewer several days after the assault. The delay with an interview allows time to process the event. For some patients, sensory memory returns. This is important in this case in order for the investigation to move forward.

Latisha did not want her mother as a support during the medical forensic evaluation, but she wants her in the room afterwards. It is important in patient-centered and trauma-informed care to include family, if safety needs are met. Patients' healing is improved with support from family. Adults need to implement the discharge planning recommendations, and the forensic nurse needs to determine if the mother is supportive of her daughter. Sexually abused adolescents whose mothers believe them and offer comfort are less likely to suffer from anger and depression.[1] Follow-up counseling was also recommended in this case, but neither Latisha nor her mother followed up with the advocacy agency.

Neurologic signs and symptoms after strangulation may include vision changes, ringing in the ears, facial or eyelid drooping, one-sided weakness, incontinence, and miscarriage. Weeks to months after an assault, a victim may have problems sleeping and experience impairment in memory and concentration. Mental health problems can include anxiety, depression, and dementia. In up to 50% of strangulation cases, there are no visible bruises. Strangulation is often used by a perpetrator to accomplish a rape or demonstrate how far he is willing to go to establish control in the relationship. Victims can be rendered unconscious in 10 seconds with as little as 4 pounds of pressure. Once the victim is released from the strangle, it can take 10 seconds or more to regain consciousness.[2]

Assess all cranial and cervical spine nerves for movement and strength, and document all observations. Include documentation of all injuries, such as red marks and scratches on the neck. Also include victim behaviors that are consistent with strangulation such as difficulty swallowing and a raspy voice.[3] The complaint of a sore throat and neck pain is often relieved by applying an ice pack to the area, reducing pain and swelling.

Photograph everything using forensic photography principles (**Appendix 1**). Quality photos diminish most arguments by a defense attorney. If an evidence technician is available, request photographs of the crime scene. This is one of the best ways to show the jury where the crime happened. The forensic nurse's photographic documentation demonstrates the outcome to the patient. In this case, Latisha presented with multiple injuries, including subconjunctival hemorrhages (red eyes) that are well documented. Comprehensive documentation is important for this case to move forward when there is no or little history and no samples that include DNA from the assailant to tie the victim and assailant to the crime scene and the elements of the crime. Follow-up photographs would be recommended to demonstrate facial features and show how the injuries healed.[4] However, in this case, the patient did not return for follow-up care.

References

1. Zajac K, Ralston ME, Smith DW. Maternal support following childhood sexual abuse: associations with children's adjustment post-disclosure and at 9-month follow-up. *Child Abuse Negl.* 2015;44:66-75.

2. Mitchell JR, Roach DE, Tyberg JV, Belenkie I, Sheldon RS. Mechanism of loss of consciousness during vascular neck restraint. *J Appl Physiol (1985).* 2012;112(3):396-402.

3. Training Institute on Strangulation Prevention. Clinical documentation of strangulation cases. Family Justice Center Web site. https://www.familyjusticecenter.org/resources/clinical-documentation-of-strangulation-cases/. Accessed February 11, 2020.

4. Secure Digital Forensic Imaging. Adult non-fatal strangulation photodocumentation protocol 2020. Family Justice Center Alliance Web site. https://www.familyjusticecenter.org/wp-content/uploads/2016/11/Secure-Digital-Forensic-Imaging-Non-Fatal-Strangulation-Protocol-2018.pdf. Accessed October 29, 2019.

Anatomic Skills 6-1

Refer to **Figures 6-1** and **6-2**. Using the letters that correspond to the structures in the photograph, label the anatomic locations.

A. ______________________________

B. ______________________________

C. ______________________________

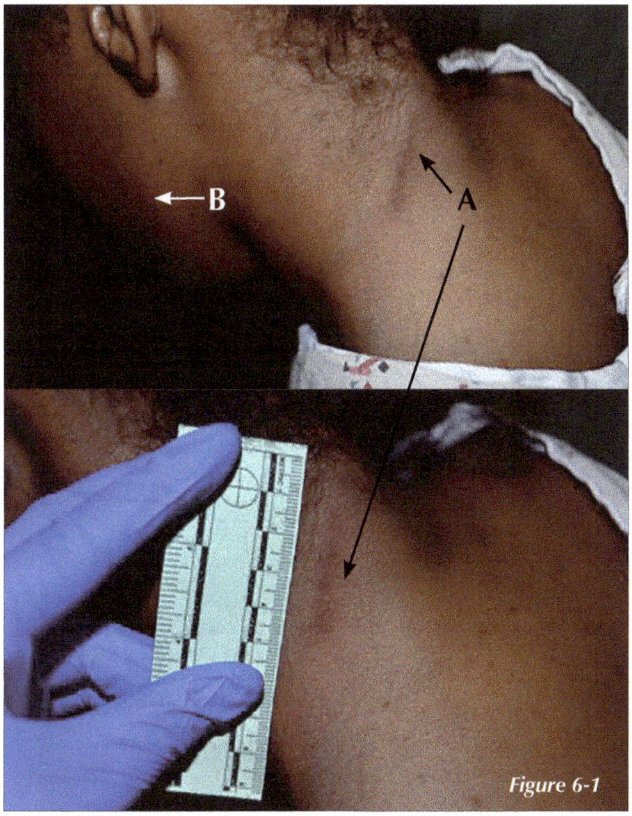

Figure 6-1

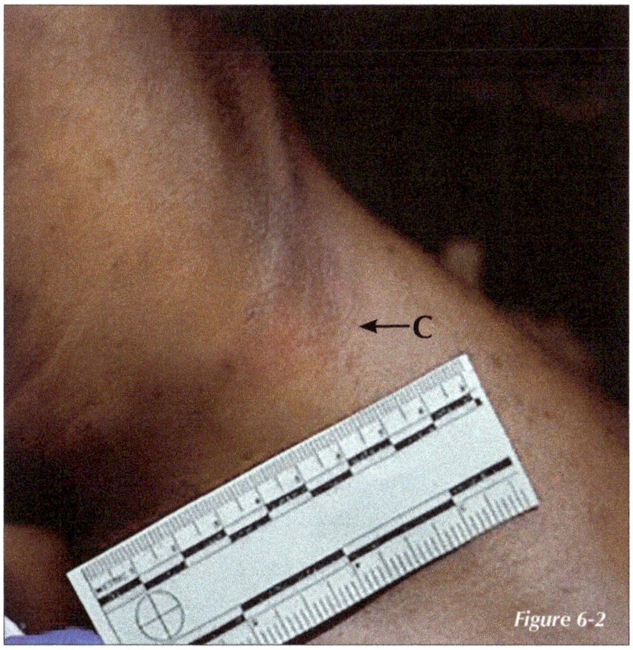

Figure 6-2

Activities

Activity 6-1. Injury Identification

Refer to **Figures 6-1** through **6-5**. Identify any injuries in respect to their anatomic location. Write objective descriptions when documenting findings.

A. ______________________________

C. ______________________________

D. ______________________________

E. ______________________________

F. ______________________________

G. ______________________________

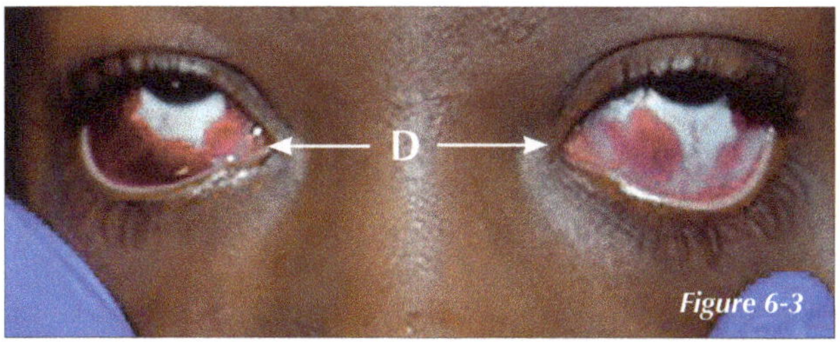

Figure 6-3

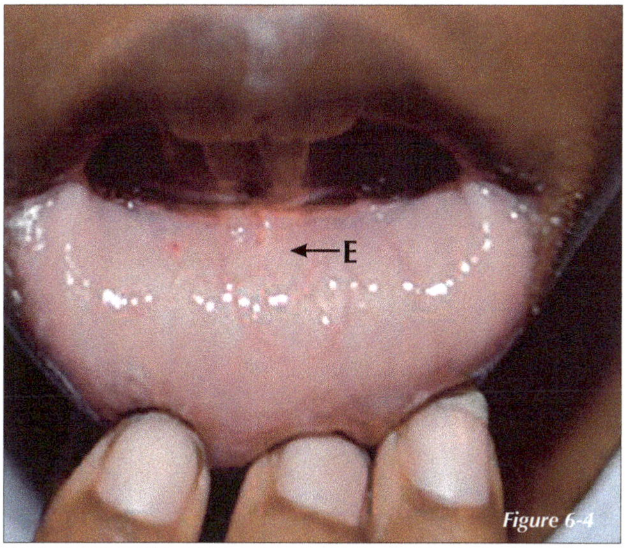

Figure 6-4

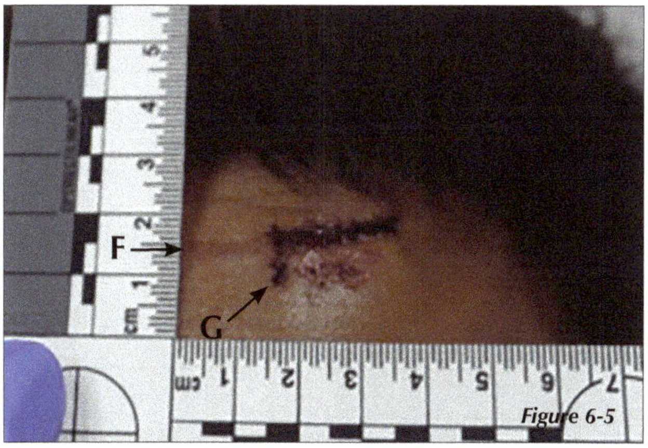

Figure 6-5

Activity 6-2. Assessment

List 3 additional questions that the forensic nurse in SANE care asks regarding the physical findings (eg, symptom Onset, Location/radiation, Duration, Character, Aggravation factors, Relieving factors, Timing, and Severity [OLDCARTS]; demonstration of method of injury [if known]; level of consciousness).

Activity 6-3. Physical Assessment

Remember that injury is progressive throughout the healing process. Because of the nature of neck and brain injury (eg, closed/open spaces with continued bleeding) there is potential for diminished function throughout the assessment. Therefore, assessment for potential serious sequelae is continuous in all patients and, when decline in function is recognized, an immediate referral to an advanced practice nurse, physician, or physician assistant is urgent and necessary. List 3 to 6 additional physical assessment procedures you should consider.

Activity 6-4. Evidence Collection

What evidence would you collect given the patient's history? What findings would promote evidence collection even if the history is deficient?

Activity 6-5. Treatment and Care

Based on the history and your findings, what treatment would you offer this patient? Would you report this case to the police or child protective services or both?

Chapter 7

24-Year-Old Female Patient Assaulted by a Former Intimate Partner

Case History

Sunny is a patient in her mid-20s. She met an old acquaintance while on vacation with her family in Mexico. She was having fun with her male friend, drinking and talking. They agreed to go back to his apartment, and while there, she reports, "He just snapped. I wasn't sure what was happening." She remembers that "all of a sudden he had his hands on my neck." She was sexually assaulted, and he dragged her by her neck into a kitchen. She describes multiple times when he put his hands on her neck, pressing down, and states that she lost consciousness twice. She describes that he strangled her with both hands from behind, and she was unable to speak and had blurry vision. She says that he looked "blank, out of control" (demeanor) and she says, "I believed I was going to die." She also says that she "thought I would be seeing my grandmother in heaven."

After admission to the emergency department, the initial workup, following best practices, includes a computed tomographic angiography (CTA), and she is observed overnight in the hospital. CTA is a noninvasive procedure that enhances certain anatomic views of vascular structures. It becomes invasive when a contrast medium is used.

> ***Clinical Pearls:***
> *Strangulation is a gendered crime. Most stranglers are men (over 90%) and most victims are women.*

Sunny returned home to the United States and reported the case the next day. The local jurisdiction is unable to charge the crime because it occurred in Mexico. There was no advocate available during the time of the examination, so the registered nurse (RN) called the hotline with Sunny to discuss safety planning. The safety planning is important because the suspect's location is unknown, and he knows where to find Sunny.

Case Discussion

Sunny's case is complex because the crime occurred in another country, outside the jurisdiction of the United States. Once Sunny arrived back in the United States and made a police report to the local law enforcement, the officers created a ***courtesy case*** file. A courtesy case asks the local jurisdiction to dispatch a law enforcement representative to meet with the patient, take a statement, authorize a medical forensic examination, write a report, and pick up the sealed evidence. The case information and kit are then transported to the jurisdiction where the crime occurred. In Sunny's case, the courtesy case evidence and documentation transfer is between the local jurisdictions in the United States and Mexico for investigation and processing.

The documentation included descriptions of external findings, which were significant. The examiner noted a variety of visible injury patterns in a number of locations on Sunny's body. When focusing on the head and neck areas and the description of a strangulation history, the medical forensic examiner noted multiple bruises to the anterior neck in a linear horizontal pattern. There was also a cluster of vertical linear abrasions to the neck that started above the horizontal bruise and stopped at the horizontal bruise, measuring 4 to 8 cm in length, and diffuse petechiae above the area of the horizontal neck bruises, covering the exposed integument.

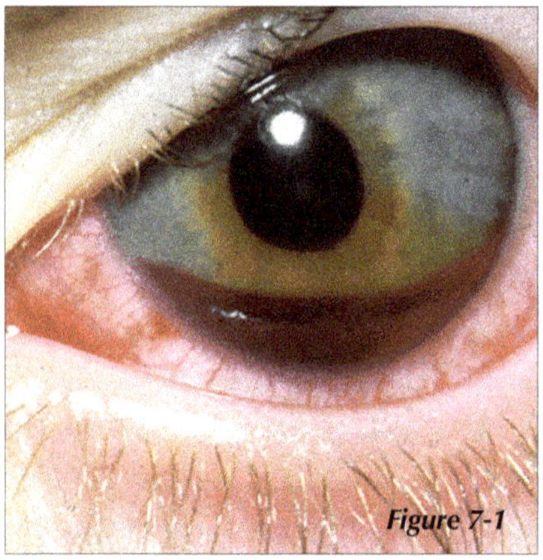

Figure 7-1. *Hyphema (Courtesy University of Michigan Kellogg Eye Center).*

Now is a good time to refer to the "how" and "what" mechanism of injury that occurred to produce petechiae. Petechiae are pinpoint spots that do not blanch with pressure, measure less than 2 to 3 mm, and appear on the skin and mucous membranes when ruptured with pressure.[1] When petechiae appear in the whites of the eyes, it is called subconjunctival hemorrhaging, and that finding was present in this case. Subconjunctival hemorrhage and petechial hemorrhage occur after a "sudden severe venous congestion to the head" causing the vessels to rupture and leak[2] and can also be found in the mouth (soft palate, tongue, cheeks, gums), nasal mucous membranes, and tympanic membranes. In this case, the carotid artery was occluded, causing an increase in negative pressure in the head. In severe cases, hyphema* is an ocular risk, necessitating avoidance of a rebleed and immediate referral for medical management to prevent blindness (**Figure 7-1**).

Discharge planning and support for this patient are important and include a variety of organizations coordinated in a community response. One is the local advocate agency that is responsible for follow up and coordination of other services, so it is important that communication remains open and collaborative between the forensic nurse program and the advocate agency and that the patient has the hotline number to call at any time.

Other agencies supporting victims include the following:

— Pathways to Safety[3] is an organization that helps Americans who have been sexually assaulted in other countries.

— Sexual Assault Support & Help for Americans Abroad (SASHAA), a program that is part of the Americans Overseas Domestic Violence Crisis Center,[4] is designed to provide advice and help to Americans who are sexually assaulted while in another country.

Advice to victims sexually assaulted out of the Unites States includes the following:

1. Get to a safe place, and call someone safe to come and be with you.

2. If you cannot find a safe place, call someone safe to come and get you.

5. If there are injuries, take pictures.

6. Call SASHAA internationally toll-free 24 hours a day, 7 days a week for further confidential advice and help.

Many law enforcement personnel do not use evidence-based processes in response to allegations of rape or sexual assault. In this case, the patient was able to return home rapidly and report to her local law enforcement in the United States and receive a courtesy medical forensic examination and a thorough medical evaluation of her injuries. Depending on the laws, the exchange of the evidence and documentation may or may not promote justice for Sunny.

References

1. McGrath A, Barrett MJ. Petechiae. Treasure Island, FL; StatPearls Publishing: 2019.

2. Tarlan B, Kiratli H. Subconjunctival hemorrhage: risk factors and potential indicators. *Clin Ophthalmol.* 2013;7:1163-1170.

3. What is sexual assault? Pathways to Safety International Web Site. https://pathwaystosafety.org/sexual-assault/. Accessed October 21, 2019.

4. American Overseas Domestic Violence Crisis Center. Catch a Fire Web site. https://www.catchafire.org/organizations/americans-overseas-domestic-violence-crisis-center_7531. Accessed October 21, 2019.

**A hyphema is a pooling or collection of blood inside the anterior chamber of the eye (the space between the cornea and the iris).*

Anatomic Skills

Anatomic Skills 7-1

Refer to **Figure 7-2**. Using the letters that correspond to the structures in the photograph, label the anatomic locations.

A. ________________________________

B. ________________________________

C. ________________________________

D. ________________________________

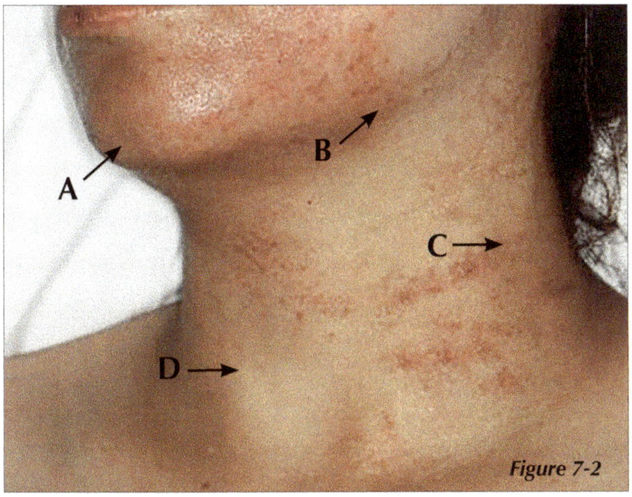

Figure 7-2

Anatomic Skills 7-2

Refer to **Figure 7-3**. Using the letters that correspond to the structures in the photograph, label the anatomic locations.

E. ________________________________

F. ________________________________

G. ________________________________

H. ________________________________

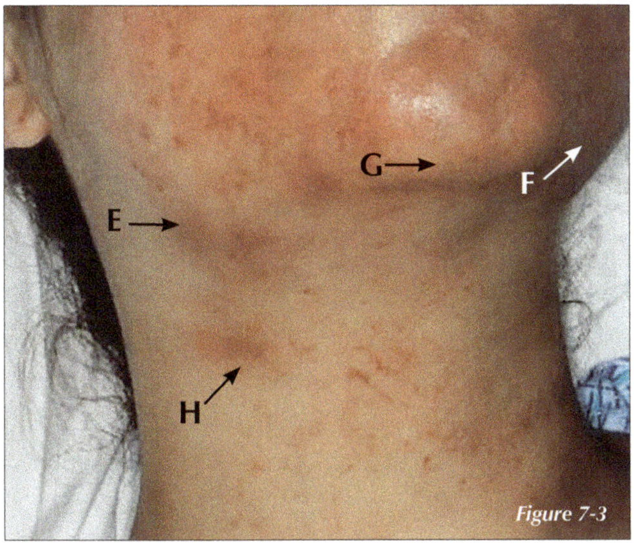

Figure 7-3

Activities

Activity 7-1. Injury Identification

Refer to **Figures 7-4** through **7-6**. Identify any injuries in respect to their anatomic location. Write objective descriptions when documenting findings.

I. ________________________________

J. ________________________________

K. ________________________________

L. ________________________________

M. ________________________________

N. ________________________________

O. ________________________________

P. ________________________________

Q. ________________________________

R. ________________________________

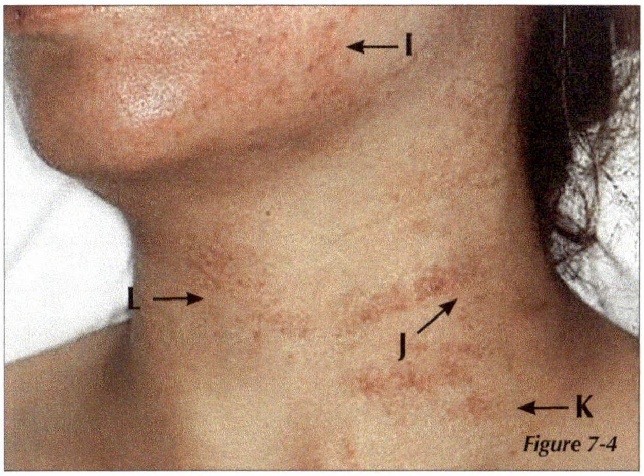

Figure 7-4

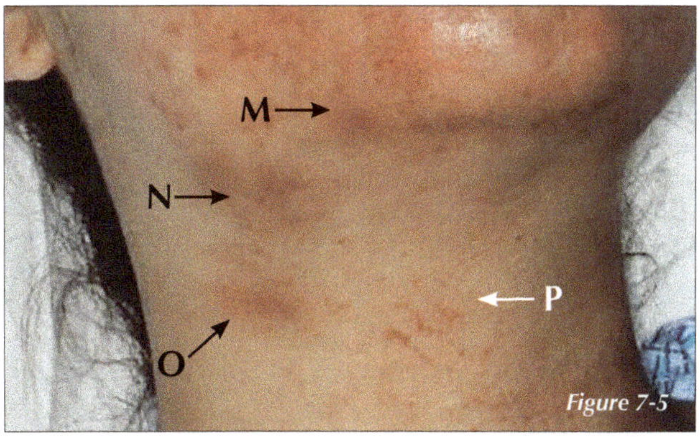

Figure 7-5

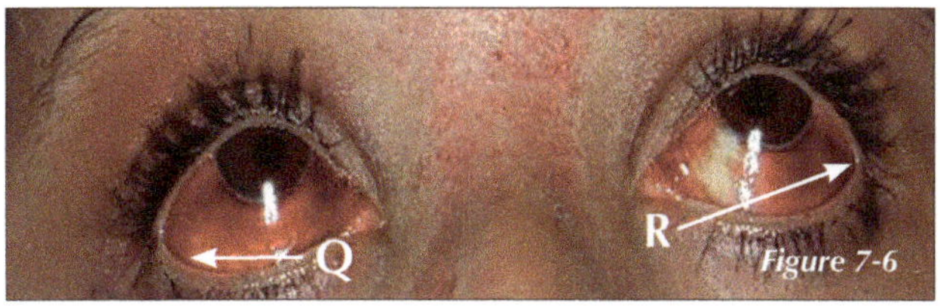

Figure 7-6

Activity 7-2. Assessment

List 3 additional questions that the forensic nurse asks regarding the physical findings (eg, symptom Onset, Location/radiation, Duration, Character, Aggravation factors, Relieving factors, Timing, and Severity [OLDCARTS]; demonstration of method of injury [if known]; level of consciousness).

Activity 7-3. Physical Assessment

Remember that injury is progressive throughout the healing process. Because of the nature of neck and brain injury (eg, closed/open spaces with continued bleeding) there is potential for diminished function throughout the assessment. Therefore, assessment for potential serious sequelae is continuous in all patients and, when decline in function is recognized, an immediate referral to an advanced practice nurse, physician, or physician assistant is urgent and necessary. List 3 to 6 additional physical assessment procedures you should consider.

Activity 7-4. Evidence Collection

What evidence would you collect given the patient's history? What findings would promote evidence collection even if the history is deficient?

Activity 7-5. Treatment and Care

Based on the history and your findings, what treatment would you offer this patient? Would you report this case to the police?

Additional Photos

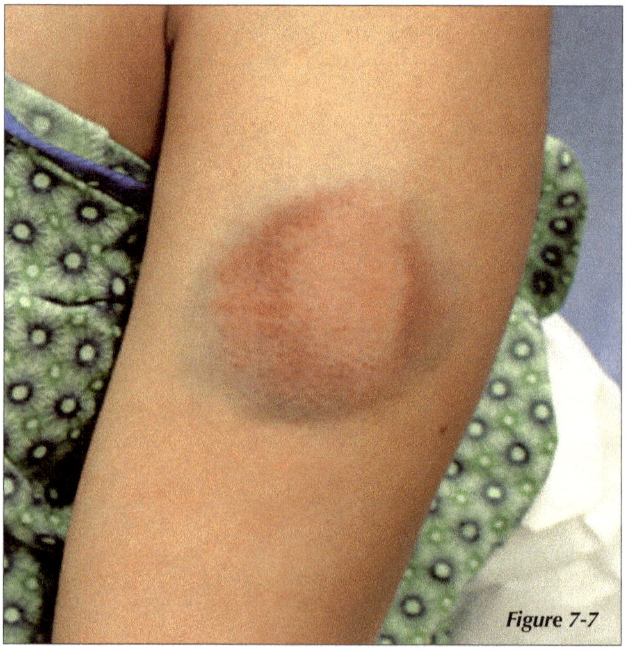

Figure 7-7

Chapter 8

65-Year-Old Female Patient Assaulted by a Former Intimate Partner

Case History

The following history was given to the forensic nurse approximately 6 hours after the assault. The patient arrives to the hospital's forensic center with a friend and describes multiple events of assault and the course of her emergency department (ED) care to the forensic nurse. The patient was seen in the ED immediately before the forensic evaluation. She was medically cleared and discharged to the offsite forensic center to be evaluated by the forensic nurse.

Linda is a 65-year-old woman who lives alone and "off the grid" without electricity. She grows most of her own food, describing her lifestyle as "living the simple life." Linda's best friend, Sam, lives about 100 miles away, but they talk weekly when Linda comes into town. Her only other mode of communication is a wired radio speaker in her truck. Sam did not hear from Linda in almost 3 weeks, so he began to worry and drove to Linda's home to check on her. Sam was concerned because of Tom, a man Linda dates from time to time. Linda mentioned to the forensic nurse during the history that Tom has "mental health issues," violent tendencies, and a history of assaulting her.

> ***Clinical Pearl:***
> *Strangulation is an ultimate form of power and control, because the batterer demonstrates his command over the victim's next breath.*

The forensic nurse also takes a history from Sam, who requires a forensic examination for injury. Sam tells the forensic nurse that when he arrived at Linda's home, he found Linda naked in the back of her truck, dazed. Her clothes were on fire in the fire pit. When Sam exited his truck, Tom surprised Sam and charged at him. Sam punched Tom in the face and continued to fight until Tom fell against the truck; he was stunned and left the property. Sam went to comfort Linda, who had multiple facial and body injuries, so he called law enforcement. Sam reports that Linda agreed to be transferred from the scene to the hospital for an ED assessment, so he accompanied her.

Linda tells the forensic nurse that on arrival to the hospital, the triage nurse noted that Linda was anxious. The midlevel provider took the medical history in which Linda reported being strangled by Tom. Linda also revealed in her medical history at the hospital, and later to the forensic nurse, that 2 weeks before this assault Tom had attacked her, causing pain in her right wrist. She had contacted law enforcement, who responded to her home. Law enforcement officials tell the forensic nurse they attempted to serve Tom with a no-contact order but were unable to locate him. Linda declined medical care at the time of the previous assault; however, today she disclosed to the emergency medical staff and the forensic nurse that she continues to have pain in her right wrist. Linda reports that the ED nurse alerted the advanced practice provider (APP), and an x-ray examination of her wrist was ordered. Linda was diagnosed with a fracture in her right wrist, and the wrist was casted. The emergency APP completed Linda's medical screening examination as required under the Emergency Medical Treatment and Labor Act and determined she is medically stable.

Linda discloses to the forensic nurse that she was strangled with one hand on the front portion of her neck. Tom also put lipstick on her face and put his other hand in her mouth to gag her. She additionally reports that Tom used her shirt to strangle her while he was sexually assaulting her and that she "wet herself." She denies a loss of consciousness but does describe "seeing spots." On a scale of 0 (no pain) to 10 (highest pain), she describes her throat pain as an 8. Linda states, "He's done this before, but he's sick...he has some mental health issues. He was just in the mental hospital and blamed me...said he was thinking I called his family to take him in. He is always really sorry when he does this...and he even buys me flowers. I need him around the land for help. I'm getting old, and he helps me chop firewood and keeps the yard up."

Linda reports that Tom has guns and threatened her with them, but says, "I don't believe he was really serious (about killing her)." She arrived in a different set of clothing because the clothes she wore during the assault were burned at the scene, but she is wearing the jewelry she had on. Linda scores 4 out of 5 on the Danger Assessment-5 (DA-5), which is administered by the forensic nurse (**Appendix 4**). A patient advocate is present and provides safety planning.

Linda reports to the forensic nurse that she declined a computed tomography angiography (CTA) because she says the ED AAP told her that she looked "okay." The forensic nurse discusses the need for observation, and when assessed during the follow-up recommendations, Sam agrees to stay with her for the next 24 hours. The forensic nurse has a standard procedure after an acute assault to have the patient observed after strangulation in case the patient comes into distress or experiences any increased neck swelling.

Sam expresses concern for Linda's health and wants her to stay in the ED overnight, but Linda declines. Advocacy services spend time with the patient to develop a safety plan, and law enforcement attempts to locate Tom but is unsuccessful. When asked by police, Linda declines to reveal Tom's location. She also decides against following up for another examination and declines any further advocacy services. Sam says he will continue to talk to Linda about the importance of her following up.

Case Discussion

It is not uncommon for patients who are experiencing violence to minimize their level of danger and rationalize continuing a relationship with the person who assaulted them. Many might ask *why?* Why would Linda continue to tolerate the abuse? An evaluation of battered women's experience with health care at the provider level revealed that "women perceived health care professionals to be disinterested or unsympathetic toward the needs of battered women, causing the women to feel ignored or trivialized."[1]

Figure 8-1. *Maslow's hierarchy of needs.*

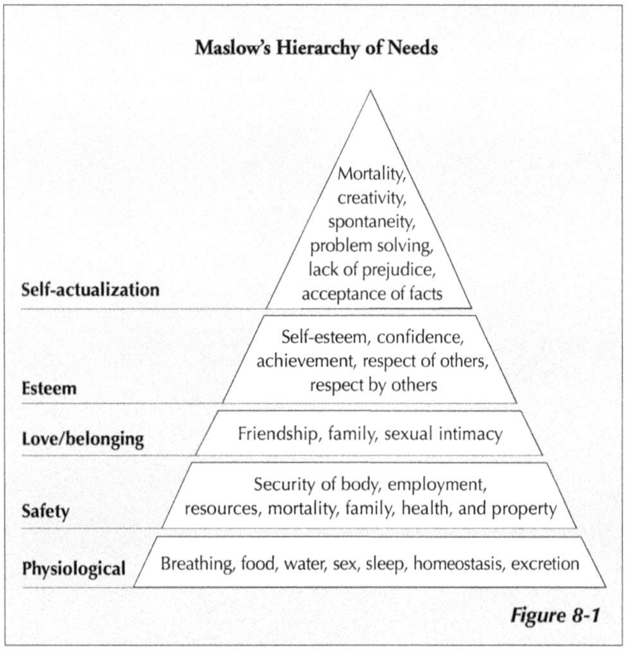

In this case, Linda lives alone with minimal resources and has no family or friends other than Sam. She was asked if she needed additional resources or shelter. She did not disclose if her living situation was by choice or out of necessity related to financial challenges. During her history, she described that she had become dependent on Tom to help her around the house to perform tasks she was no longer able to complete. Necessities motivate people, and according to Maslow's hierarchy of needs (**Figure 8-1**), this includes physiologic (basic) needs. Physiologic needs include air, food, shelter, clothing, and sleep. Maslow explains that to move to up the hierarchy, one must have those needs met first. In Linda's situation, Tom helped chop firewood for her, and he tended to her garden. He also burned Linda's clothing, showing her that he had control over her shelter and clothing. In the history, Linda described 2 different strangulation events, showing an increased threat to her safety because of Tom's assertion of power over her physiologic need for oxygen.

As trauma-informed health care providers, it is important to understand that "why" questions could hinder the health care provider–patient relationship. Rather than asking patients "why," another tactic to use is open-ended interviewing. Even if Linda declines services now, in the future, she may accept services from providers who respect her decisions by using patient-centered and trauma-informed strategies in the care of patients at risk of lethal relationships. Therefore, a basic understanding of intimate partner violence dynamics is essential for the first responder.

The physical symptoms described by Linda are consistent with her history of external pressure being applied to the neck. Her symptoms included urinary incontinence, reports of "seeing spots," and throat pain. Linda disclosed to the nurse that she did not consent to a CTA of the neck because the APP told her she "looked fine." The forensic nurse explained what a CTA is and how important this would be to make sure her neck and vessels were okay. The forensic nurse also discussed with Linda the importance of CTA given that she lives many miles from the hospital. The gold standard for care of a patient post-strangulation is a CTA of the neck.[2] The forensic nurse gave Linda discharge instructions that outlined the dangers and symptoms of strangulation. The patient should then be given the choice to return to the ED and offered crime victim compensation resources.

To achieve power and control, Tom used blaming, intimidation, coercion, and threat tactics (**Appendix 17**), and Linda was isolated because of her living situation. Once physical or sexual violence is introduced into a relationship, that abusive relationship becomes harder to exit. Abusers make behavior choices, and changes in behavior occur when the abuser is provided choices with accountability. When the abuser is not held accountable, violence often increases.[3] Linda also reported that Tom had a gun and had threatened her with it; however, she did not believe he would hurt her with it.[4] The forensic nurse used the DA-5, and the patient scored 4 out of 5.[4,5]

Linda's score on the DA-5 indicates she is at a highly predictive risk for serious assault or homicide and needs a full Danger Assessment (**Appendix 3**). The patient was in direct contact with her assigned advocate but continued to decline services. Linda's case is complex, requiring consideration of not only continued abuse and assault but also medical vulnerability if the unseen injuries are more serious (eg, dissection of the artery or veins). If the patient did not decline the evaluation, she should have a complete workup, including CTA of her neck, a follow-up examination, and an appointment with her advocate, who could have possibly assisted her with resources.

References

1. Patch M, Anderson JC, Campbell JC. Injuries of women surviving intimate partner strangulation and subsequent emergency health care seeking: an integrative evidence review. *J Emerg Nurs*. 2018;44(4):384-393.
2. Recommendations for the medical/radiographic evaluation of acute adult, non-fatal strangulation. Training Institute on Strangulation Prevention Web site. https://www.strangulationtraininginstitute.com/wp-content/uploads/2015/07/Recommendations-for-Medical-Radiological-Eval-of-Non-Fatal-Strangulation-v17.9.pdf. Accessed August 27, 2019.
3. Wolf-Smith JH, LaRossa R. After he hits her. *Fam Relat*. 1992;41(3):324-329.
4. Campbell JC. Danger assessment-5. Johns Hopkins School of Nursing Web site. https://learn.nursing.jhu.edu/instruments-interventions/Danger%20Assessment/DA-5_2.26.15.pdf. Accessed August 27, 2019.
5. Snider C, Webster D, O'Sullivan CS, Campbell J. Intimate partner violence: development of a brief risk assessment for the emergency department. *Acad Emerg Med*. 200916(11):1208-1216.

Anatomic Skills

Anatomic Skills 8-1

Refer to **Figure 8-3**. Using the letters that correspond to the structures in the photograph, label the anatomic locations.

A. ______________________________

B. ______________________________

C. ______________________________

D. ______________________________

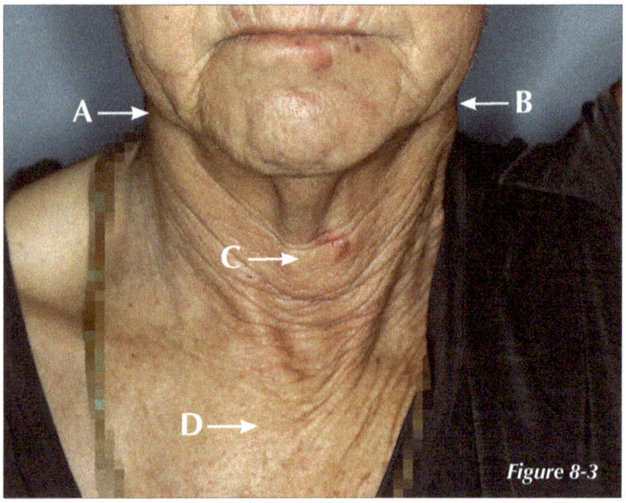

Figure 8-3

Anatomic Skills 8-2

Refer to **Figure 8-4**. Using the letters that correspond to the structures in the photograph, label the anatomic locations.

E. ______________________________

F. ______________________________

G. ______________________________

H. ______________________________

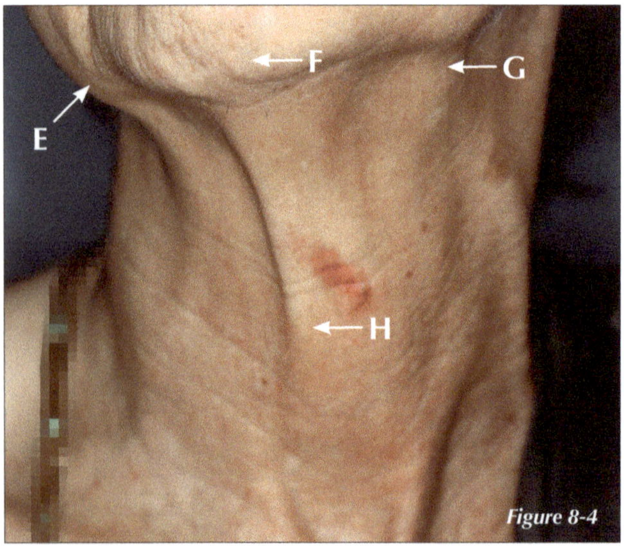

Figure 8-4

Activities

Activity 8-1. Injury Identification

Refer to **Figures 8-5** to **8-8**. Identify any injuries in respect to their anatomic location. Write objective descriptions when documenting findings.

I. ______________________________

J. ______________________________

K. ______________________________

L. ______________________________

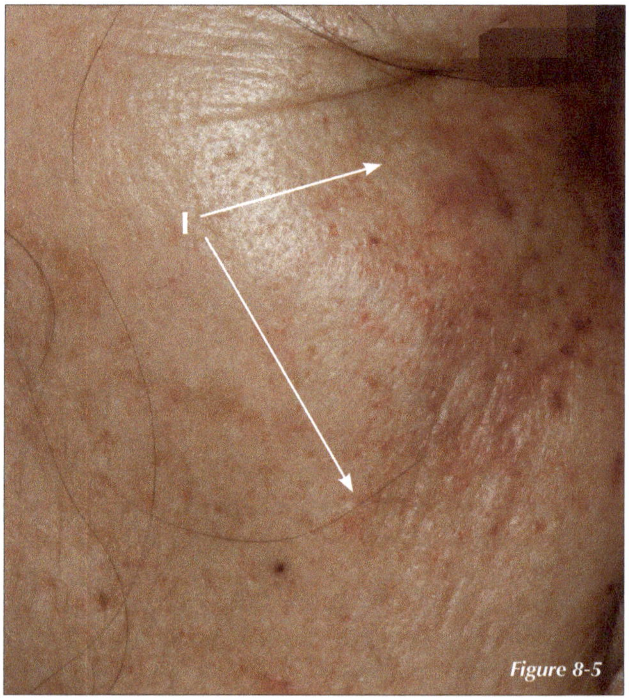

Figure 8-5

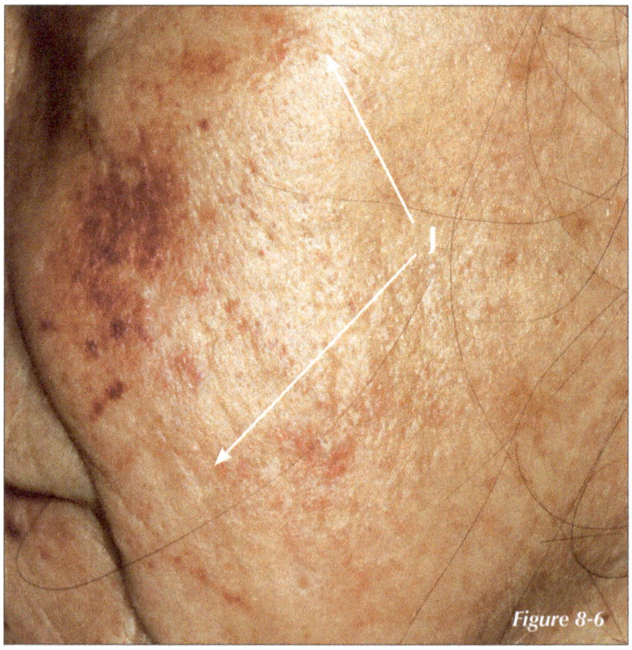

Figure 8-6

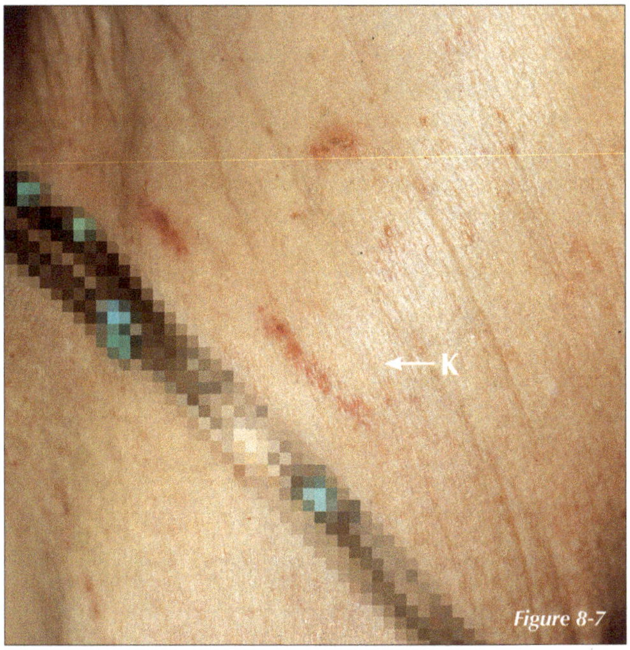

Figure 8-7

Activity 8-2. Assessment

List 3 additional questions that the forensic nurse in SANE care asks regarding the physical findings (eg, symptom Onset, Location/radiation, Duration, Character, Aggravating factors, Relieving factors, Timing, and Severity [OLDCARTS]; demonstration of method of injury [if known]; level of consciousness).

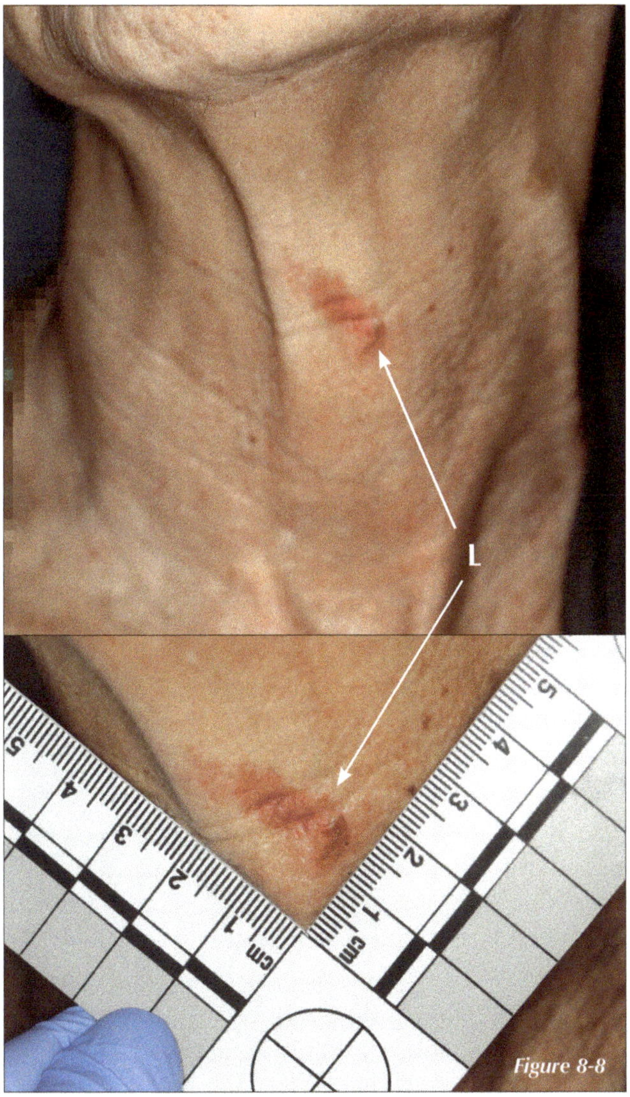

Figure 8-8

Activity 8-3. Physical Assessment

Remember that injury is progressive throughout the healing phases. Because of the natural of neck and brain injury (eg, closed/open spaces with continued bleeding), there is potential for diminished function throughout the assessment. Therefore, assessment for potential serious sequelae is continuous in all patients and, when decline in function is recognized, an immediate referral to an advanced practice nurse, physician, or physician assistant is urgent and necessary. List 3 to 6 additional physical assessment procedures you should consider.

Activity 8-4. Evidence Collection

What evidence would you collect given the patient's history? What findings would promote evidence collection even if the history is deficient?

Activity 8-5. Treatment and Care

Based on the history and your findings, what treatment would you offer this patient? Would you report this case to the police or adult protective services?

Activity 8-6. Lethality Assessment

During care and as part of discharge planning, all patients who are suspected to be victims of domestic violence should be assessed for risk of immediate danger. List 4 indicators of escalating danger in a person who has experienced domestic violence. What questions should you ask a patient to assess his or her risk of immediate danger?

Chapter 9

31-Year-Old Female Patient Assaulted by a Former Intimate Partner

Case History

Mary is a 31-year-old woman. Mary and Joe dated for several years. During their turbulent relationship, her 2 children went to live with their father in another state. About a month ago, Joe and Mary had a falling out, and Mary filed domestic violence charges after Joe assaulted her. The judge issued a no-contact court order. Since then, Mary has spent a lot of time with her mother. Mary and her mother were at a party together, and Joe showed up. He was drunk and started a fight with Mary and her mother. Witnesses said that during the assault, Joe grabbed and strangled Mary at least 5 different times with 1 hand, 2 hands, and his forearms. Mary screamed, "He said he's going to kill me now." Joe dragged Mary into the bathroom. The witnesses dialed 911, and Joe left. Witnesses shared their experience with the first responders (law enforcement officers and emergency management services [EMS] from the fire department). EMS transported Mary via ambulance to the emergency department (ED), accompanied by her mother, who was visibly shaken. Mary reports that Joe also sexually assaulted her during this strangulation event.

> ***Clinical Pearl:***
> *The cost of misreporting or misunderstanding strangulation crimes is incredibly high, because strangulation frequently foreshadows an escalating use of violence and homicidal intent.*

The forensic nurse consulted with the advocate to provide services to Mary, which includes use of the sexual assault evidence collection kit. Mary tells the forensic nurse, "I was at a motel partying with my mom… (gasping air) when my ex-boyfriend, Joe, (gasping air) attacked me (gasping air). He's done this before, and (gasping air) I didn't say anything." She complains that she "lost consciousness," now has a raspy voice, and has continual "throat pain, headache, and neck pain." On inspection, Mary has scratch marks on her neck, and her fingernail is broken. She also has injuries on her lower forearms and hands.

The forensic nurse conducts a medical forensic interview, and Mary gives permission for the medical forensic examination to include sexual assault and strangulation assessment with photographs. She also gives permission for the advocate to be present during the examination. During the detailed history gathered by the forensic nurse, Mary discloses that she urinated on herself. She states, "I was mortified. I didn't know what to do. I don't have health insurance and didn't go to a doctor when he did this before. My mom insisted we come to the hospital… is she okay?" The patient will need specific follow-up instructions for both sexual assault and strangulation.[1]

Mary's mother is waiting in the lobby, complaining of chest pain. The triage nurse is considering a medical examination for Mary's mother. Support for Mary's mother is also necessary after medical clearance, because she is concerned that Joe will come to the house and harm both of them. An advocate or social worker assists the mother in safety planning and obtaining a restraining order.

Case Discussion

The Training Institute on Strangulation Prevention provides the following statistics[1]:

1. A woman who has suffered a nonfatal strangulation incident with her intimate partner is 750% more likely to be killed by the same perpetrator with a gun.[2,3]

2. In 2017, 44 police officers were shot and killed across the United States in the line of duty. Thirty-three of those officers were killed by a perpetrator with a public record history of at least 1 nonfatal strangulation incident.[4]
3. The majority of strangulation attacks do not leave any visible external injuries on the victim. This is important because people often do not know this and feel if there are no marks, there is no evidence. The injuries may also be subtle and therefore overlooked by the untrained eye. Skin tone can also affect how easily injuries are seen, so a methodic, head-to-toe examination is extremely important.[5]
4. Strangulation has been identified as one of the most lethal forms of domestic violence and sexual violence; unconsciousness may occur within seconds and death within minutes.
5. Strangulation is an ultimate form of power and control because the batterer demonstrates his command over the victim's next breath.[6]
6. When domestic violence perpetrators strangle their victims, not only is this a felonious assault or possibly an attempted murder, but too often it can lead to hypoxic brain injury and a subsequent fatal outcome.

By 2019, 48 states passed laws to prosecute strangulation and suffocation assaults as a felony. Additionally, the 2013 reauthorization of the Violence Against Women Act added strangulation and suffocation to federal law, and strangulation and suffocation were added to the Uniform Code of Military Justice in 2019.

Injury is progressive throughout the healing phases. Because of the nature of neck and brain injury (eg, closed/open spaces with continued bleeding), there is the potential for diminished function throughout the assessment. Therefore, assessment for potential serious sequelae is continuous in all patients, and when decline in function is recognized, an immediate referral to an advanced practice nurse, physician, or physician assistant is urgent and necessary.

Insurance coverage for medical sequelae is used first under states' compensation plans. Victim witness funds, while available, require the patient to apply, typically through the district attorney's office. In these cases, there is a community advocate who assists Mary. Inevitably, there are medical charges for the radiographs, computed tomographic angiography scan, and other screenings order by the advanced practice provider in the ED. If the patient does not have insurance to cover the medical charges, referrals to victim's compensation are a safety net and very important.[7]

References

1. Mengo C, Gidycz C. When abused women decide to seek help from a victims assistance program: their perceived needs and self-reported mental health symptoms. *Violence Vict.* 2019;34(4):613-634.
2. K Stavra. "All abusers are not equal": new IPV research reveals an indicator of deadly abuse. Training Institute on Strangulation Prevention Web site. https://www.strangulationtraininginstitute.com/all-abusers-are-not-equal-new-ipv-research-reveals-an-indicator-of-deadly-abuse/. Published January 8, 2020. Accessed May 21, 2020.
3. Glass N, Laughon K, Campbell J, et al. Non-fatal strangulation is an important risk factor for homicide in women. *J Emerg Med.* 2008;35(3):329-335.
4. Gwinn C, Strack G, Mack M. Law reform targets the crime of strangulation. *Domestic Violence Report.* 2014;19(6):81-100.
5. Rozzi HV, Riviello R. How to evaluate strangulation. American College of Emergency Physicians Web site. https://www.acepnow.com/article/how-to-evaluate-strangulation/. Published April 17, 2019. Accessed May 21, 2020.
6. Floyd B. Strangulation: a concerning type of domestic abuse. Training Institute on Strangulation Prevention Web site. https://www.strangulationtraininginstitute.com/strangulation-concerning-type-domestic-abuse/. Published October 6, 2016. Accessed May 21, 2020.
7. Daigle LE, Guastaferro WP, Azimi A. Victims' compensation as a tool of therapeutic justice: examining the physical and mental health needs of victim compensation applicants and the role of health in receiving compensation. *Violence Vict.* 2016;31(5):837-853.

Anatomic Skills 9-1

Refer to **Figures 9-1** to **9-3**. Using the letters that correspond to the structures in the photograph, label the anatomic locations.

A. ______________________________

B. ______________________________

C. ______________________________

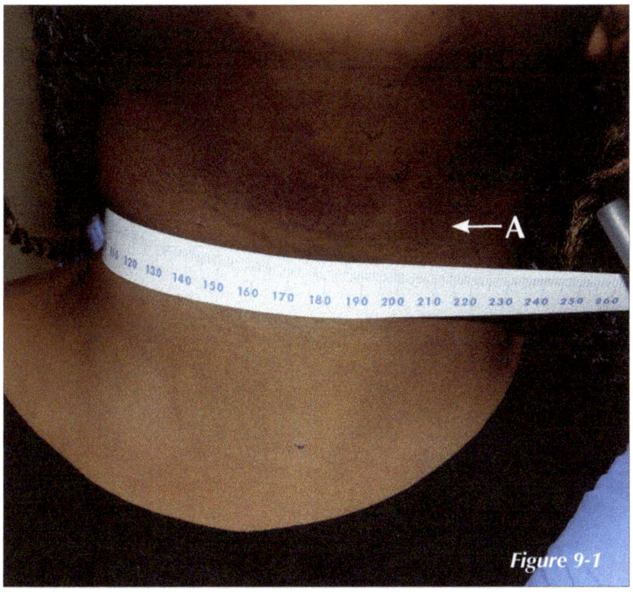

Figure 9-1

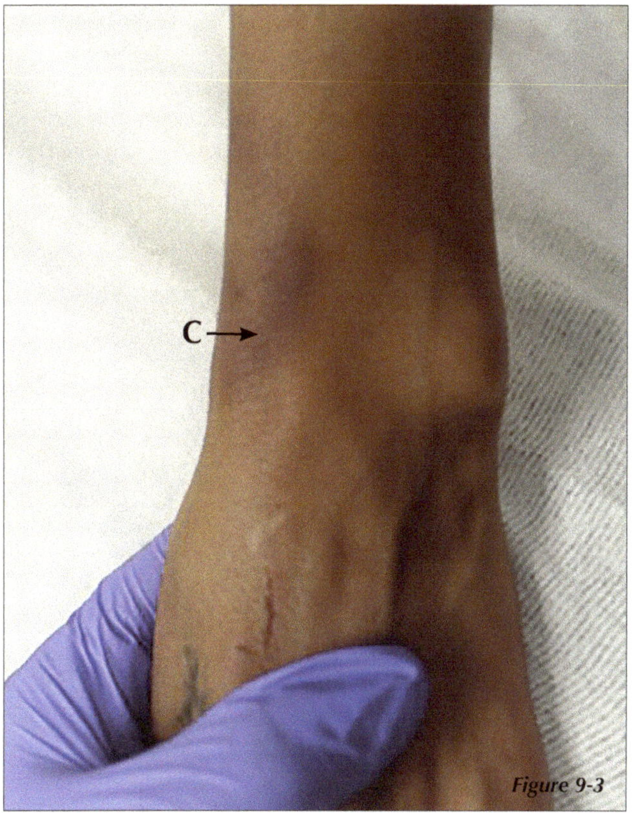

Figure 9-3

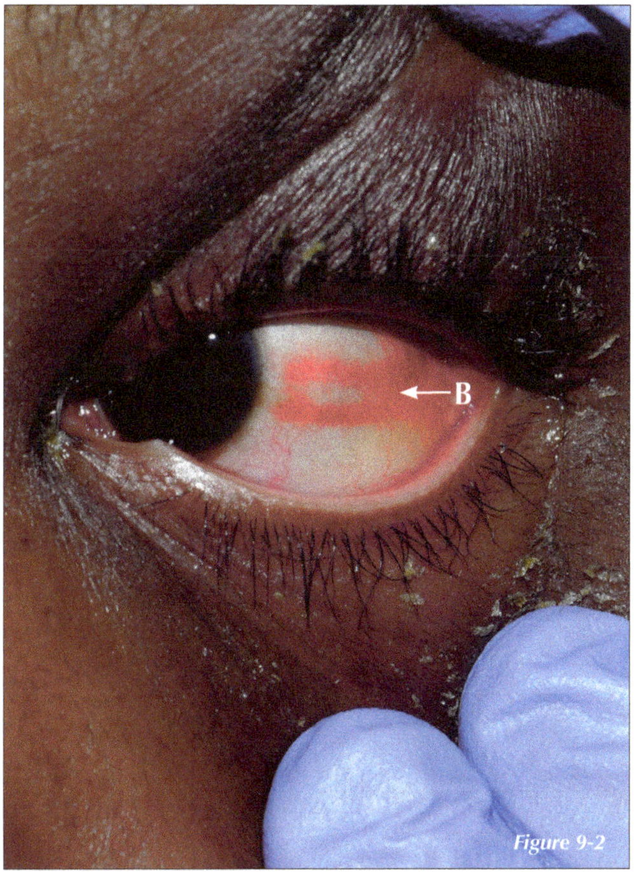

Figure 9-2

Activities

Activity 9-1. Injury Identification

Refer to **Figures 9-2** and **9-3**. Identify any injuries in respect to their anatomic location. Write objective descriptions when documenting findings.

B. ______________________________

C. ______________________________

Activity 9-2. Assessment

List 3 additional questions that the forensic nurse asks regarding the physical findings (eg, symptom Onset, Location/radiation, Duration, Character, Aggravation factors, Relieving factors, Timing, and Severity [OLDCARTS]; demonstration of method of injury [if known]; level of consciousness).

____

____

____

____

____

____

____

____

Activity 9-3. Physical Assessment

Remember that injury is progressive throughout the healing process. Because of the nature of neck and brain injury (eg, closed/open spaces with continued bleeding) there is potential for diminished function throughout the assessment. Therefore, assessment for potential serious sequelae is continuous in all patients and, when decline in function is recognized, an immediate referral to an advanced practice nurse, physician, or physician assistant is urgent and necessary. List 3 to 6 additional physical assessment procedures you should consider.

Activity 9-4. Evidence Collection

What evidence would you collect given the patient's history? What findings would promote evidence collection even if the history is deficient?

Activity 9-5. Treatment and Care

Based on the history and your findings, what treatment would you offer this patient? Would you report this case to the police?

Activity 9-6. Lethality Assessment

During care and as part of discharge planning, all patients who are suspected to be victims of domestic violence should be assessed for risk of immediate danger. List 4 indicators of escalating danger in a person who has experienced domestic violence. What questions should you ask a patient to assess his or her risk of immediate danger?

Chapter 10

22-Year-Old Female Patient Assaulted by a Former Intimate Partner

Case History

Esther met David in college. He demanded all her time when she was not in class, and she loved the attention. Esther became more and more isolated from her friends, and by her senior year, she was only going to work and to school. David became increasingly possessive of her, looking at her bills and checking her mail. He insisted on knowing the password for her phone, and he regularly monitored her texts to her family. When Esther turned 22 years old, David talked her into moving in with him. The night she moved into his place, Esther arrived in the emergency department (ED) with law enforcement. Neighbors had called the police because the yelling and threats were so loud, they became afraid for Esther's safety. When law enforcement arrived, they saw that Esther had injuries, so David was arrested.

In the ED, Esther tells the triage nurse that her boyfriend, David, got home from work and immediately accused her, saying, "I heard you've been talking to Grant." Esther explains to the nurse that Grant is a "guy from school." Esther says, "I didn't know what he was talking about!" Esther then reports that when David heard the denial, he grabbed her phone and started looking through her texts. Esther says, "I was climbing on him trying to get my phone back and yelling at him. He saw other guys' names from my classes and work, and he got really, really mad and pushed me down on the couch. I was sitting up, and he was pushing my head back until I was hanging over the back of the couch, and then he 'choked' me." When asked to describe the choking, Esther states, "He had his 2 hands around my neck and was squeezing so hard. He looked like the devil. He was calling me a whore." Esther reports that she could not breathe and "was trying to talk, and it came out in squeaks without words." She states, "He was choking me for a long time, and then he started laughing." When he let go, Esther says she was trying to catch a breath. She says she was crying. She turned away from him on the couch and was holding her neck. She says David then "bear hugged" her from behind and "started biting me, and I started screaming." A neighbor rang the doorbell multiple times and yelled that he had called the cops. Esther says, "When David heard that, he got up, got my purse and jacket, opened the door, and told me to get out." Esther explains that he punched her in the face, pushed her out the door, and locked it behind her. When asked about her neck injuries and the bite marks, Esther admits that she told the patrol officer that they were from consensual sexual activity and says, "I didn't want to get David in trouble." The patrol officer noticed that she was coughing and holding her neck and encouraged her to be seen in the ED. She was brought by ambulance to the ED and discharged after being medically cleared. She left the hospital, declining the care of the forensic nurse.

> ***Clinical Pearl:***
> *The association between strangulation and other lethal criminal acts is clear, and many states increase penalties on conviction when strangulation is clearly documented in the medical record.*

Esther's symptoms worsen 2 days later, and she calls the officer who brought her to be seen by the forensic nurse. When asked about the subsequent symptoms she experienced following the fight, Esther says that she is now coughing and "clearing her throat a lot." She says that her back and neck are "real sore" and her voice is "a little deeper than usual."

During the examination, the forensic nurse observes irregular bruising on both sides of Esther's neck, linear abrasions on her neck and chest, bruising and swelling of her lips, and self-inflicted bite marks on her tongue. Esther states she does not remember biting her tongue, but "all I could think about then was that I couldn't breathe! And didn't feel pain." She states that she is sure she "didn't pass out because I was staring at David the whole time while he was choking me, and that's why he was laughing at me! He said my eyes were bugging out!" The forensic nurse notices she has multiple double-arched bite marks on her posterior neck and back. Esther says that she reached out to her older sister, who has taken her in and is helping her "get over David."

Later, the forensic nurse heard that Esther moved back into David's home. David appeared in court, Esther dropped the charges, and she did not appear for the scheduled follow-up appointment with the advocate and forensic nurse.

Case Discussion

This case presents a complexity that forces the generalist forensic nurse to consider not only the biology of trauma and healing and the psychological conflicts that occur in domestic violence before elopement from the relationship, but also the social risk that occurs when data predicts mortality (eg, increased risk of homicide when strangulation is used in intimate partner violence).[1,2] The forensic nurse has basic nursing knowledge about assessment of hypoxic and anoxic brain injury and the neurologic outcomes. In order to determine the difference, the patient answers questions, and the forensic nurse evaluates the demeanor of the patient to inform the documentation. In this case, the patient reports (subjective history) that she experienced strangulation and battering (eg, documentation in quotes removes interpretation and bias of what is said).

OLDCARTS is an acronym to guide a complete subjective documentation. The forensic nurse evaluation of objective findings is an accurate description of what is seen (gross, enlarged, and/or microscopic), touched (palpation), heard (auditory or auscultation), or smelled/tasted (particularly useful in stranger assaults). Together, the subjective history and objective findings create a narrative that informs and guides advanced practice providers' care, which includes a basic workup and implementing the best practices of contrast angiographic studies.

In this case, the patient has multiple pattern injuries, with some evidence of underlying structural injury to the larynx, a hoarse voice, poor memory of how injuries occurred (tongue), and fear of worsening outcomes (eg, if she accuses her partner, she is uncertain about his reaction, which drives her decisions about health care; therefore she left the ED once cleared). Once Esther was away from her assailant and with her sister, she developed worsening symptoms (increasing signs and symptoms of airway obstruction) and support for leaving her partner. With the sister, she agreed to a thorough medical-legal evaluation. After the generalist forensic nurse's evaluation, she consulted with an advanced practice provider who completed the medical work-up that included contrast imaging of the neck.

Forensic nursing practice often occurs independently through memorandums or dependently through reassignment of duties in an organization. To protect the patient, the generalist forensic nurse without advanced practice credentials and licensure needs standing and signed medical protocols for management of patients with a strangulation history to ensure that the occasional dissected carotid is not missed and recovery from hypoxic and anoxic brain injury is adequately addressed throughout recovery. These protocols are as simple as referral to a hospital with recommendations from the community agency (who holds the Mutual Aid Memorandum of Understanding), to beginning the process of imaging and laboratory work for the advanced practice provider in the institution where the generalist forensic nurse works. Diagnosis warrants an ICD-9 or ICD-10 code for asphyxia or assault.[3] Keep in mind that medical workups are covered by insurance, and if the patient is uninsured, the Crime Victim's Compensation fund will cover additional medical expenses.[4]

Finally, the patient needs a medical home to follow the healing process and inevitable chronic disease and mental health outcomes, and collaboratively, the medical home needs partnerships with community agencies serving the domestic violence victims/survivors and their children. Frequently, the YWCA or Family Justice Centers exist in urban areas, and rural agencies are sparse. Regardless, it is incumbent on the forensic nurse to identify and refer to the agencies that serve survivors.

References

1. Glass N, Laughon K, Campbell J, et al. Non-fatal strangulation is an important risk factor for homicide in women. *J Emerg Med.* 2008;35(3):329-335.
2. Messing JT, Patch M, Wilson JS, Kelen GD, Campbell J. Differentiating among attempted, completed, and multiple nonfatal strangulation in women experiencing intimate partner violence. *Womens Health Issues.* 2018;28(1):104-111.
3. Centers for Medicare & Medicaid Services. 2020 ICD-10-CM. https://www.cms.gov/Medicare/Coding/ICD10/2020-ICD-10-CM. Accessed May 05, 2020.
4. The Office for Victims of Crime. Crime victims fund. https://www.ovc.gov/pubs/crimevictimsfundfs/index.html. Accessed May 05, 2020.

Anatomic Skills

Anatomic Skills 10-1

Refer to **Figure 10-1**. Using the letters that correspond to the structures in the photograph, label the anatomic locations.

Arrow A. ______________________________

Arrow B. ______________________________

Arrow C. ______________________________

Arrow D. ______________________________

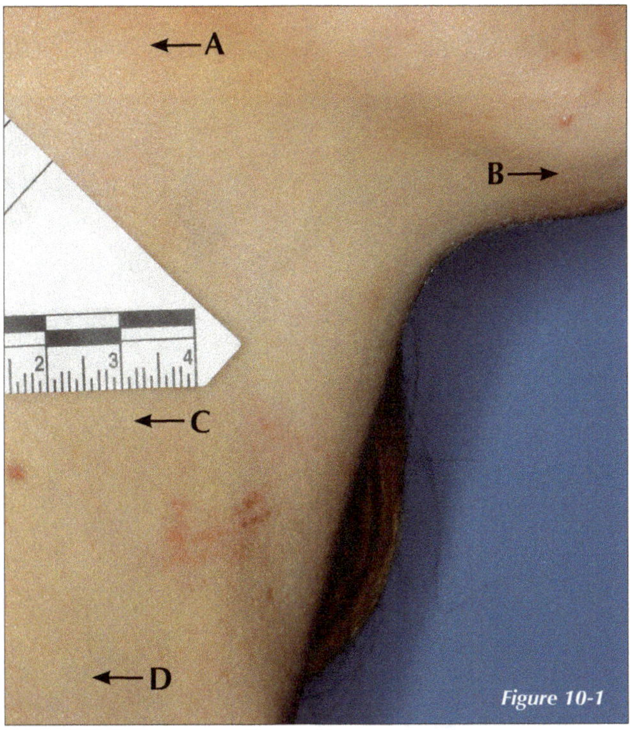

Figure 10-1

Anatomic Skills 10-2

Refer to **Figure 10-2**. Using the letters that correspond to the structures in the photograph, label the anatomic locations.

Arrow E. ______________________________

Arrow F. ______________________________

Arrow G. ______________________________

Arrow H. ______________________________

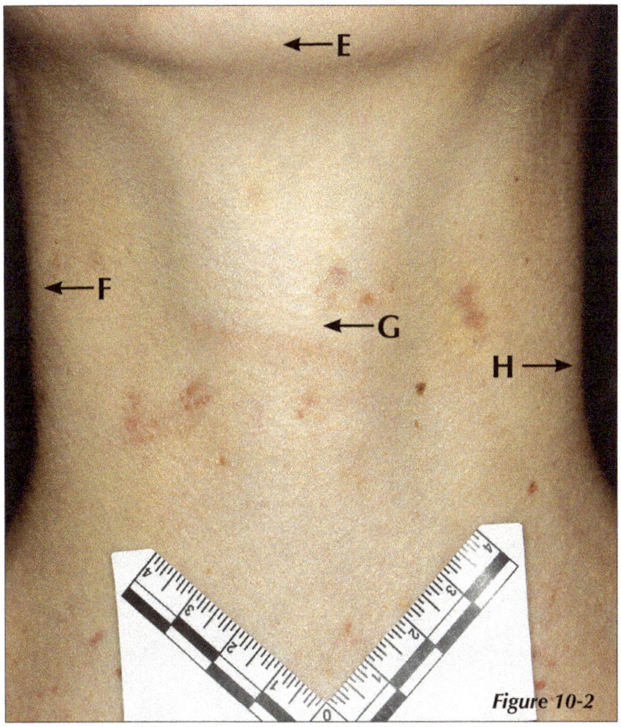

Figure 10-2

Activities

Activity 10-1. Injury Identification

Refer to **Figures 10-3** through **10-8**. Identify any injuries in respect to their anatomic location. Write objective descriptions when documenting findings.

Arrow I. ____

Arrow J. ____

Arrow K. ____

Arrow L. ____

Arrow M. ____

Arrow N. ____

Arrow O. ____

Arrow P. ____

Arrow Q. ____

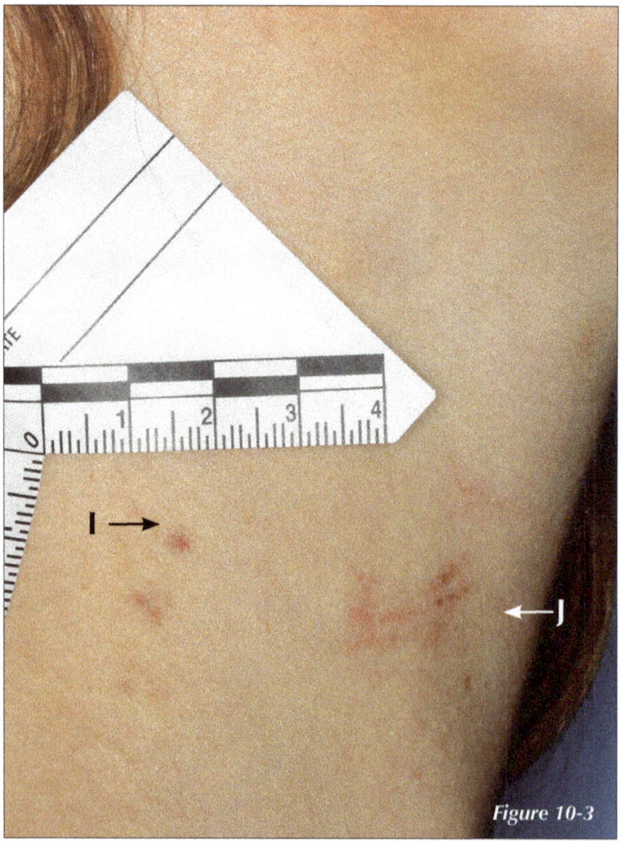

Figure 10-3

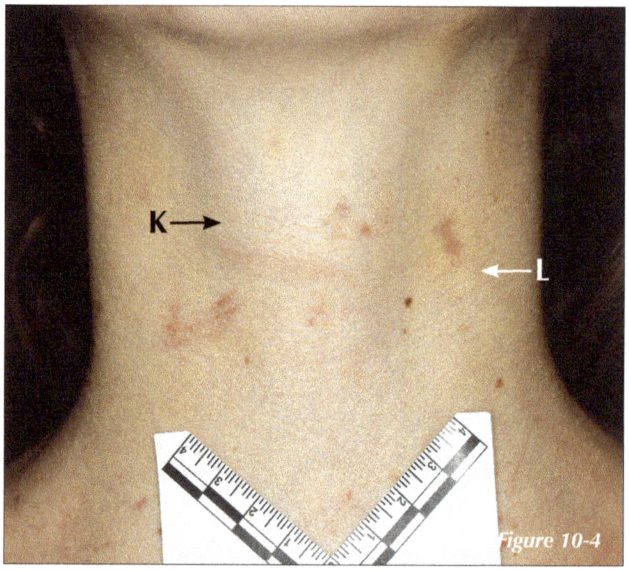

Figure 10-4

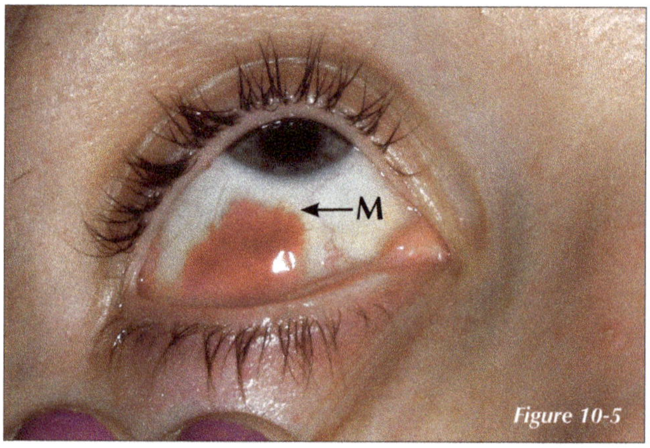

Figure 10-5

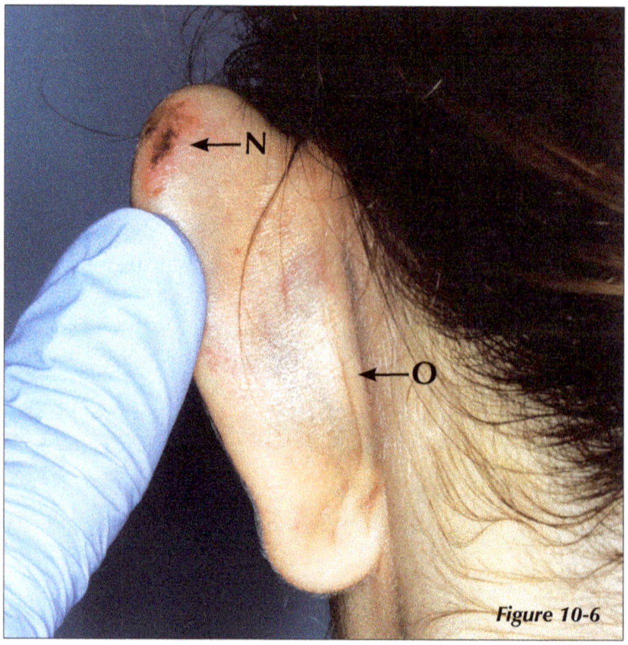

Figure 10-6

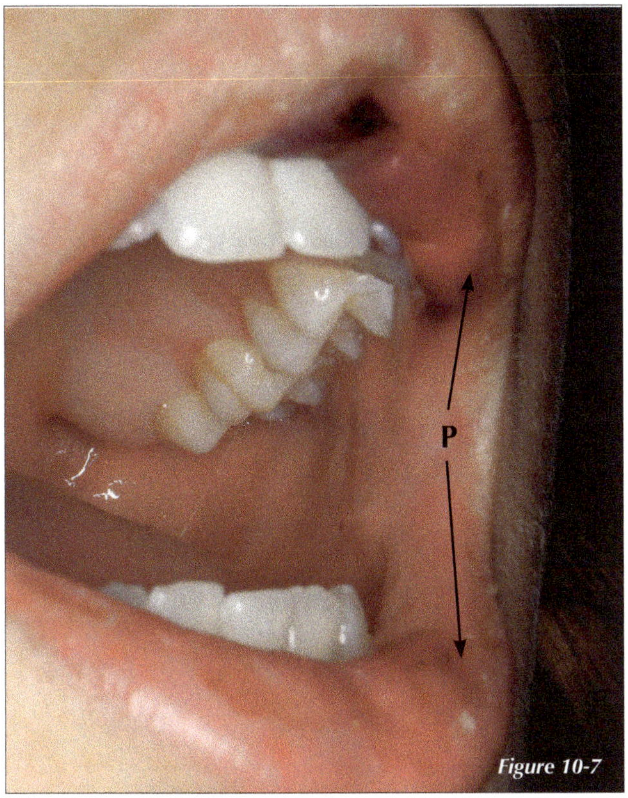

Figure 10-7

Activity 10-2. Assessment

List 3 additional questions that the forensic nurse in SANE care asks regarding the physical findings (eg, symptom Onset, Location/radiation, Duration, Character, Aggravating factors, Relieving factors, Timing and Severity [OLDCARTS]; demonstration of method of injury [if known]; level of consciousness).

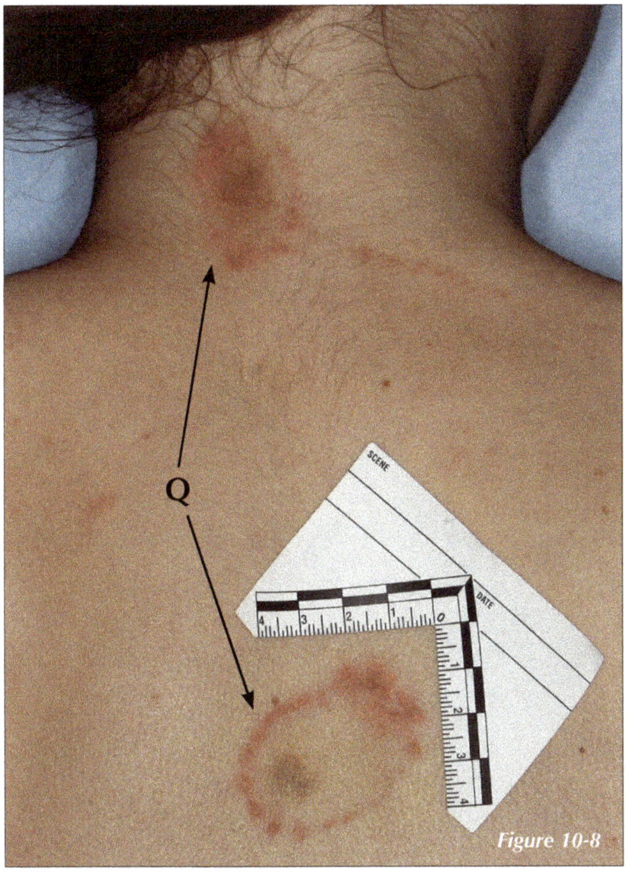

Figure 10-8

Activity 10-3. Physical Assessment

Remember that injury is progressive throughout the healing phases. Because of the nature of neck and brain injury (eg, closed/open spaces with continued bleeding), there is potential for diminished function throughout the assessment. Therefore, assessment for potential serious sequelae is continuous in all patients, and when decline in function is recognized, an immediate referral to an advanced practice nurse, physician, or physician assistant is urgent and necessary. In addition, if the patient is in need of emergent care, take note of existing injury at time of arrival because lifesaving measures will alter the body's appearance. List 3 to 6 additional physical assessment procedures you should consider.

Activity 10-4. Evidence Collection

What evidence would you collect given the patient's history? What findings would promote evidence collection even if the history is deficient?

Activity 10-5. Treatment and Care

Based on the history and your findings, what treatment would you offer this patient? Would you report this case to the police?

Activity 10-6. Lethality Assessment

During care and as part of discharge planning, all patients who are suspected to be victims of domestic violence should be assessed for risk of immediate danger. List 4 indicators of escalating danger in a person who has experienced domestic violence. What questions should you ask a patient to assess his or her risk of immediate danger?

Chapter 11

70-year-old Male Patient Assaulted by an Employee

Case History

John is a 70-year-old man living on the family farm. His wife died 15 years earlier. His 33-year-old daughter, Jenny, lived with him until recently when she moved out of the house. Although retired, John grows and sells flowers. He has many acres of land and uses temporary staff to care for and harvest the plants when they reach maturity. His head ranch hand, Michael, entered his home and asked where Jenny was. John would not reveal his daughter's location, and Michael became very angry. John told Michael that Jenny said she was uncomfortable around Michael and did not like to be around him. Michael became more enraged. Michael put his right hand around John's neck and pushed him into the wall. John tells the forensic nurse, "I couldn't talk or breathe, and the pressure was unbearable for a few seconds." When asked how he escaped, John says, "I pulled at Michael's fingers to get them off my neck," and then "I twisted my body until Michael let go."

John ran upstairs yelling, "Michael, get out of my house!" John says that Michael followed him upstairs threatening, "If you don't tell me where Jenny is, you'll be sorry." John reports that he was scared because Michael had never acted this way before. John ran into his upstairs bedroom and closed and locked the door. He says he told Michael he was going to call the police if Michael did not leave. John says, "Michael began to curse and pound on the door, so I ran out on the balcony." He closed the sliding door, realizing his phone was still inside the bedroom. He says he was so scared he contemplated jumping off the second story balcony. Because there was concrete on the ground under the balcony he hesitated, and at that moment Michael was able to break open the door. Michael came out onto the balcony and dragged John back into the bedroom. He pushed John down to the ground, knelt over him, and placed both hands around his neck while yelling and spitting in his face. John states he could not "breathe or make any sounds," and he started "to see black and felt warm." John remembers he attempted to "turn over thinking I could crawl away," but Michael put John in "a choke hold," and John "felt a sting" on his back.

> ***Clinical Pearl:***
> *Strangulation is a lethal form of assault with a variety of hypoxic and anoxic symptoms, necessitating careful history taking and documentation.*

The next thing John remembers is that he was standing up, and Michael was telling him he would die next time if he did not tell him where Jenny was. John then told Michael that Jenny was in the guest house. He says, "She wasn't, but I thought maybe Michael would go look for her and I could get away." Michael ran downstairs and toward the guest house. John followed and jumped into his truck and started driving down the driveway. John states the gates to the farm were closed and he "couldn't remember which button to press to open the gate, so I rammed my truck through the gates." He says he was afraid to slow down because he thought Michael would be running after him. He knew he left his cell phone in the house, so he drove 2 miles down the road to his neighbor's house to call the police.

The neighbor saw John and called the police and for an ambulance. When the ambulance arrived, John was transported to the hospital. He had a complete trauma workup and was admitted. The forensic nurse was called 12 hours after the incident. When asked about specific symptoms he experienced, John states he feels that his mouth is "full of spit," and it is painful to swallow. He states his voice is "much more raspy" than usual, his neck and back hurt, and he feels "like I can't really turn my head." He also states his mouth and back are "burning." He says he is not sure if he lost consciousness and knows he did not urinate, but when asked if he noticed his underwear was wet, he remembers that it was when the emergency department (ED) staff took it off. He says he "feels foggy" and states there "are some things I just can't make myself remember." The forensic nurse notes that John has signs of light erythema across both sides of his neck with linear abrasions on the anterior neck and chest. Multiple small, round bruises are observed within the hair of his beard around the jawline. He has a subconjunctival hematoma in the left eye and states, "I don't remember, but I don't think Michael punched or slapped me." John states that one of his front teeth is "wiggling," and bruising is noted on the left buccal area. He has a double-arched bite mark on his upper middle back and some bruising on his arms and shoulders. During the examination John states, "I thought this was it, I was going to be with my wife in heaven, but I never told him where Jenny really was."

John is discharged from the hospital after 2 days and is seen for a follow-up examination 7 days after the assault because he "needed to get all his doctor appointments taken care of." John says he still has headaches, "foggy moments," and his neck continues to be stiff and "is still swollen." His left neck shows a significant amount of dark bruising, and swelling is noted on his right and front neck. His neck circumference is measured at a 1-cm increase from the initial examination, and he is referred back to the ED.

Case Discussion

During an assault, manual strangulation does not require planning or additional weapons to control a victim. This case presents an elderly male patient who had no suspicion that the suspect would be violent with him. There are special considerations a health care provider must take into account when assessing a male victim. Does the patient have facial hair? If so, how would you assess for injury underneath the facial hair? Does the health care professional have an inherent bias about men as victims? Does society expect that men should be better equipped to protect themselves? According to the Center for Disease Control and Prevention,[1] approximately 1 in 10 men in the United States experience sexual violence, physical violence, and/or stalking by an intimate partner during their lifetime and report some form of intimate partner violence (IPV)–related impact. Commonly reported IPV-related impacts among male victims are fear, concern for safety, and symptoms of posttraumatic stress disorder, among others. In this case history it appears there could be additional dangers to the patient's daughter. The nature of the suspect's relationship with the patient's daughter is unknown. The patient diverted the suspect by sending him to find his daughter in a false location in order to escape.

The patient described a choke hold and a sting to his back. The patient did not know what caused the sting, so it is important for the examiner to inspect the patient from head to toe. The patient denies that he urinated or lost consciousness but reports his underwear was wet in the emergency room. The examiner should assess the circumference of the neck during the initial examination and repeat during the follow-up. It is concerning that the patient reports increased secretions, so the examiner should also assess if the patient is able to manage his own secretions and report any findings to the emergency medical care team. Because there is a possible period of amnesia, loss of consciousness, and involuntary urination, accompanied by presyncopal symptoms, is it imperative to assess for and discuss with the patient the significance of these symptoms (**Appendix 14**).

References

1. Violence prevention: intimate partner violence, sexual violence, and stalking among men. Centers for Disease Control and Prevention Web site. https://www.cdc.gov/violenceprevention/datasources/nisvs/men-ipvsvandstalking.html. Updated October 25, 2018. Accessed December 6, 2019.

Anatomic Skills

Anatomic Skills 11-1

Refer to **Figure 11-1**. Using the letters that correspond to the structures in the photograph, label the anatomic locations.

A. ____________________

B. ____________________

C. ____________________

D. ____________________

Anatomic Skills 11-2

Refer to **Figure 11-2**. Using the letters that correspond to the structures in the photograph, label the anatomic locations.

E. ____________________

F. ____________________

G. ____________________

H. ____________________

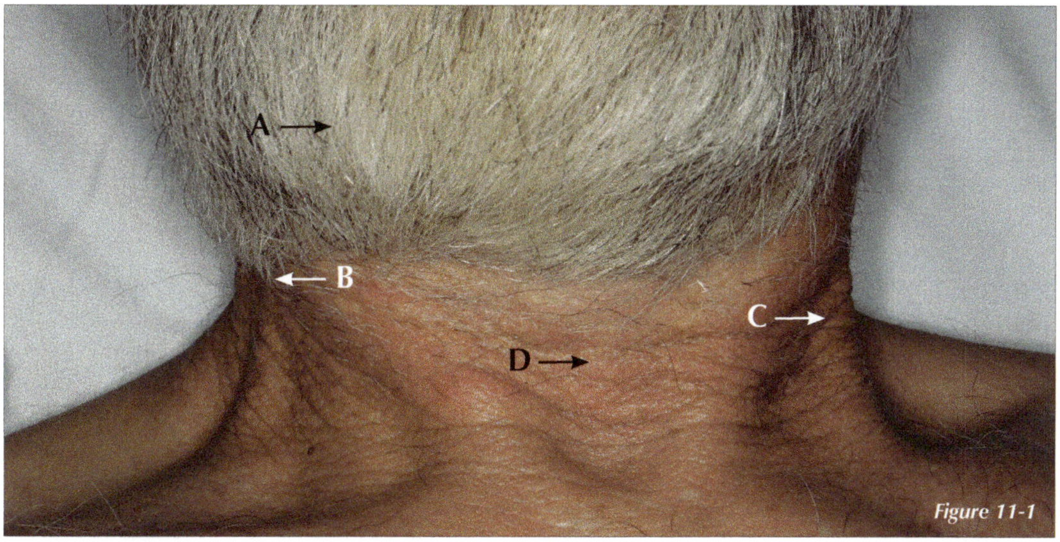

Figure 11-1

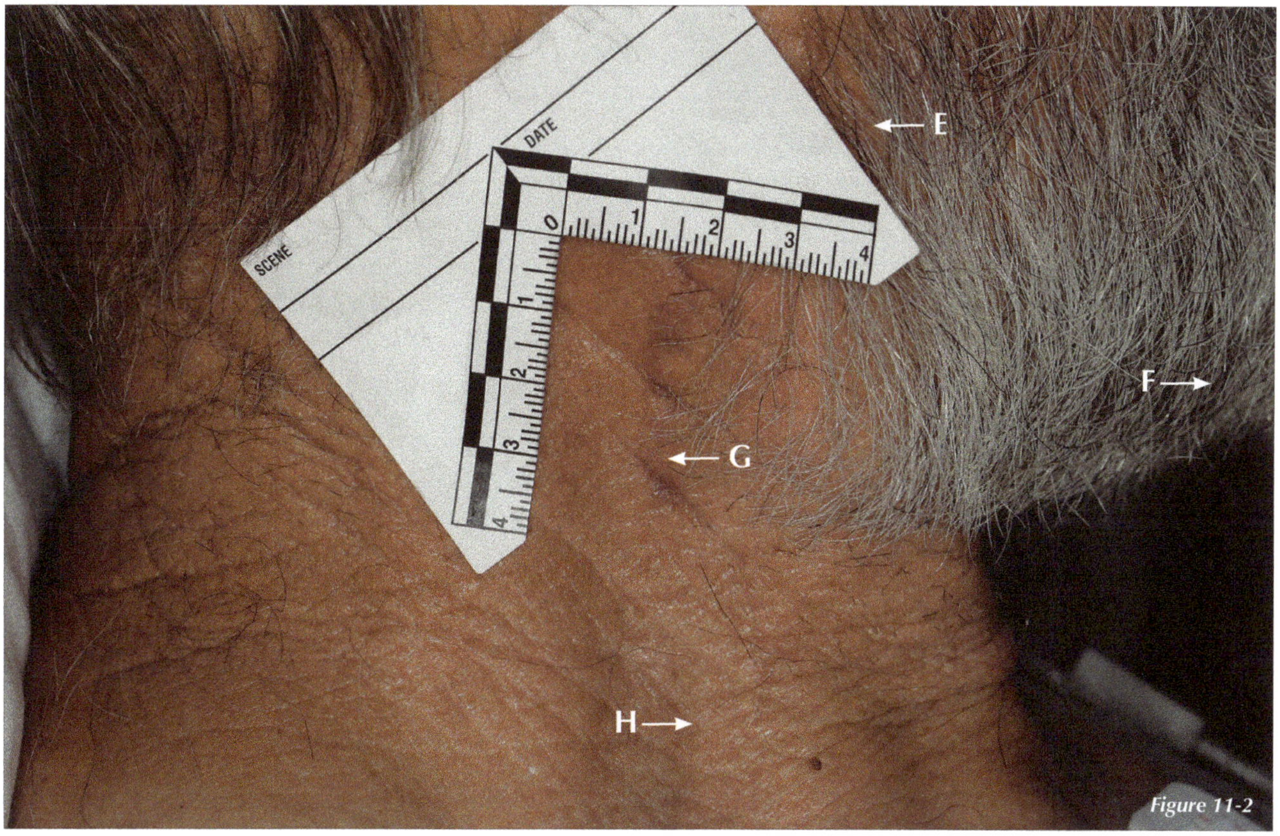

Figure 11-2

Activities

Activity 11-1. Injury Identification

Refer to **Figures 11-3** through **11-8**. Identify any injuries in respect to their anatomic location. Give objective descriptions when documenting findings.

I. ______________________________

J. ______________________________

K. ______________________________

L. ______________________________

M. ______________________________

N. ______________________________

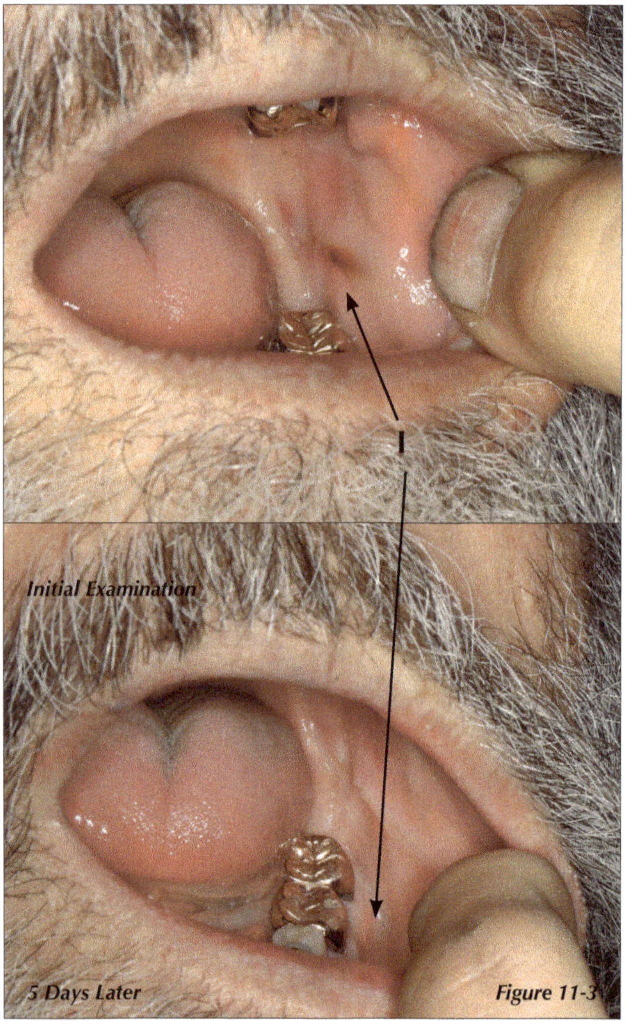

Figure 11-3

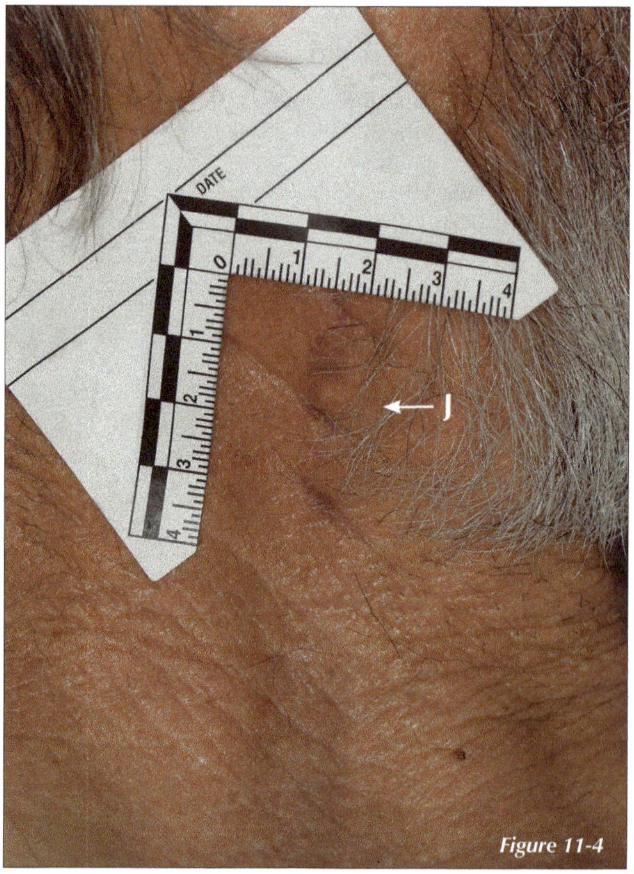

Figure 11-4

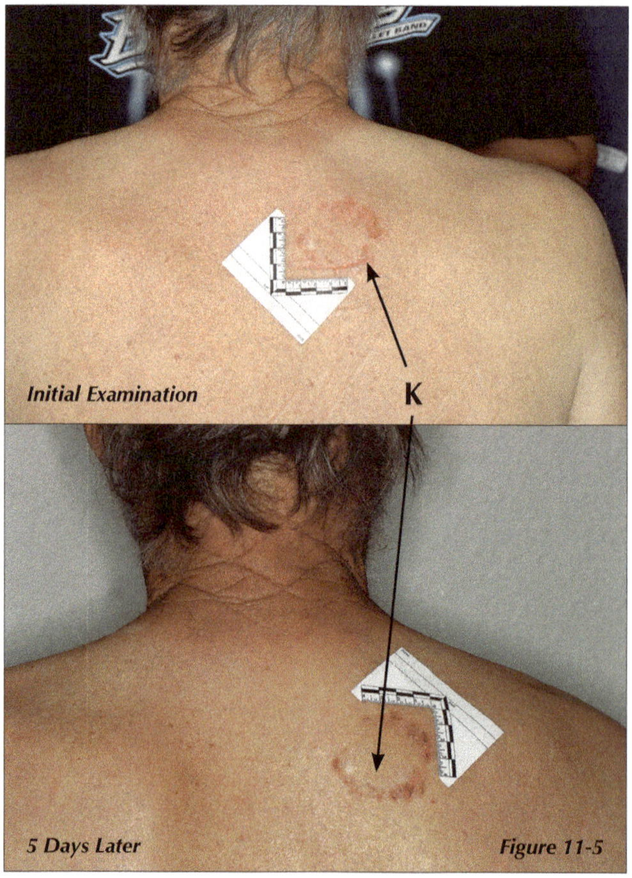

Figure 11-5

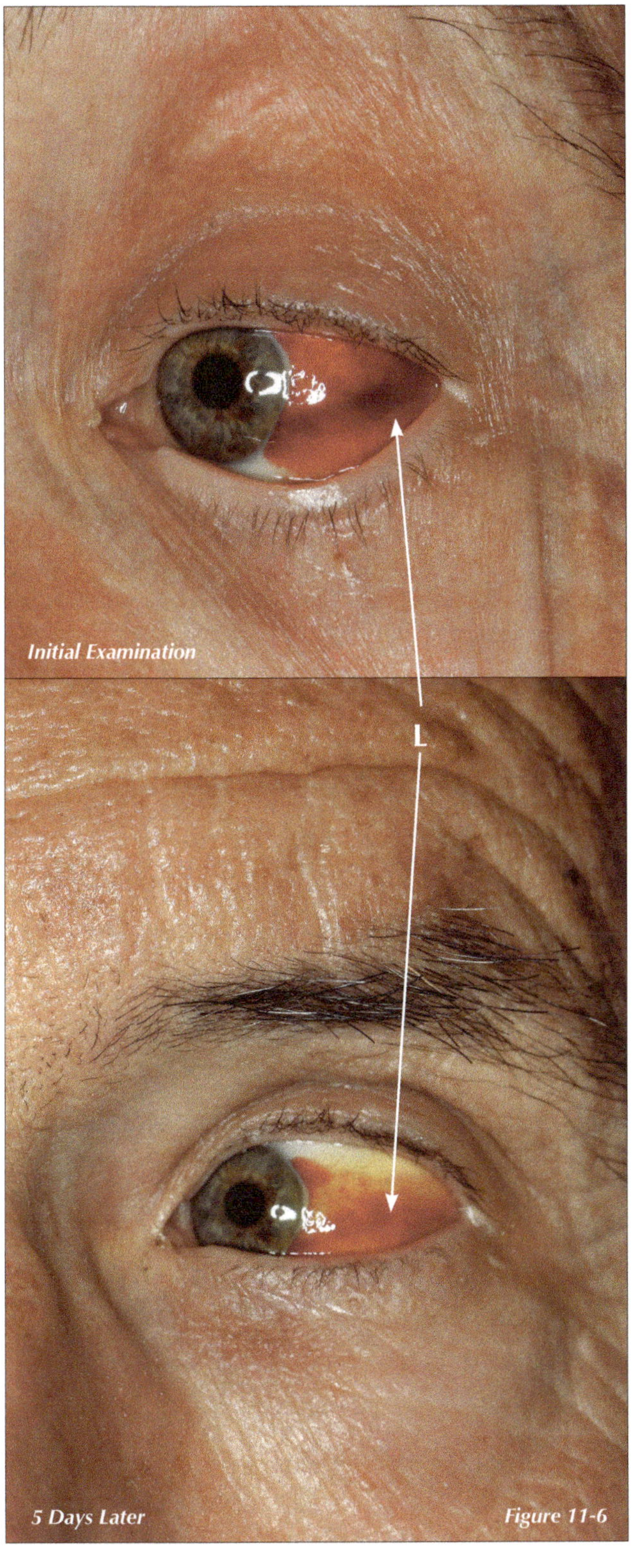

Initial Examination

5 Days Later

Figure 11-6

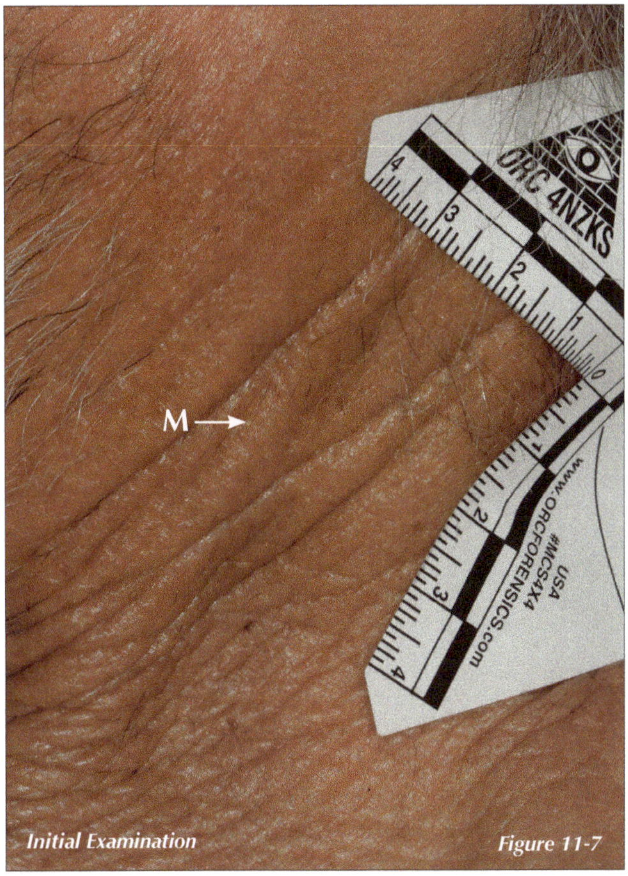

Initial Examination

Figure 11-7

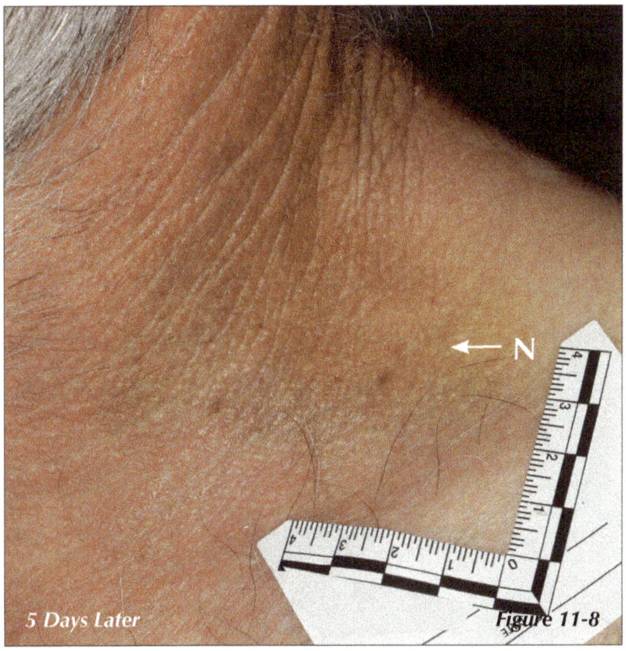

5 Days Later

Figure 11-8

Activity 11-2. Assessment

List 3 additional questions that the forensic nurse in SANE care asks regarding the physical findings (eg, symptom Onset, Location/radiation, Duration, Character, Aggravating factors, Relieving factors, Timing and Severity [OLDCARTS], demonstration of method of injury [if known], level of consciousness).

Activity 11-3. Physical Assessment

Remember that injury is progressive throughout the healing phases. Because of the nature of neck and brain injury (eg, closed/open spaces with continued bleeding as noted with the increasing diameter of the neck 7 days later), there is potential for diminished function throughout the assessment. Therefore, assessment for potential serious sequelae is continuous in all patients, and when decline in function is recognized, an immediate referral to an advanced practice nurse, physician, or physician assistant is urgent and necessary. List 3 to 6 additional physical assessment procedures you should consider.

Activity 11-4. Evidence Collection

What evidence would you collect given the patient's history? What findings would promote evidence collection even if the history is deficient?

Activity 11-5. Treatment and Care

Based on the history and your findings, what treatment would you offer this patient? Would you report this case to the police or adult protective services?

Chapter 12

56-Year-Old Female Patient Assaulted by an Ex-Husband

Case History

Nina received final divorce papers while Guy was in jail for previous domestic violence assaults. Nina thought he was still in jail because she had not seen him for 6 months. However, last week, Guy began stalking her. Nina says that Guy had recently contacted her friend and said he wanted to get back together with Nina. He also asked the friend where Nina was staying. Nina believes that the red car parked outside her quilting group had been following her, and she has had hang-up calls on her phone recently. She believes Guy is responsible for both. Nina states she was leaving her home to go to the store and noticed the red car parked across the street. She turned to go back into the house, and Guy came up from behind. He grabbed her by her neck with one hand and her hair with the other and pushed her toward the door. She states he was squeezing her neck so hard that she "thought his fingers would rip her head off." He told her, "Open the door. We are both going in!" Nina says, "I started to scream," but Guy continued to push her into the house. Guy threw her on the ground by her neck. Nina says she landed on her back on the floor and thinks she hit her head. Nina says, "Guy kicked me in the ribs and told me that I was his and I could never be with anyone else." Nina says she sat up but was still on the ground. She says, "I told Guy that I didn't want to be with him anymore" and that it was not right "how he treated me."

> ***Clinical Pearl:***
> *Forty-eight states, 20 tribes, and 2 United States territories have passed laws to prosecute strangulation and suffocation assaults as a felony.*

She says, "His eyes looked like the devil, and he jumped on top of me, pushing my head down to the ground with one hand." Once on the ground, he put both hands around her neck. "He was sitting on my stomach and had all his weight on my neck." Nina says that on a scale of 0 to 10, the pressure on her neck was a "10." She could not breathe or speak, and she began to see "floating lights." She says that "he was yelling at me, but I could not hear what he was saying to me." She says she was trying to pull his fingers off her neck, but she could not move them. She believes he was holding her neck for about 20 seconds. Nina begins to cry and says, "I thought I would never see my children and grandbaby ever again. I thought he was going to kill me."

The next thing Nina remembers is sitting on the couch while Guy was "doing something in the bedroom." She does not remember how she got onto the couch. She says that she could hear her neighbor outside barbecuing and ran out the front door, yelling for her neighbor. The neighbor ran toward her as Guy was coming out the door. Nina told the neighbor to call the police. Guy ran to his car and drove away.

After a comprehensive medical evaluation, Nina was discharged from the emergency department (ED). She is seen for a medical forensic examination after discharge. During the medical forensic history, Nina says that the doctor asked her what happened, but she tells to the nurse, "I didn't tell him the whole story." She says, "They did some x-rays of my arm and head." She states her whole body hurts, her voice "sounds funny," and she feels like her tongue is "a giant ball." She states it is hard to talk because she thinks she may have bit her tongue but does not remember it. She says it is hard to swallow, and she hears a high-pitched squeak in her right ear. When Nina is asked if she urinated during the assault, she says "no." Law enforcement reports that her shorts were wet when they arrived at the home, and she changed out of them before the paramedics came. When asked about her wet shorts, Nina says, "Oh, maybe I did pee a little, because I was really scared. I don't remember."

The nonfatal strangulation photography protocol was followed (**Appendix 1**). Nina demonstrated on a mannequin head the positions of her assailant's hands during the strangulation event (**Figure 12-1-a** and **b**).

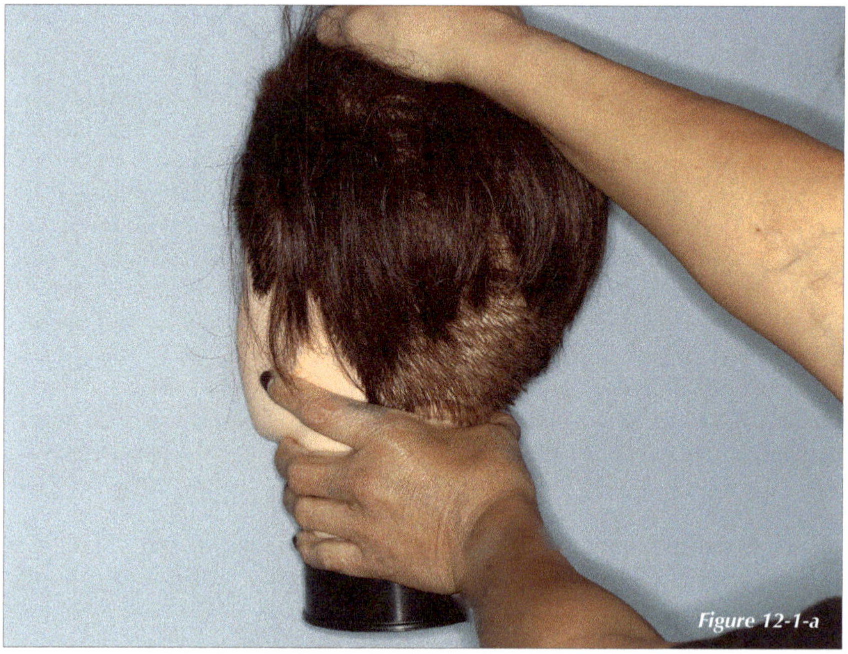

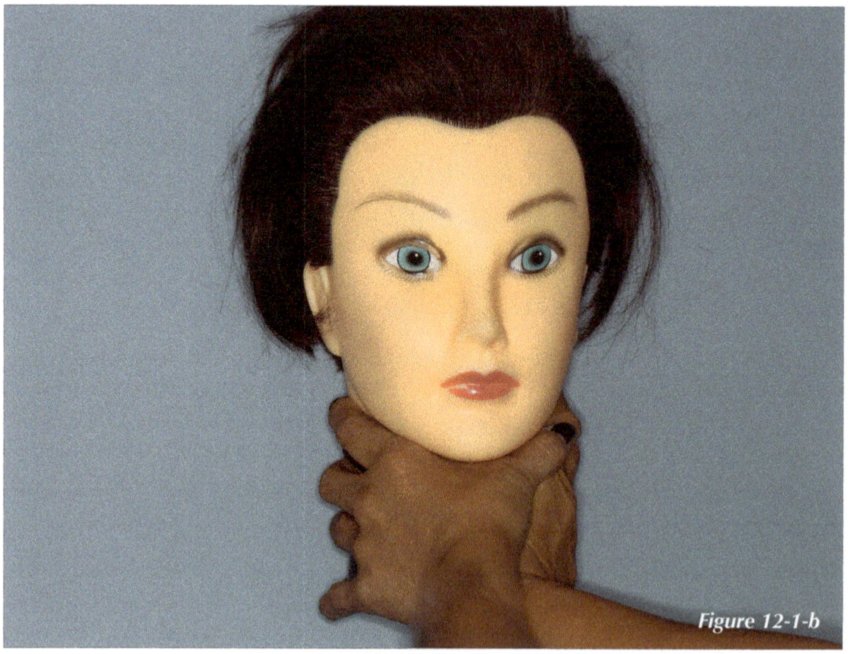

Figure 12-1-a. *Hand positions of the first strangulation event when Nina was "pushed" into the house.*

Figure 12-1-b. *Hand positions during the second strangulation event when Nina was on her back, on the ground.*

Case Discussion

After reading the case history, the examiner should be able to recognize not only the immediate physical danger based on the mechanism of injury described from the strangulation, but also the dangers of stalking. Not only was the abuser stalking Nina himself, but it appears that he was also stalking by proxy. He called Nina's friend to gather information and to convince her friend that he wanted to get back together with Nina. It is unclear from the history if the friend did in fact disclose any information, but involving a third party to track and gather information shows a level of escalating dangerous behavior.[1]

The patient in this case described concerns that she was followed to a friend's home and also that she was receiving hang-up calls. The victimization of stalking has complex psychosocial traumatic effects on the patient.[2] The warning signs of stalking could be missed by medical professionals without proper training or screening tools, which could lead to future physical harm of the patient. Stalking cases should be properly dealt with in the criminal justice system using protection orders and by advocacy while safety planning.[3]

It is not uncommon for a patient to minimize symptoms of abuse. Most often, after a strangulation assault, patients will downplay the fact that they urinated on themselves. It is important for the health care provider to be patient and ask information-gathering questions in a trauma-informed manner. It might be helpful for the health care provider to ask about clothing first, with a simple noninvasive question such as, "Can you tell me if you are wearing the same clothing you were wearing at the time of the assault?" If not, asking, "Can you tell me if you remember anything different about your clothing?" might allow the health care provider to gather more objective data. The patient might not remember urinating on herself and therefore might not be able to answer that question, but if the patient remembers wet clothing, this could be indicative of urination during the strangulation assault. This patient described episodes of memory loss and pain to the neck. It is unclear by this history if the patient received a computed tomographic angiogram. It would be important for the medical professional to clarify what tests she received. The patient did not disclose the full history in the ED, so the emergency provider might not have the full assault history. The forensic nurse examiner has trauma-informed interview training and should review the medical safety based on the new information received during the history.

The patient will need a head-to-toe medical forensic examination, and because she did not disclose her entire assault history in the ED, she may need to be referred back to the ED so that the evaluation can be based on the full extent of her assault. This patient will also need a Danger Assessment, safety planning, and advocacy resources.

References

1. Logan T, Cole J, Shannon L, Walker R. *Partner Stalking: How Women Respond, Cope, and Survive*. New York, NY: Springer Publishing Company; 2006.

2. Korkodeilou J. 'No place to hide': stalking victimisation and its psycho-social effects. *International Review of Victimology*. 2017;23(1):17-32.

3. Melton HC. Stalking in the context of intimate partner abuse: in the victim's words. *Feminist Criminology*. 2007;2(4):347-363.

Anatomic Skills

Anatomic Skills 12-1

Refer to **Figure 12-2**. Using the letters that correspond to the structures in the photograph, label the anatomic locations.

A. ______________________________

B. ______________________________

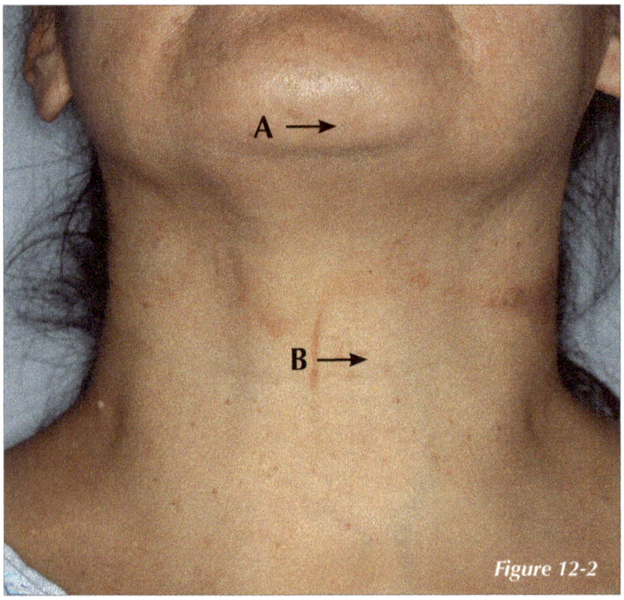

Figure 12-2

Anatomic Skills 12-2

Refer to **Figure 12-3**. Using the letters that correspond to the structures in the photograph, label the anatomic locations.

C. ______________________________

D. ______________________________

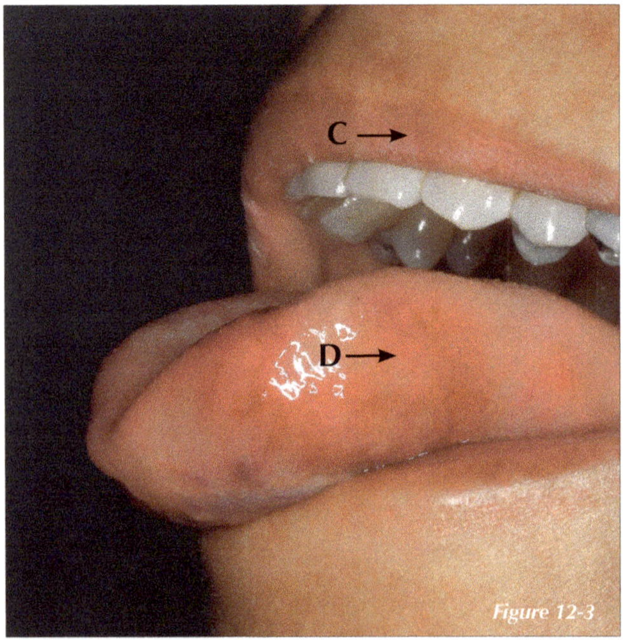

Figure 12-3

Activities

Activity 12-1. Injury Identification

Refer to **Figures 12-4** through **12-7**. Identify any injuries in respect to their anatomic location. Give objective descriptions when documenting findings.

E. ______________________________

F. ______________________________

G. ______________________________

H. ______________________________

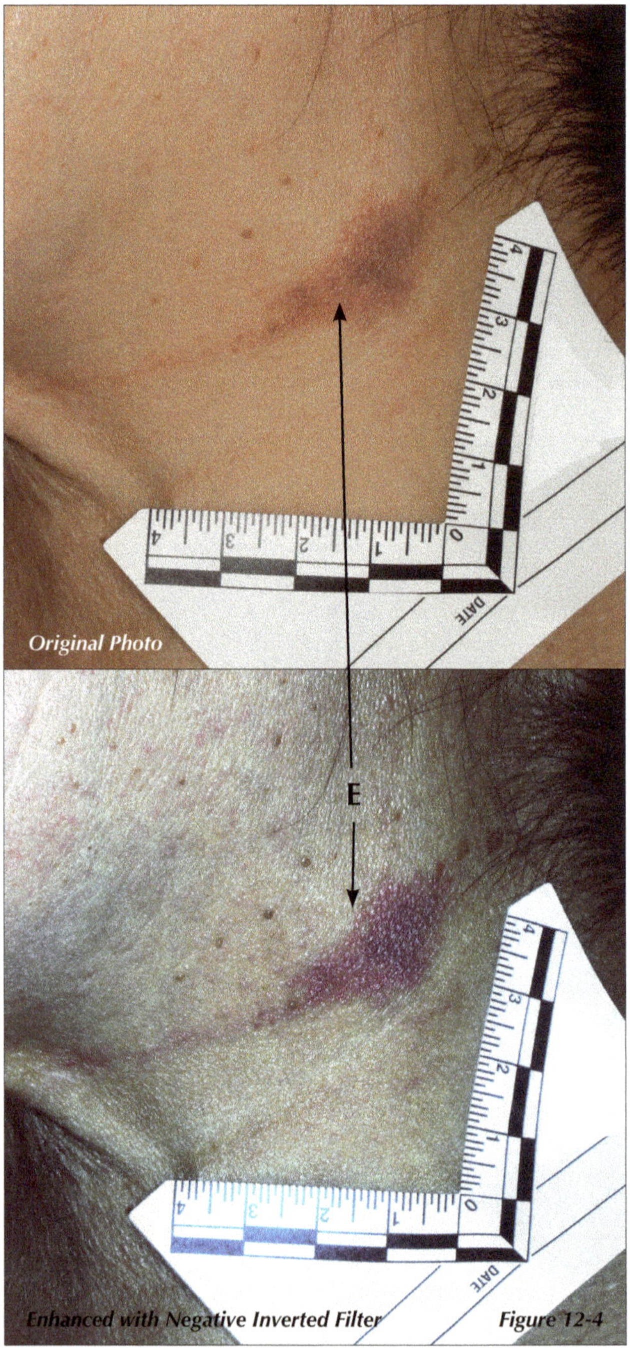

Figure 12-4

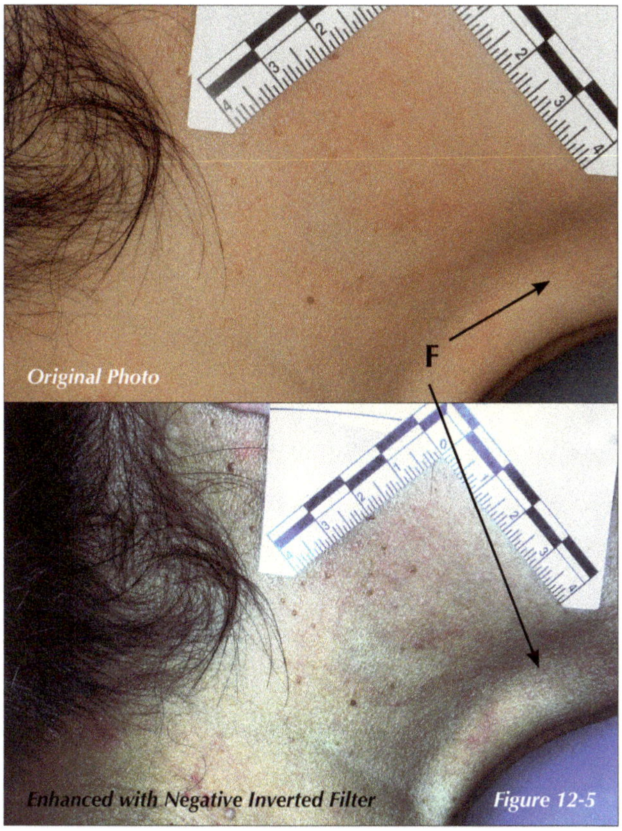

Figure 12-5

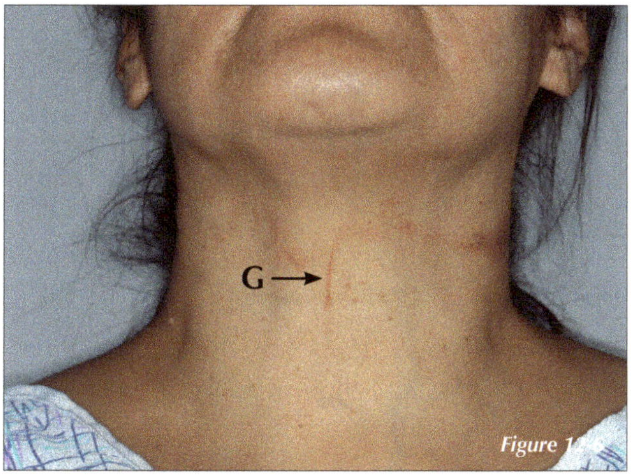

Figure 1

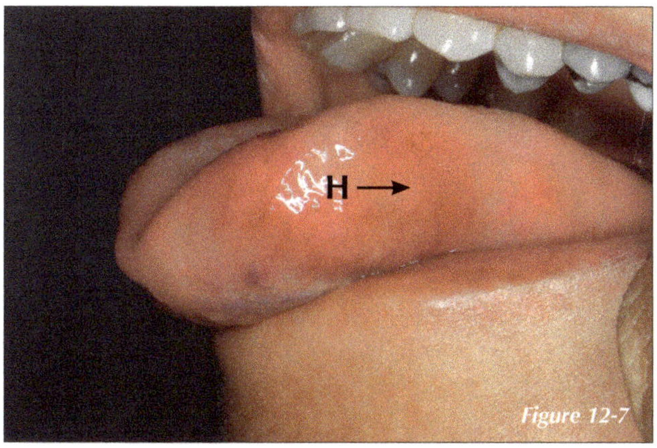

Figure 12-7

Activity 12-2. Assessment

List 3 additional questions that the forensic nurse asks regarding the physical findings (eg, symptom Onset, Location/radiation, Duration, Character, Aggravating factors, Relieving factors, Timing and Severity [OLDCARTS]; demonstration of method of injury [if known]; level of consciousness).

Activity 12-3. Physical Assessment

Remember that injury is progressive throughout the healing phases. Because of the nature of neck and brain injury (eg, closed/open spaces with continued bleeding), there is potential for diminished function throughout the assessment. Therefore, assessment for potential serious sequelae is continuous in all patients, and when decline in function is recognized, an immediate referral to an advanced practice nurse, physician, or physician assistant is urgent and necessary. List 3 to 6 additional physical assessment procedures you should consider.

Activity 12-4. Evidence Collection

What evidence would you collect given the patient's history? What findings would promote evidence collection even if the history is deficient?

Activity 12-5. Treatment and Care

Based on the history and your findings, what treatment would you offer this patient? Would you report this case to the police?

Activity 12-6. Lethality Assessment

During care and as part of discharge planning, all patients who are suspected to be victims of domestic violence should be assessed for risk of immediate danger. List 4 indicators of escalating danger in a person who has experienced domestic violence. What questions should you ask a patient to assess his or her risk of immediate danger?

Chapter 13

30-Year-Old Female Patient Assaulted and Strangled by an Intimate Partner

Case History

Victoria and Julio have known each other since childhood. They became romantically involved when they both arrived in the same United States community with work visas. Today, Victoria, who is a 30-year-old Hispanic woman, reports she was physically assaulted and strangled by Julio. She states, "I know why he's mad… I'm dating another man. When I saw him, he was yelling and screaming about me being a whore! I tried to walk away, and he attacked me from behind. He put his arm around my neck." She thinks Julio lifted her off the ground with his arm, and she could not breathe because of the pressure on her neck. She says she attempted to pull his arm away from her neck and dug her fingernails into his arm and her neck. Victoria reports that she blacked out and thinks she fell face-first onto the floor, creating a lip/tooth injury. Victoria reports that after waking up she was strangled a second time with associated unconsciousness and states she urinated "on myself." She complains of pain on the left side of her head, face, left shoulder, left neck, and upper chest. When asked if there was more to report, Victoria states, "That's all I remember." A translator was used in this case as Victoria was more comfortable using her native language.

Case Discussion

Victoria has a high risk for a carotid artery dissection for 2 reasons: (1) the application of compressive forces on the neck from the application of the forearm and (2) the stretching of the neck when she was lifted up by the neck. The history of being rendered unconscious twice with associated loss of bladder control indicates a prolonged period of anoxia. Urination is associated with a minimum of 15 seconds of continual pressure to the arteries taking oxygenated blood to the brain.[1] Many victims with anoxic brain injuries, manifested by the loss of consciousness and urination, require long-term follow-up for possible anoxic brain damage.

> ***Clinical Pearl:***
> *When domestic violence perpetrators strangle their victims, not only is this a felonious assault or possibly an attempted murder, but too often it can lead to a fatal outcome.*

In this case, follow up with a health care provider should be included in the discharge instructions. This case will be complicated by the fact that the victim and the assailant are both in the United States on work visas. Many immigrants are afraid to admit they have been a victim of a crime in part because they believe they will be deported from the United States if they report the crime. United States law provides several protections for legal and undocumented immigrants who are victims of a crime. There are specific protections for victims of domestic violence, human trafficking, and other certain crimes. U nonimmigrant status (or U visa) offers immigration protection for victims and is also a tool for law enforcement. To obtain U status, the victim must obtain a certification from law enforcement. However, law enforcement officials should note that providing a certification does not grant a benefit; only US Citizenship and Immigration Services can grant or deny this benefit.[2] Case management is needed in this case because of the multidimensional issues relating to background, language barriers, and potential for lack of follow-up health care.

References

1. Kabat H, Anderson JP. Acute arrest of cerebral circulation in man. *Arch Neuro Psychiatr.* 1943;50(5):510–528.
2. Immigration options for victims of crimes. Department of Homeland Security Web site. https://www.dhs.gov/immigration-options-victims-crimes. Updated April 18, 2019. Accessed January 6, 2019.

Anatomic Skills 13-1

Refer to **Figure 13-1**. Using the letters that correspond to the structures in the photograph, label the anatomic locations.

A. ______________________________

B. ______________________________

C. ______________________________

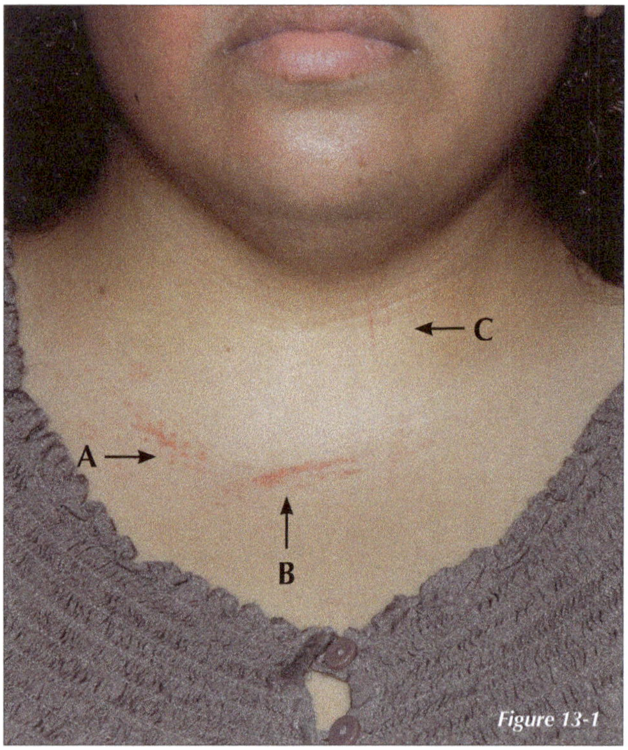

Figure 13-1

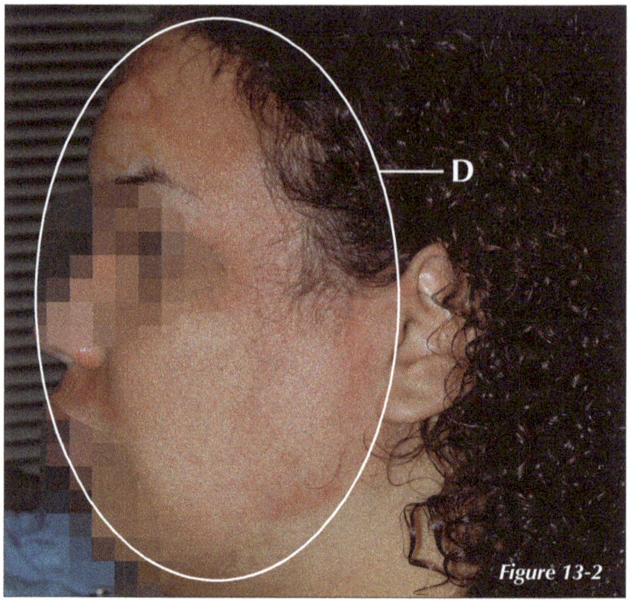

Figure 13-2

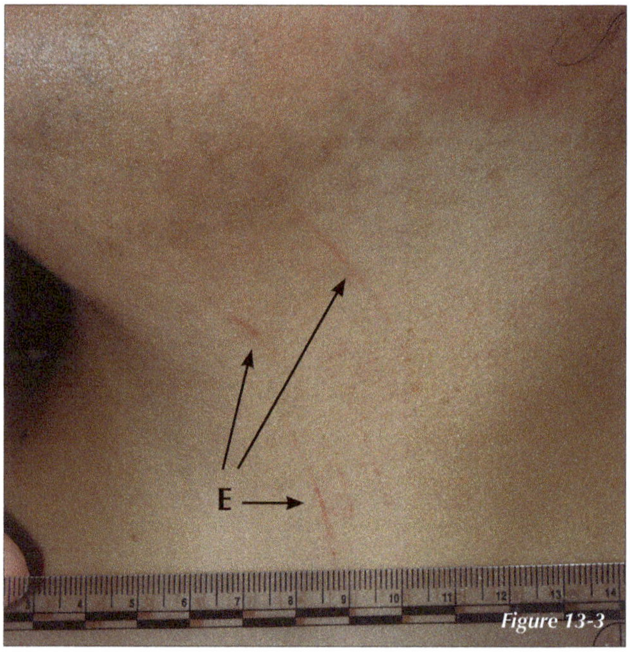

Figure 13-3

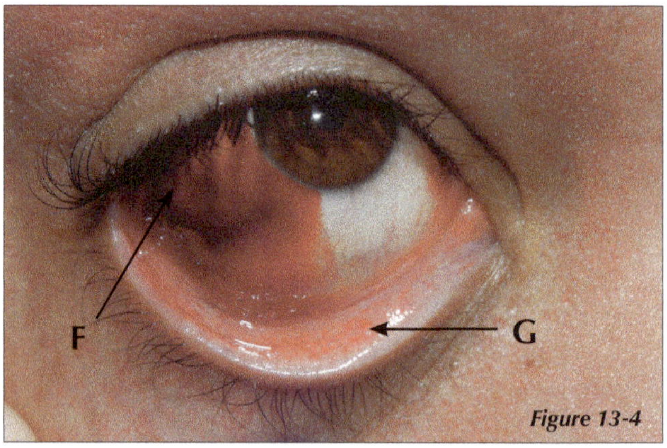

Figure 13-4

Activities

Activity 13-1. Injury Identification

Refer to **Figure 13-2** through **13-9**. Identify any injuries in respect to their anatomic location. Write objective descriptions when documenting findings.

D. ______________________________

E. ______________________________

F. ______________________________

G. ______________________________

H. ______________________________

I. ______________________________

J. ______________________________

K. ______________________________

L. ______________________________

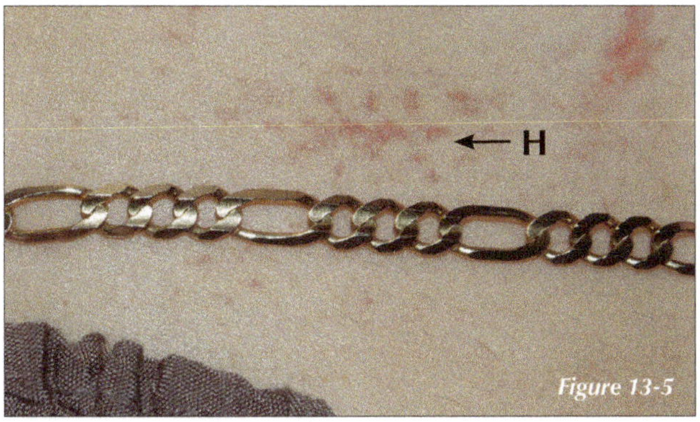

Figure 13-5

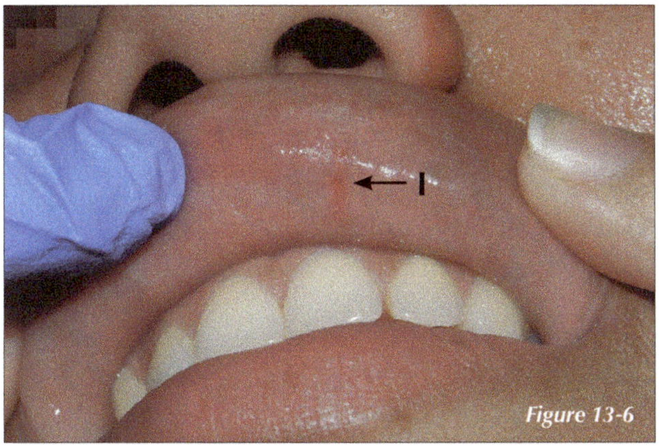

Figure 13-6

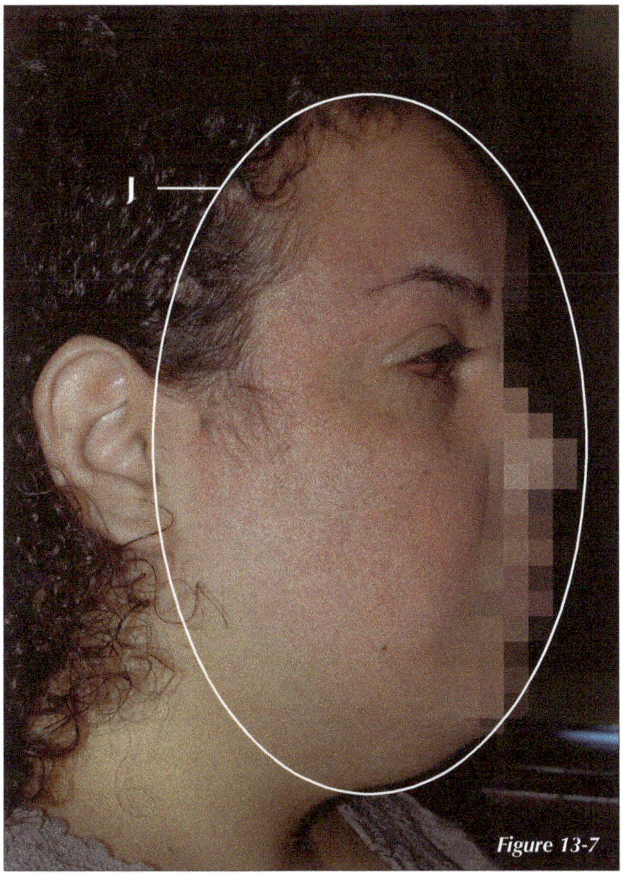

Figure 13-7

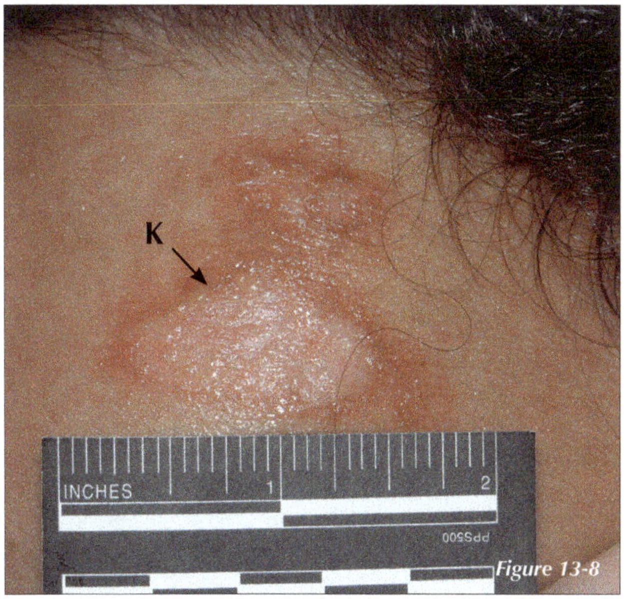

Figure 13-8

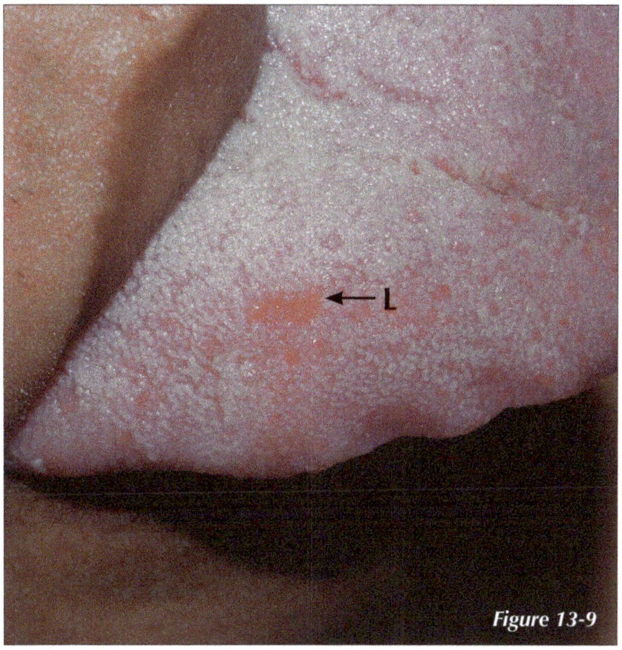

Figure 13-9

Activity 13-2. Petechial Hemorrhages

What is the presence of petechial hemorrhages over the entire face called? What is the presence of petechial hemorrhages over the entire face associated with?

Activity 13-3. Assessment

List 3 additional questions that the forensic nurse in SANE care asks regarding the physical findings (eg, symptom Onset, Location/radiation, Duration, Character, Aggravating factors, Relieving factors, Timing and Severity [OLDCARTS]; demonstration of method of injury [if known]; level of consciousness).

Activity 13-4. Physical Assessment

Remember that injury is progressive throughout the healing phases. Because of the nature of neck and brain injury (eg, closed/open spaces with continued bleeding), there is potential for diminished function throughout the assessment. Therefore, assessment for potential serious sequelae is continuous in all patients, and when decline in function is recognized, an immediate referral to an advanced practice nurse, physician, or physician assistant is urgent and necessary. List 3 to 6 additional physical assessment procedures you should consider.

Activity 13-5. Evidence Collection

What evidence would you collect given the patient's history? What findings would promote evidence collection even if the history is deficient?

Activity 13-6. Treatment and Care

Based on the history and your findings, what treatment would you offer this patient? Would you order a computed tomographic angiogram? Would you report this case to the police?

Activity 13-7. Lethality Assessment

During care and as part of discharge planning, all patients who are suspected to be victims of domestic violence should be assessed for risk of immediate danger. List 4 indicators of escalating danger in person who has experienced domestic violence. What questions should you ask a patient to assess his or her risk of immediate danger?

Chapter 14

25-Year-Old Female Patient Assaulted by a Stranger

Case History

Jackie is a 25-year-old single woman who works in a retail store. She states, "I've never had sex with a man. I'm a lesbian." She currently is staying in a hotel while her apartment is being remodeled. She reports that on Friday night, she heard a lot of talking in the hotel's common area, so she went there to "see what was going on." She told the responding law enforcement officer that she began drinking beers with the group. She reports that she thinks she had 5 or 6 beers. She does not remember much after drinking the beer until she woke up with no clothes on in another hotel room. She complains that her throat is sore, and now she can barely talk. She went back to her hotel room and called her friend, who went over and insisted on calling law enforcement. Both her friend and the officer encouraged Jackie to go to the hospital. At the hospital, Jackie tells the nurse, "My throat is very sore," and the nurse observes her having difficulty swallowing. The nurse also notes that there are marks on her neck.

Since Jackie has no memory of what happened, a full medical-legal evaluation is offered as a service she may want to consider. At a minimum, she is a victim of stranger physical assault, and she has visible and auditory injury. Jackie was given all options for reporting to law enforcement and undergoing the medical-legal examination. She tells the forensic nurse that she wishes to move forward with the medical-legal examination. Police are notified that Jackie wants to file a report, and a case number is obtained from the responding officer.

> ***Clinical Pearl:***
> *Strangulation is a lethal form of assault with a variety of hypoxic and anoxic symptoms, necessitating careful history taking and documentation.*

Jackie's friend is there to support her during the examination. During the interview, Jackie has little memory of the events that happened, and she tells the nurse, "I don't remember anything."

The examiner takes swabs of the perioral area, oral cavity, and neck. Palpation and sample collections help nurses assess elicited pain reactions, which are important to note during examination. Jackie does complain of pain in the neck area with movement and again during the nurse's swabbing. Superficial bruising is visible.

Head and neck photographs, using the principles of forensic photography, are part of the initial assessment (**Appendix 1**). Jackie has a hard time opening her mouth fully and cries out in pain when she tries to. The nurse applies a small ice pack after photography, assessment, and sample collection specifically to minimize post-injury swelling. The sexual assault evaluation proceeds after Jackie's airway is stable and treatment is initiated.

Case Discussion

In this case, discussion of strangulation guidelines with the physician was initiated by the nurse before starting the sexual assault evaluation and evidence collection. Early discussion allows time for the orders to be processed so procedures are seamless. After the examinations, it is important for the forensic nurse to discuss plans for discharge and follow-up. Because Jackie has a friend with her, she plans to go back to the hotel to gather her belongings and stay with her friend. A 2-week follow-up with her health care provider is also recommended.

To promote inclusion and equity in health care, it was important for the health care provider to acknowledge Jackie's sexual orientation. The Centers for Disease Control and Prevention reports that many health care providers do not routinely discuss sexual orientation or gender identity (SO/GI) with patients; consequently, many health care facilities do not have systems to collect structured SO/GI data from all patients (**Figure 14-1**). Without this information, lesbian, gay, bisexual, transgender, and queer (LGBTQ) patients and their specific health care needs cannot be identified, the health disparities they experience cannot be addressed, and provision of important health care services may not be available. This population's special needs include appropriate preventive screenings, assessments of risk for sexually transmitted infections and HIV, discussions about parenting, and effective interventions for behavioral health concerns related to the experiences of anti-LGBTQ stigma.[1] An opportunity for transgender persons to share information about their SO/GI in a welcoming and patient-centered environment demonstrates acceptance and opens the door to a more trusting patient-provider relationship. The National Academy of Medicine[2] and the Joint Commission[3] recommend SO/GI data collection as a way to learn about which populations are being served and to measure the quality of care provided to LGBTQ persons. Some patients may question the relevance of being asked about their sex listed at birth or their sexual orientation. The meaningful integration of sex and gender throughout each stage of the research process results in better quality evidence to inform health care for all,[4] and providers need this information to recommend appropriate preventive care.[3] For some, sexual orientation and gender identity may be fluid across time, so periodic reassessment is recommended.

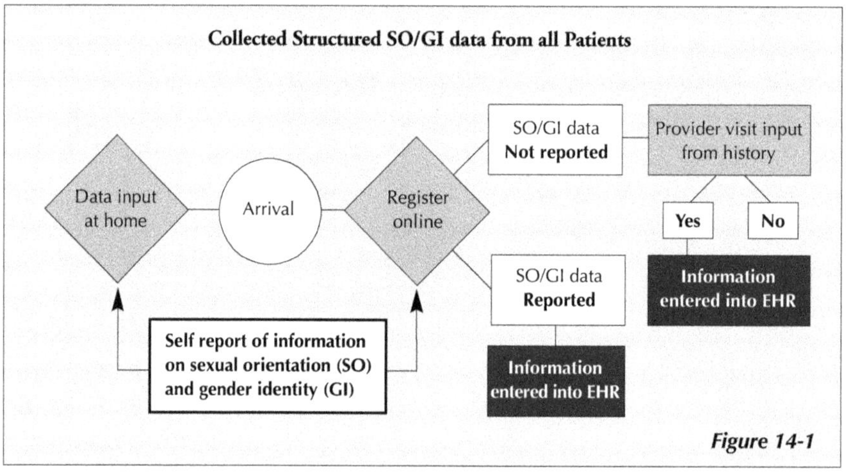

Figure 14-1. *Sample process for collecting sexual orientation and gender identity data from patients in the clinical setting. (Courtesy CDC, Atlanta, GA.)*

References

1. Centers for Disease Control and Prevention. Collecting sexual orientation and gender identity information. Centers for Disease Control and Prevention Web site. https://www.cdc.gov/hiv/clinicians/transforming-health/health-care-providers/collecting-sexual-orientation.html. Updated October 21, 2019. Accessed December 26, 2019.

2. National Academy of Medicine. *The Health of Lesbian, Gay, Bisexual, and Transgender (LGBT) People: Building a Foundation for Better Understanding.* Washington, DC: National Academies Press; 2011.

3. Deutsch MB, Buchholz D. Electronic health records and transgender patients—practical recommendations for the collection of gender identity data. *J Gen Intern Med.* 2015;30(6):843-847.

4. Day S, Mason R, Tannenbaum C, Rochon PA. Essential metrics for assessing sex & gender integration in health research proposals involving human participants. *PLoS One.* 2017;12(8):e0182812.

Anatomic Skills

Anatomic Skills 14-1

Refer to **Figure 14-2**. Using the letters that correspond to the structures in the photograph, label the anatomic locations.

A. ______________________________

B. ______________________________

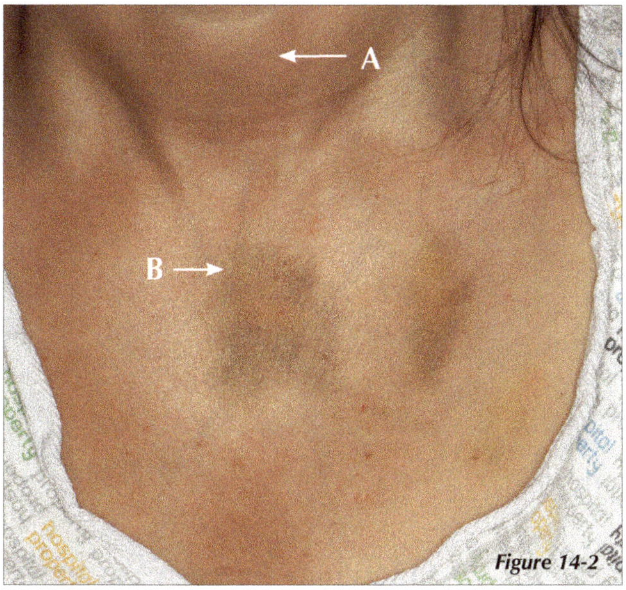

Figure 14-2

Anatomic Skills 14-2

Refer to **Figure 14-3**. Using the letters that correspond to the structures in the photograph, label the anatomic locations.

C. ______________________________

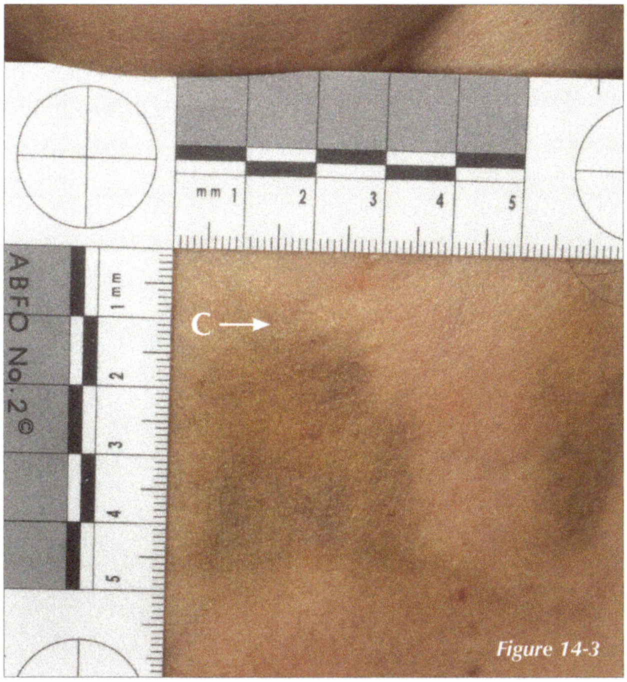

Figure 14-3

Activities

Activity 14-1. Injury Identification

Refer to **Figure 14-4-a** and **b**. Identify any injuries in respect to their anatomic location. Give objective descriptions when documenting findings.

D. ______________________________

E. ______________________________

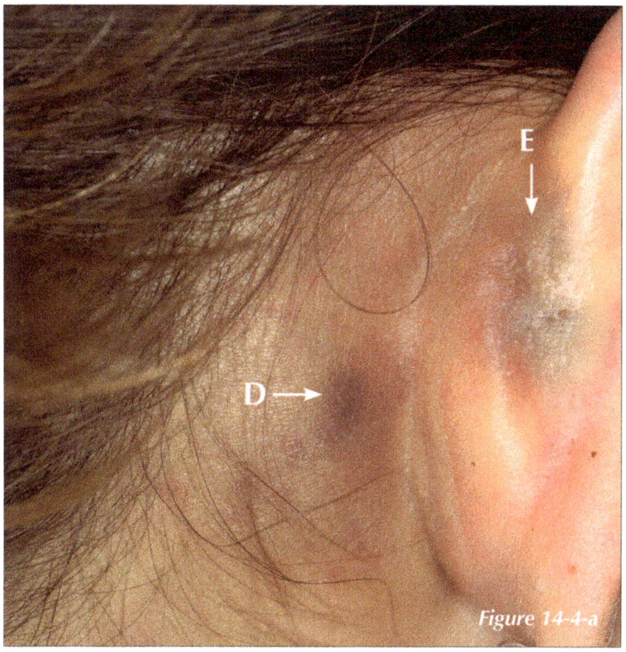

Figure 14-4-a

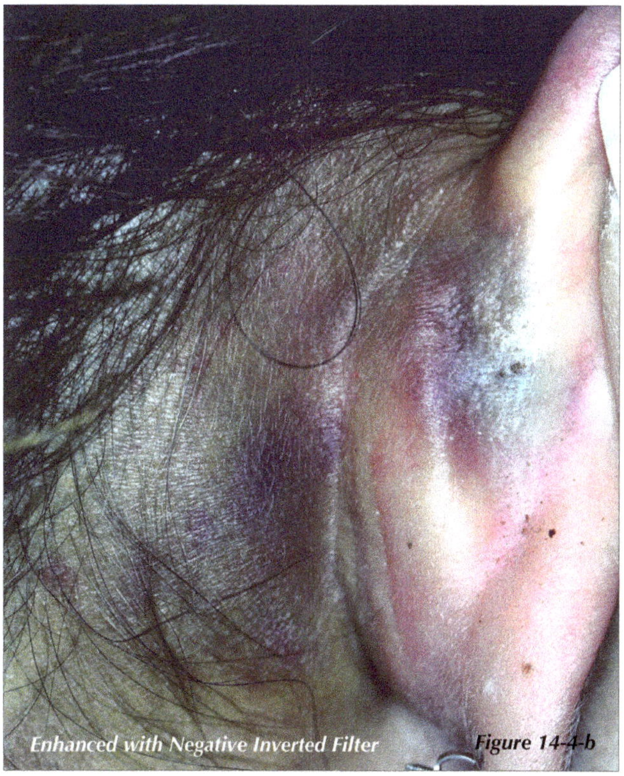

Figure 14-4-b

Activity 14-2. Injury Identification

Refer to **Figure 14-5-a** and **b**. Identify any injuries in respect to their anatomic location. Give objective descriptions when documenting findings.

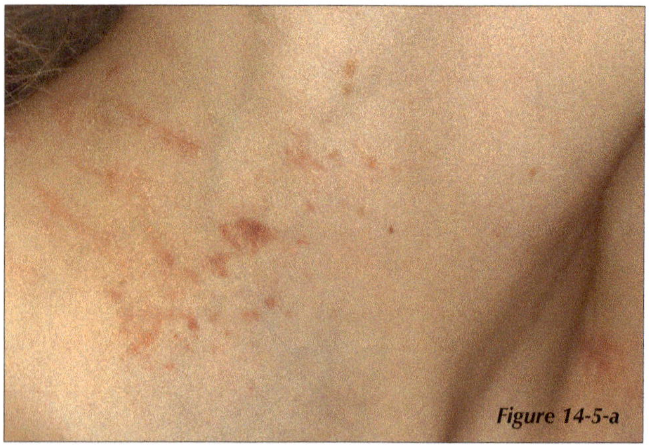

Figure 14-5-a

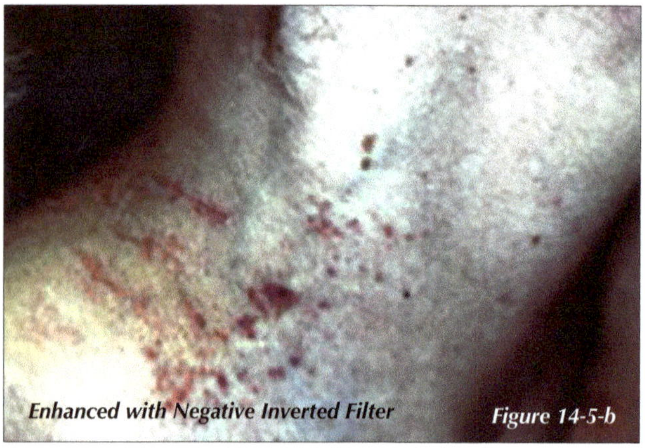

Figure 14-5-b

Activity 14-3. Assessment

List 3 additional questions that the forensic nurse in SANE care asks regarding the physical findings (eg, symptom Onset, Location/radiation, Duration, Character, Aggravating factors, Relieving factors, Timing, and Severity [OLDCARTS], demonstration of method of injury [if known], and level of consciousness).

Activity 14-4. Physical Assessment

Remember that injury is progressive throughout the healing phases. Because of the nature of neck and brain injury (eg, closed/open spaces with continued bleeding), there is potential for diminished function throughout the assessment. Therefore, assessment for potential serious sequelae is continuous in all patients, and when decline in function is recognized, an immediate referral to an advanced practice nurse, physician, or physician assistant is urgent and necessary. List 3 to 6 additional physical assessment procedures you should consider.

Activity 14-5. Evidence Collection

What evidence would you collect given the patient's history? What findings would promote evidence collection even if the history is deficient?

Activity 14-6. Treatment and Care

Based on the history and your findings, what treatment would you offer this patient? Would you report this case to the police?

Chapter 15

46-Year-old Female Patient Assaulted and Strangled by Her Husband

Case History

Clare is a 46-year-old woman who presents to the emergency department (ED) via emergency medical services. She reports that her husband attacked her and that she was struck in the face with multiple punches; kicked in the face, head and ear; could not breathe; and was strangled until she lost consciousness. She states her husband was on top of her and was pushing on her neck with his left hand (**Figure 15-1**). Clare complains of severe right facial pain, right cheek numbness, chest pain, and right wrist pain. During the examination, Clare admits to the forensic nurse that she was incontinent of stool. She reports previous domestic assaults stating, "This is my third black eye. That's why I couldn't go to my family's house on Easter." Clare also says she has been strangled before by her husband and was unable to breathe. Radiologic procedures in the ED include a computed tomography angiography (CTA) of the neck, computed tomography (CT) of the face, CT of the head, and x-rays of the chest and right wrist.

> ***Clinical Pearl:***
> *The majority of strangulation attacks do not leave any visible external injuries on the victim.*

Case Discussion

Clare not only sustained blunt force trauma to the face from blows and kicks, she also sustained a prolonged anoxic insult resulting in the loss of rectal tone and defecation. Defecation is associated with a minimum of 30 seconds of continual pressure to the arteries that provide oxygenated blood to the brain.[1] The right cheek numbness is from damage to the right infraorbital nerve associated with her right orbital blowout fracture. Her CTA was negative. Clare will need follow-up with ophthalmology and oral surgery.

Figure 15-1. *Reconstruction of how pressure was applied to Clare's neck.*

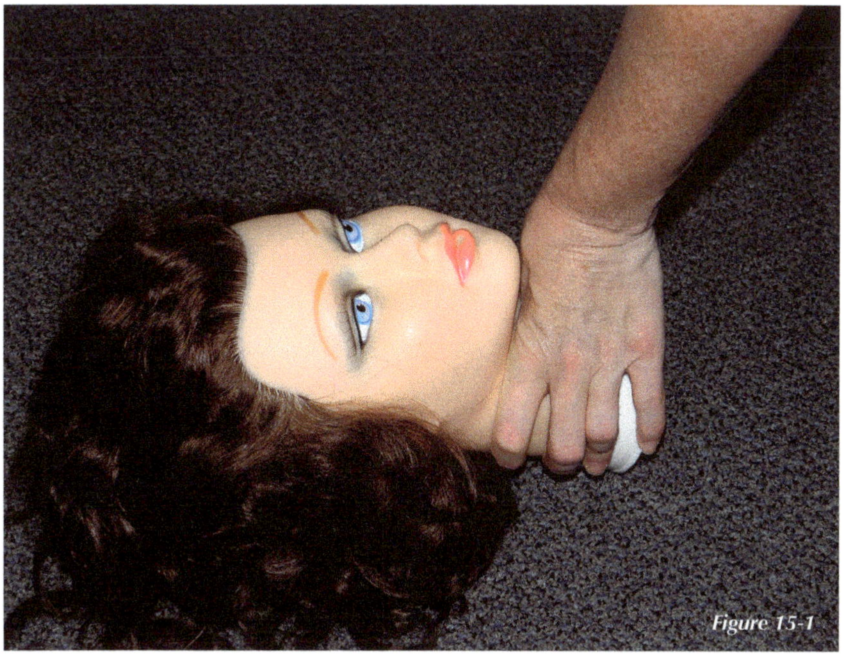

Discharge planning is important in this case, because a restraining order is needed. There is no one with Clare the ED, so it is important to discuss the support system she has and if any family is close by. She is discharged and will need someone to stay with her tonight. It is recommended that someone stay with her for 24 hours minimum. In this case, the police have arrested the husband, and he is in jail. Clare agrees to be contacted by the advocate who will talk with her the next day and assist her in obtaining the restraining order.

References

1. Kabat H, Anderson JP. Acute arrest of cerebral circulation in man. *Arch Neurol Psychiatr.* 1943;50(5):510-528.

Anatomic Skills 15-1

Refer to **Figure 15-2**. Using the letters that correspond to the structures in the photograph, label the anatomic locations.

A. ____________________

B. ____________________

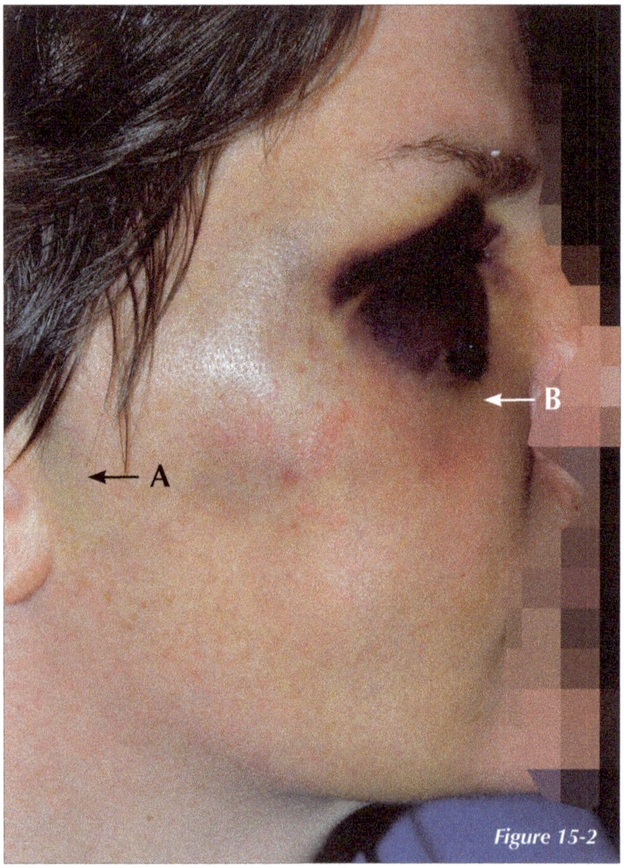

Figure 15-2

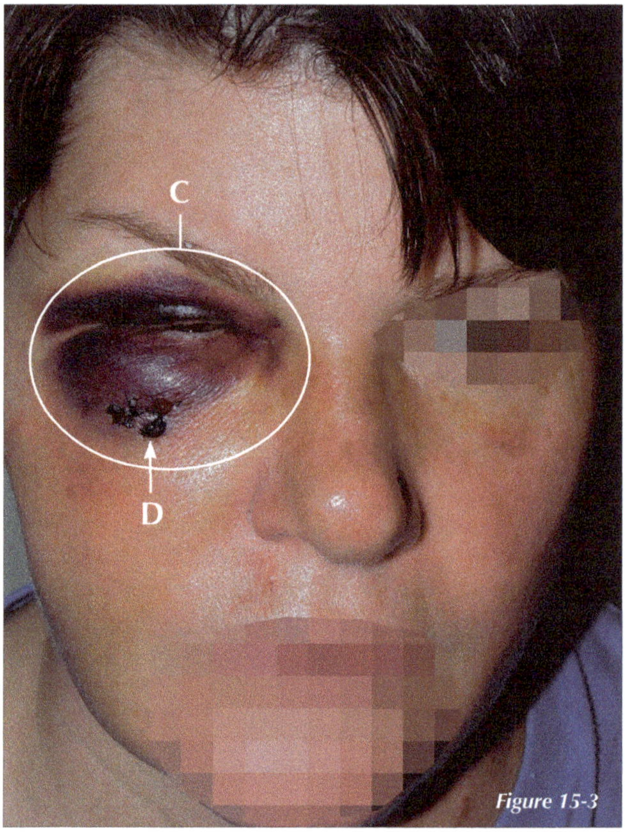

Figure 15-3

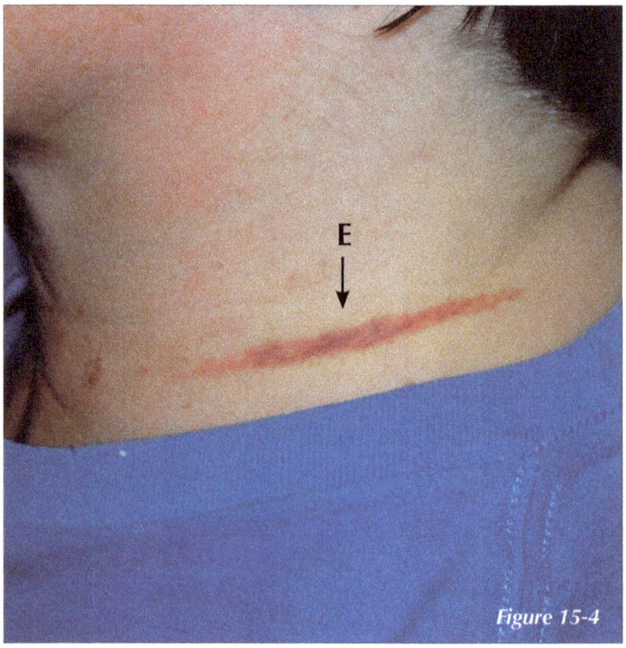

Figure 15-4

Activities

Activity 15-1. Injury Identification

Refer to **Figures 15-3** through **15-8**. Identify any injuries in respect to their anatomic location. Give objective descriptions when documenting findings.

C. ____________________

D. ____________________

E. ____________________

F. ____________________

G. ____________________

H. ____________________

I. ____________________

J. ____________________

K. ____________________

L. ____________________

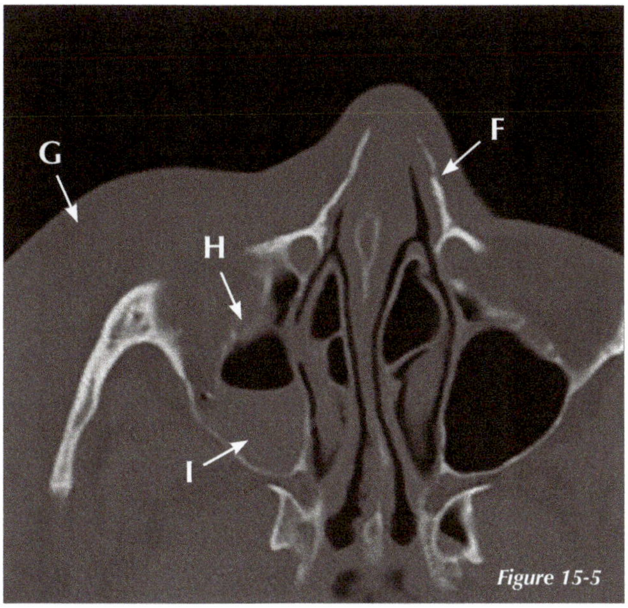

Figure 15-5

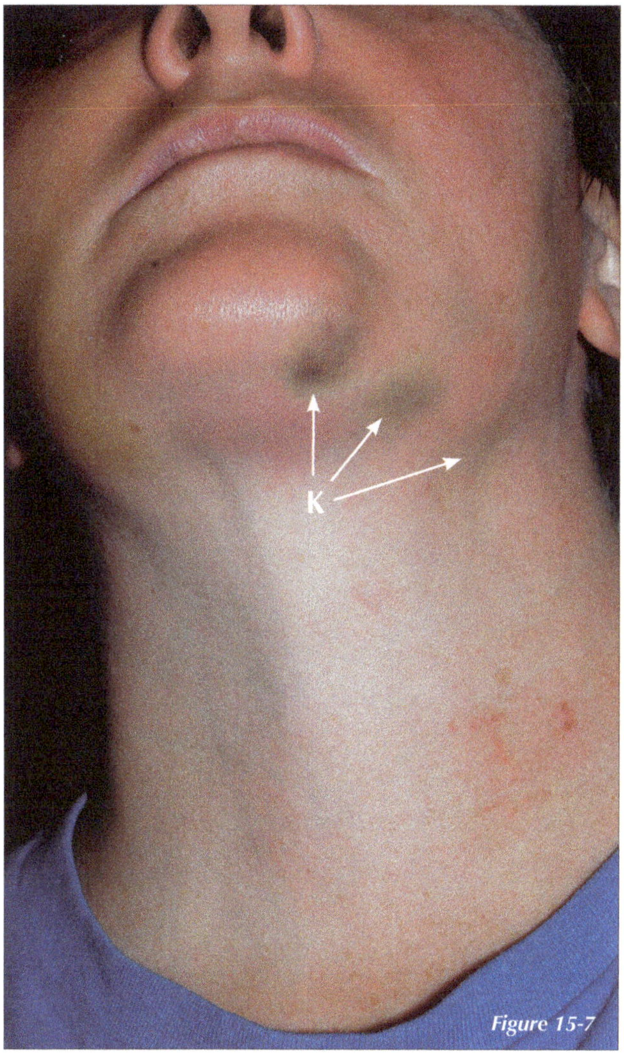

Figure 15-7

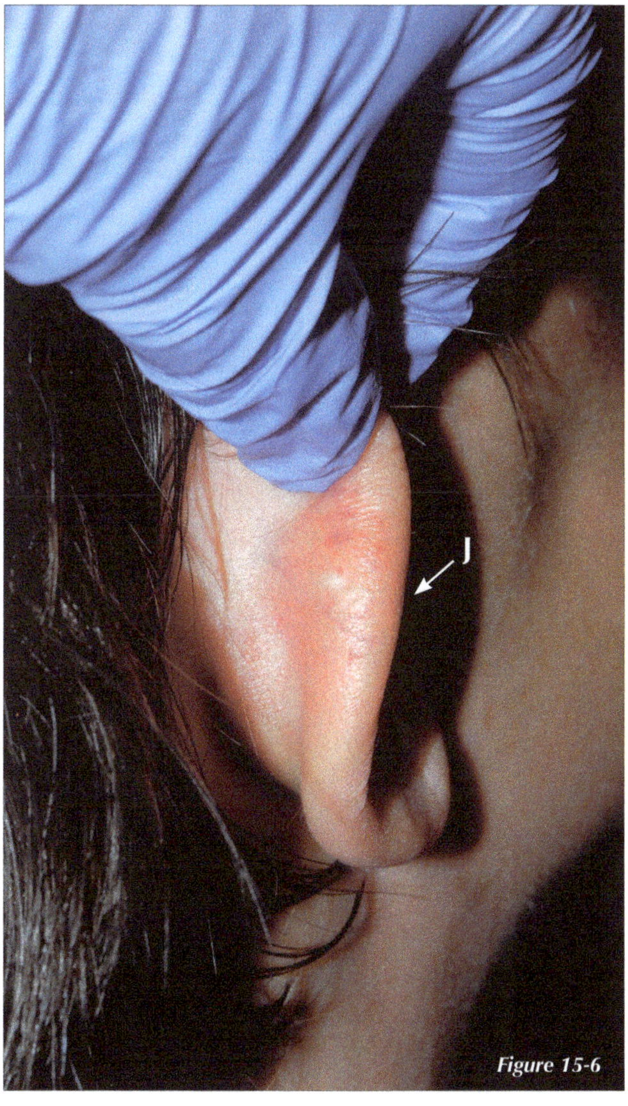

Figure 15-6

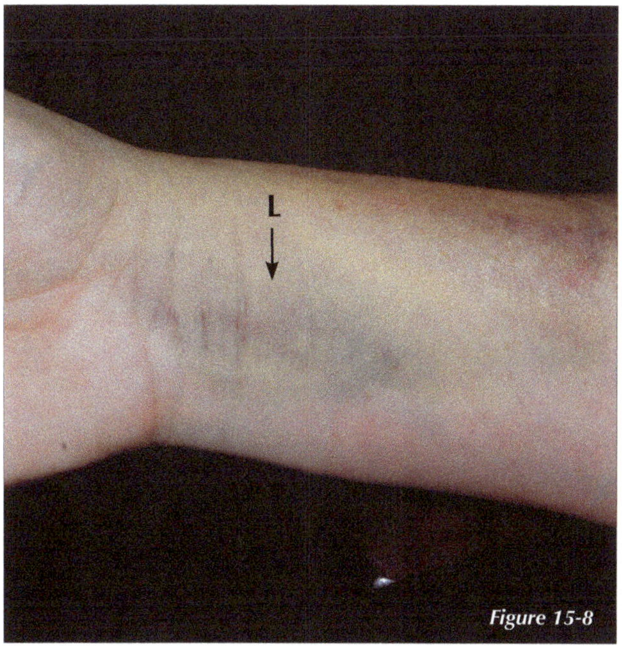

Figure 15-8

Activity 15-2. Assessment

List 3 additional questions that the forensic nurse asks regarding the physical findings.

Activity 15-3. Physical Assessment

Remember that injury is progressive throughout the healing phases. Because of the nature of neck and brain injury (eg, closed/open spaces with continued bleeding), there is potential for diminished function throughout the assessment. Therefore, assessment for potential serious sequelae is continuous in all patients, and when decline in function is recognized, an immediate referral to an advanced practice nurse, physician, or physician assistant is urgent and necessary. List 3 to 6 additional physical assessment procedures you should consider.

Activity 15-4. Evidence Collection

What evidence would you collect given the patient's history? What findings would promote evidence collection even if the history is deficient?

Activity 15-5. Treatment and Care

Based on the history and your findings, what treatment would you offer this patient? Would you report this case to the police?

Activity 15-6. Lethality Assessment

During care and as part of discharge planning, all patients who are suspected to be victims of domestic violence should be assessed for risk of immediate danger. List 4 indicators of escalating danger in a person who has experienced domestic violence. What questions should you ask a patient to assess his or her risk of immediate danger?

Section III

Appendix

Appendix 1. Nonfatal Strangulation Photography*

Introduction

Health care providers working in the field of clinical forensic medicine often examine individuals who are victims of domestic violence and nonfatal strangulation. The use of this protocol promotes the continuing development of the highly specialized skills necessary for an effective evaluation and documentation of presenting symptoms from a person who has experienced a domestic violence and/or a nonfatal strangulation assault. This protocol is beneficial in assisting first responders, nurses, physicians, nurse practitioners, physician assistants, emergency department (ED) health care providers, attorneys, and law enforcement in the assessment and documentation of domestic violence and nonfatal strangulation cases in their communities.

Recommended Equipment

— Protective portable camera case (meets or exceeds IP67 • MIL C-4150J • Def Stan 81-41/STANAG 4280).

— Digital SLR camera capable of capturing RAW and JPG files (with appropriate accessories, depending on the camera system used).

— Hand-held camera remote.

— Foot pedal-controlled camera remote.

— Low-profile, quick-release camera stand with ball-head function.

— Photomacrographic scales.

— A computer (64-bit with 6 GB RAM) with 1.0 TB or greater of accessible local storage space. The best place to store forensic data is on a local, secure computer network. Never store digital evidence in the Cloud.

— Computer software and storage capable of reading and managing vast amounts of digital data.

— Computer software capable of securing and encrypting vast amounts of digital images and video at AES 256-bit federal military-level encryption standards.

— High-speed connection to the Internet (not less than 10 Mbps download and 5 Mbps upload).

— Nested, end-to-end encrypted asynchronous file transfer technologies.

— Optional 24-inch or larger HDTV or screen with an HDMI connector.

Procedure

1. ***The bookend:*** The very first photo the medical forensic provider should capture is that of a bookend card (ie, a photograph of identifiable information of a subject to mark the beginning and end of a photodocumentation series), a patient's ID wristband, or a photo of a printed evidence label. Bookends are used to signify the beginning and end of a series of photographs representing 1 encounter with a patient. The bookend should include the following information: case number, patient name, date and time of the examination, and provider's name and title/license (**Appendix Figure 1**). (Note: A copy of the SDFI bookend card can be downloaded at no charge at http://www.sdfi.com/downloads/SDFI_1Up_Bookend_Card_Page_Scaling_None.pdf.)

Appendix Figure 1. *Bookend card.*

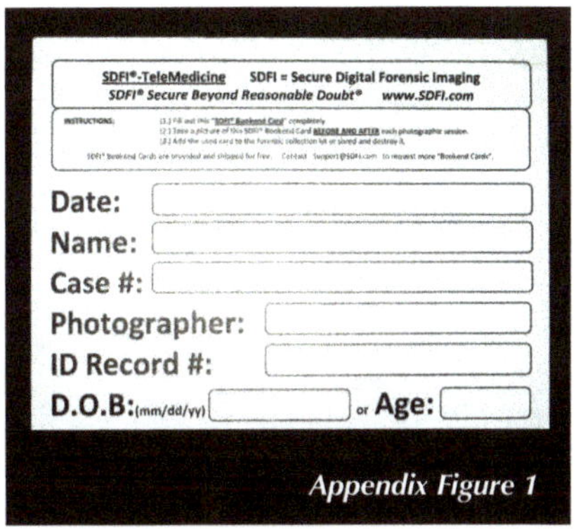

**Reprinted with permission from SDFI-Telemedicine LLC.*

2. ***General condition:*** Photograph the full body using an overlapping photographic storyboard (**Appendix Figure 2-a** through **t**). A storyboard is a stepped method for documenting all areas and angles on a person presenting for evaluation. The storyboard is a series of overlapping photos of a subject, displayed in sequence, to show that each image in the series is a part of the whole. This series of photos will identify the patient and is useful in determining the general condition and presentation of the patient at the time of examination. The purpose of establishing photographs is to present the investigator with a continuous, overlapping perspective of the entire body.

   All swabbing for trace or biological evidence from the face structures is completed after initial storyboard photography. After the first series of photographs identifying the general presentation condition of the patient, swab for trace and biological evidence around mouth, ears, and neck, as well as other fluorescent areas. After swabbing, if the patient is wearing makeup, have the patient remove it gently with a wipe in preparation for an additional storyboard of the head and neck without makeup.

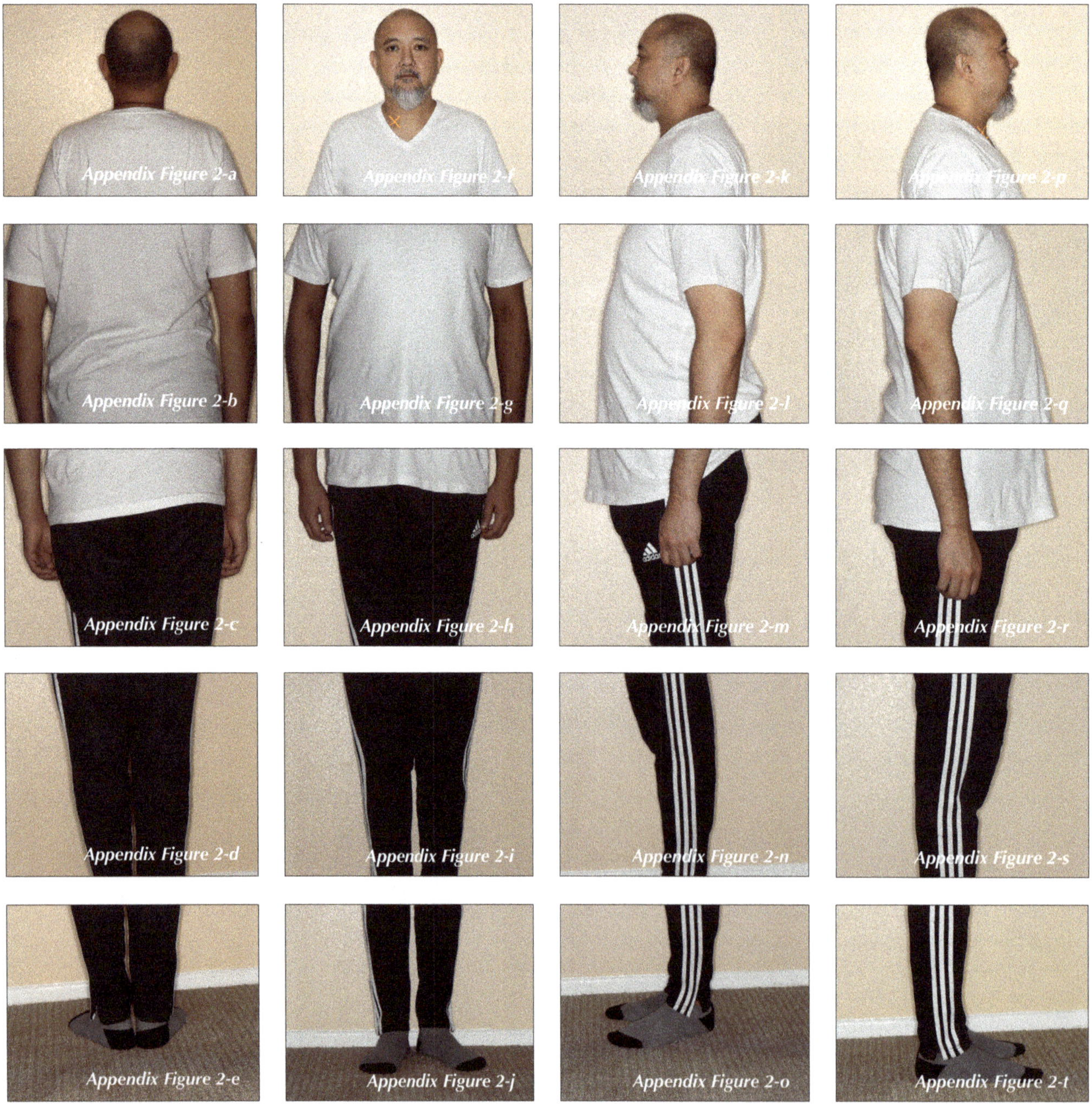

Appendix Figure 2-a through t. *Full-body photographs. (Note: Subject is a model commissioned for photographic demonstration. He is not a patient nor an assault victim.)*

3. Capture a series of mid-distance and close-up photos of all non-genital areas of interest from the head-to-toe assessment using the rule of thirds, fourths, and fifths. The rule uses photographs to identify landmarks, closer photos to identify areas of interest, and the closest photos with and without a reference (eg, ABFO ruler, coin, other standardized object). It is a guideline in composing a series of far-away, mid-distance, and close-up photographs.

   The mid-distant example picture **Appendix Figure 3-a** features the area of interest at the center of the image (shown as an orange X) and at the same time shows the front of the neck and both shoulders. This orientation photo will indicate where the area of interest is located on the body.

   Next, take a close-up photo of the area of interest on the person's body, first with a measuring device or an object of known size in the picture (**Appendix Figure 3-b**), then one without a measuring device (**Appendix Figure 3-c**). Stand directly in front of the area and take the picture at a 90-degree angle to the area of interest.

   After taking the close-up photos of a particular non-genital area of interest, capture an extreme close-up of that area (**Appendix Figure 3-d**). When taking extreme close-up pictures, make sure that the area of interest fills the viewfinder without cutting any part of it out of the frame. If it is too large, use the storyboard methods to capture overlapping sections to create the entire area. On rounded surfaces, stand directly in front of the area and take the picture at a 90-degree angle until all areas are photographed with 90-degree angles. Repeat taking a series of pictures of all areas of interest that are non-genital.

Appendix Figure 3-a. *Mid-distant orientation photo.*

Appendix Figure 3-b. *Close-up with measurement.*

Appendix Figure 3-c. *Close-up without measurement.*

Appendix Figure 3-d. *Extreme close-up.*

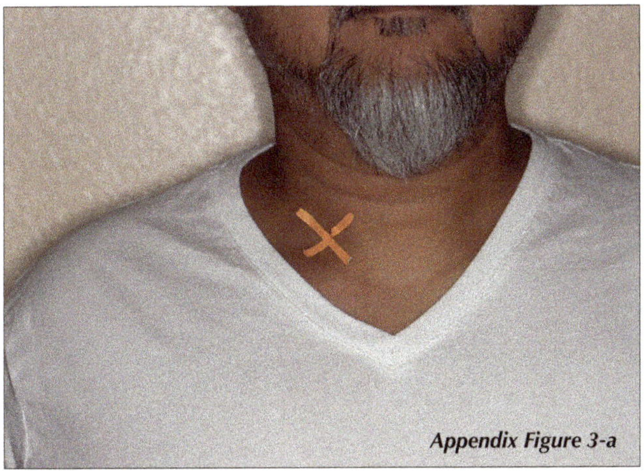

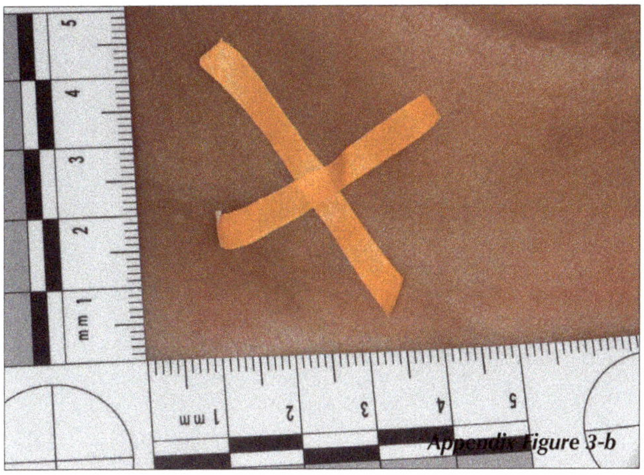

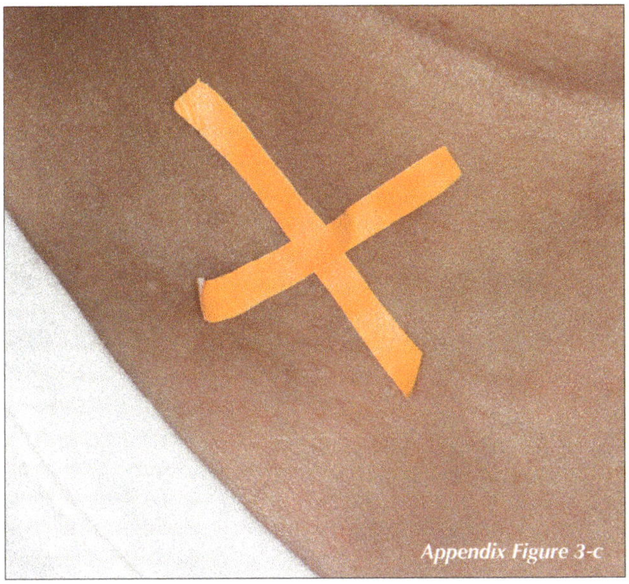

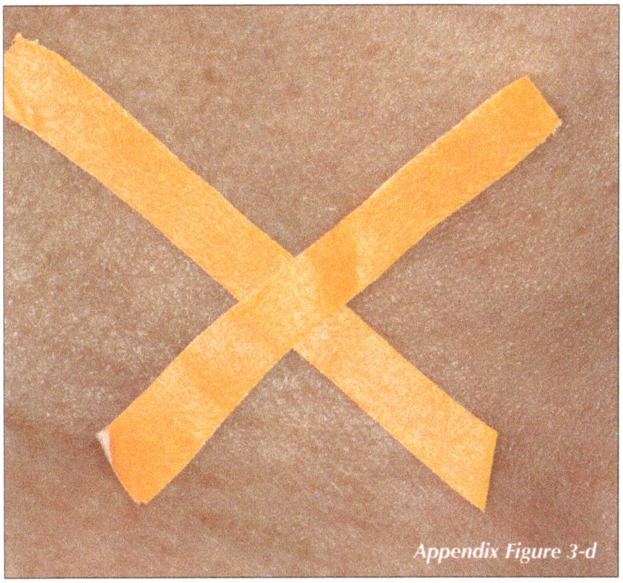

4. Capture a series of mid-distant photos of the front, back, left side, and right side of the face/head, upper chest/neck, upper back/nape, and shoulders. Capture another photo of the front of the neck with the head tilted back to expose the full neck and the area under the chin. This allows augmentation of the neck and head (**Appendix Figure 4-a** through **3-e**). Follow the storyboard and the rule of thirds, fourths, and fifths if there is an area of interest.

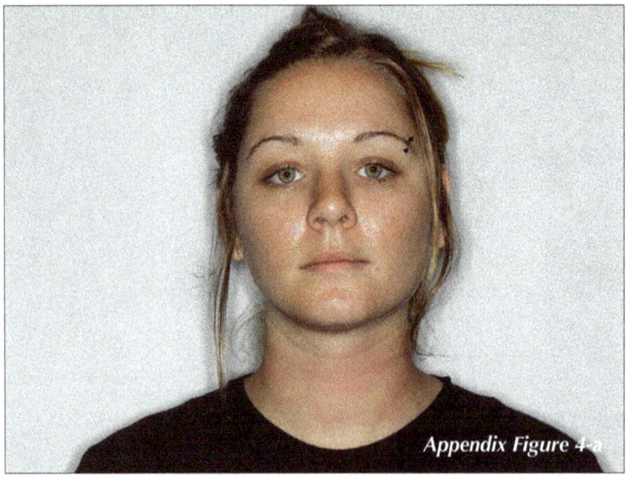
Appendix Figure 4-a

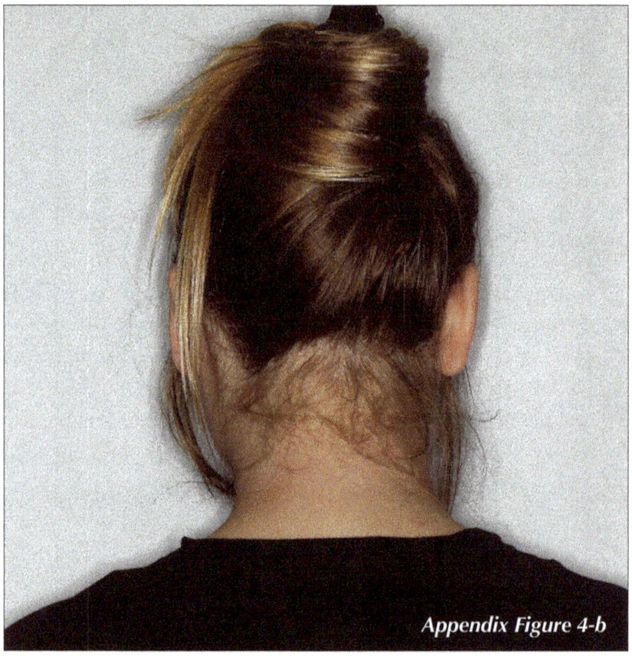
Appendix Figure 4-b

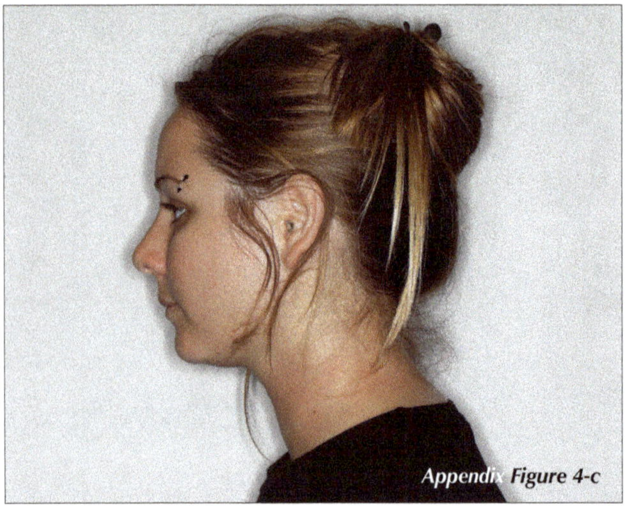
Appendix Figure 4-c

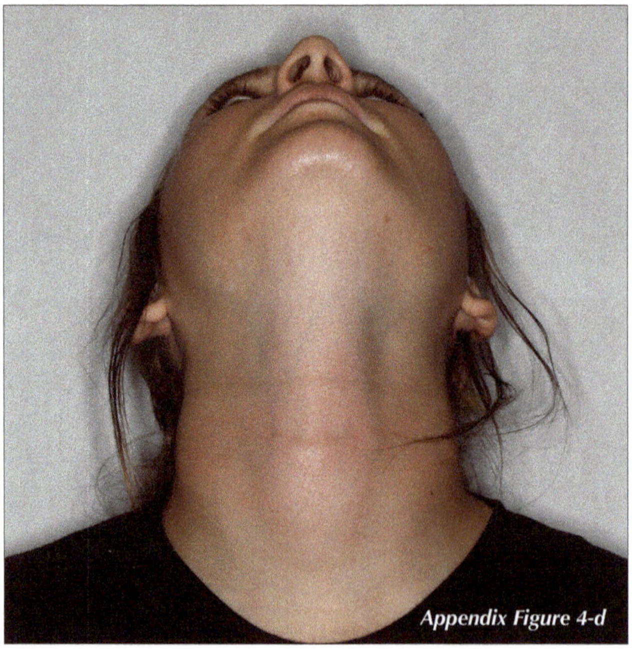
Appendix Figure 4-d

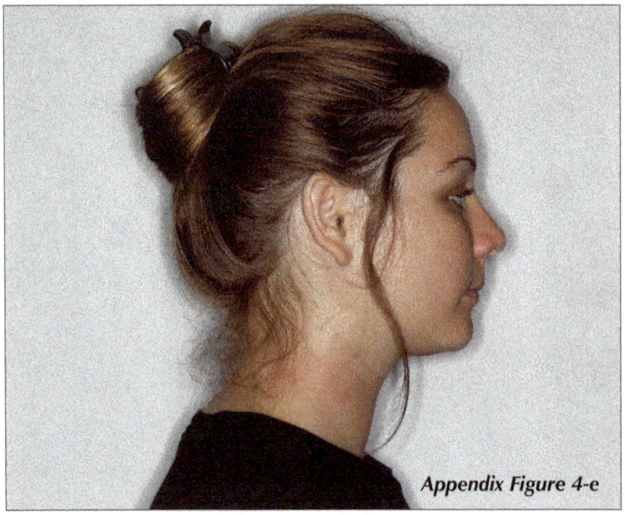
Appendix Figure 4-e

Appendix Figures 4-a through e. *A series of mid-distance photos. (Note: Subject is a model commissioned for photographic demonstration. She is not a patient nor an assault victim.)*

5. Using the final steps of the rule of thirds, fourths, and fifths, capture a series of close-up photos of any visible areas of interest on the front, left side, right side, and back of the neck. Take the photos with a scale first and then without. Conduct an assessment for other visible areas of interest that might be located on the earlobes, scalp, jawline, submandibular area, and chin (**Appendix Figure 5-a** through **j**).

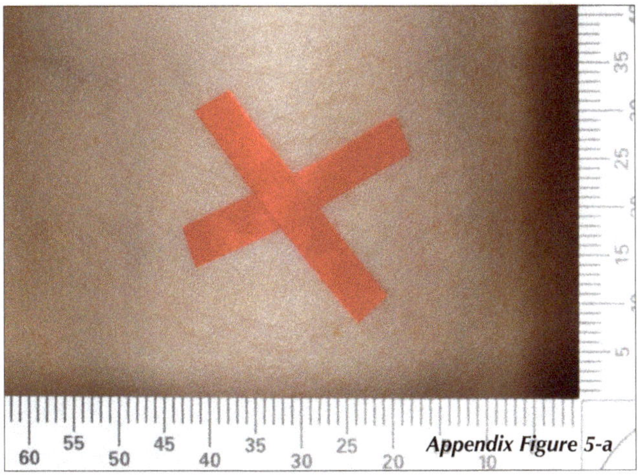

Appendix Figure 5-a

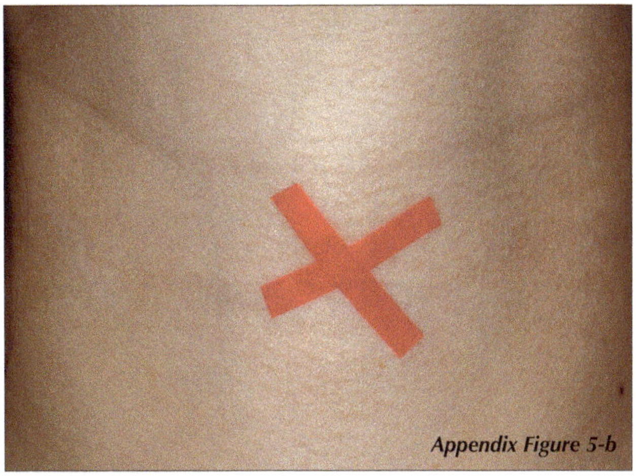

Appendix Figure 5-b

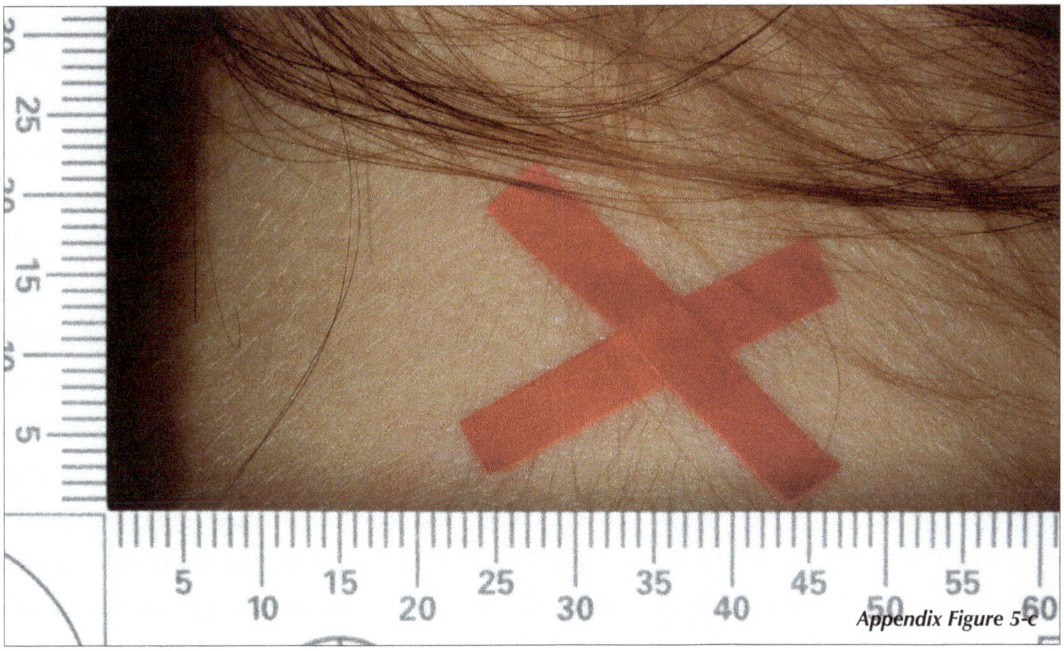

Appendix Figure 5-c

Appendix Figure 5-a and b. *Front of the neck, with and without scale.*

Appendix Figure 5-c and d. *Back of the neck, with and without scale.*

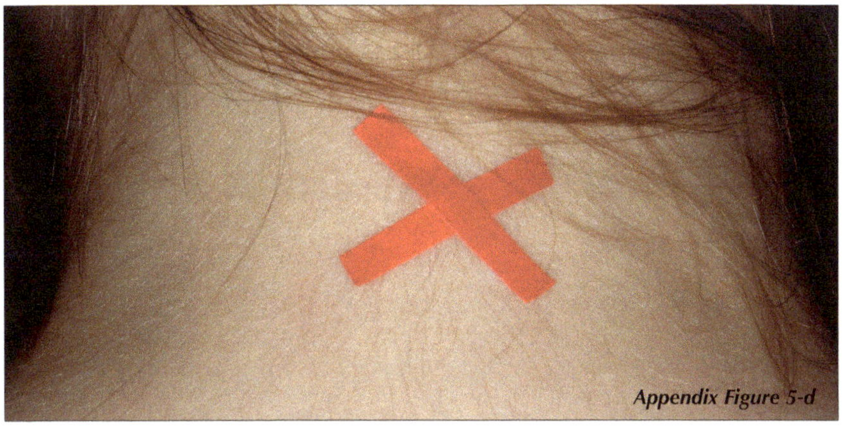

Appendix Figure 5-d

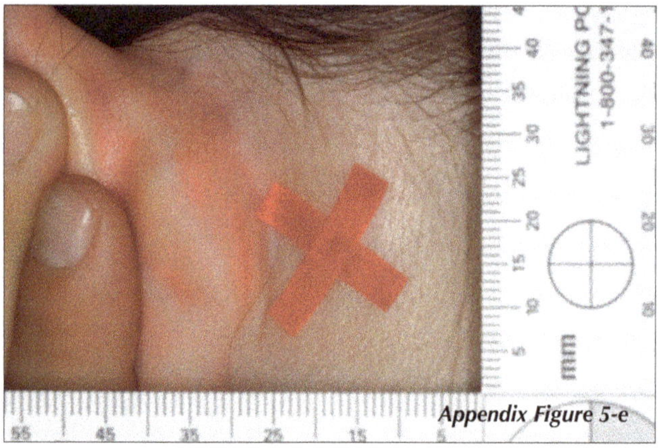

Appendix Figure 5-e

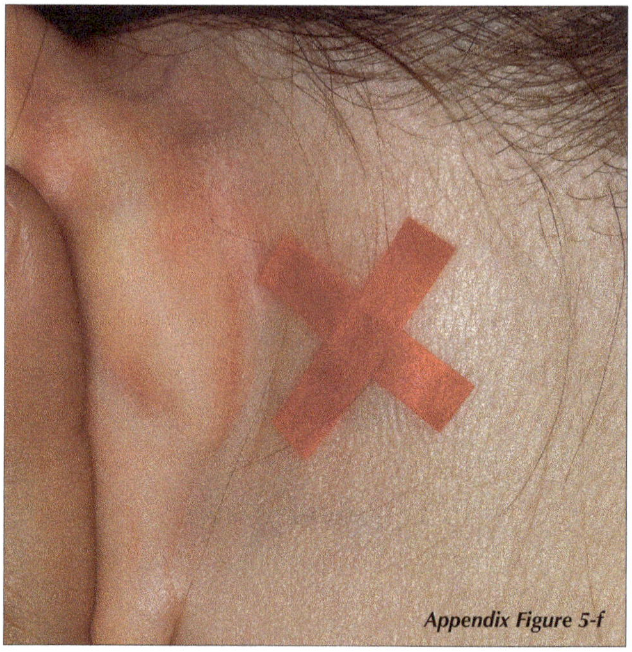

Appendix Figure 5-f

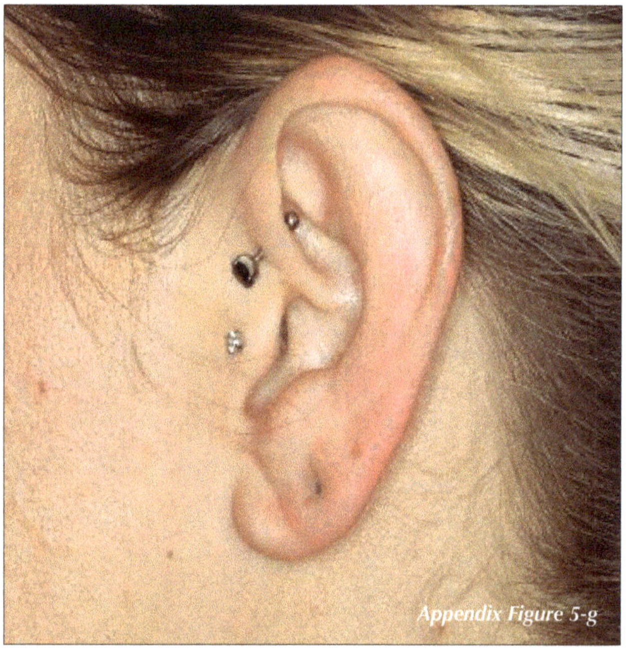

Appendix Figure 5-g

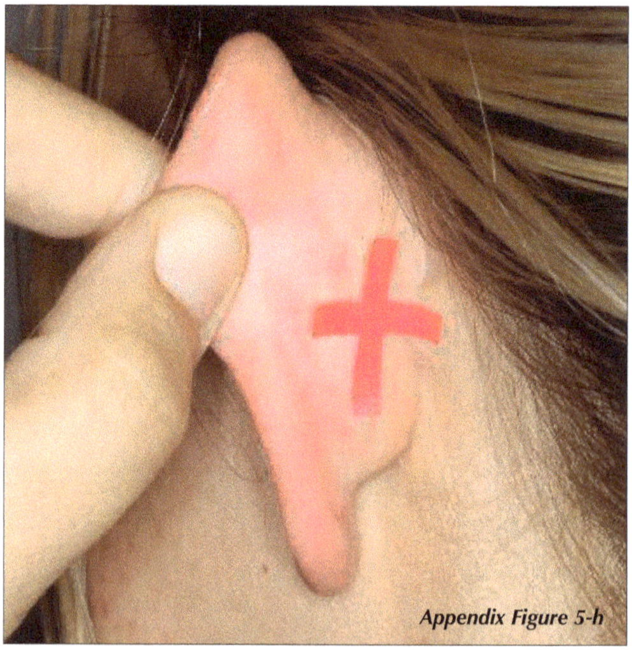

Appendix Figure 5-h

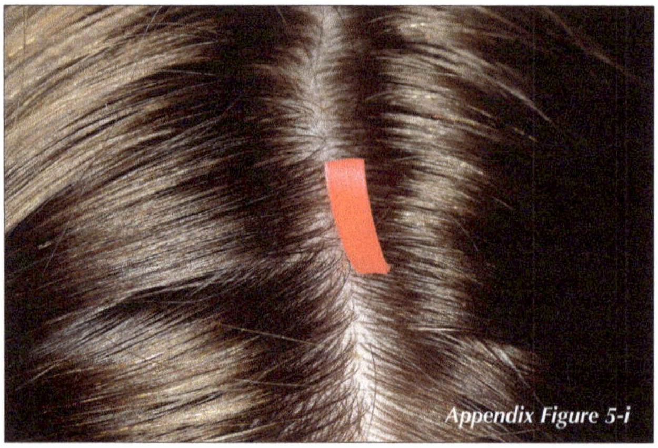

Appendix Figure 5-i

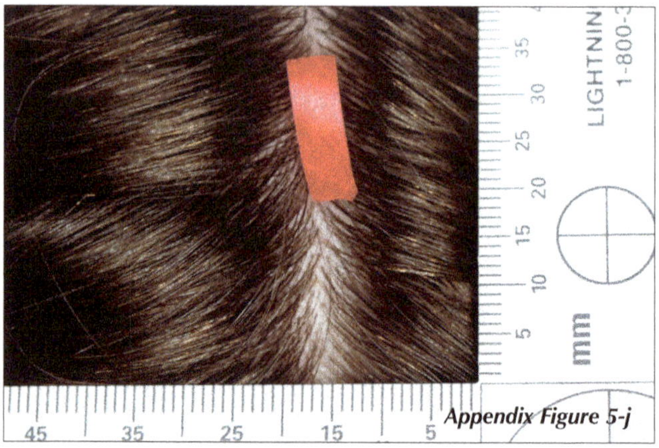

Appendix Figure 5-j

Appendix Figure 5-e and f. Behind the ears, with and without scale.

Appendix Figure 5-g and h. Inner and outer earlobes.

Appendix Figure 5-i and j. Scalp, with and without scale.

6. Capture a series of close-up photos of the eyes in all 9 gaze positions as shown below. The examiner looks for petechial hemorrhages or subconjunctival hemorrhages (**Appendix Figure 6-a** through **i**) and neurologic abnormalities of cranial nerves III, IV, and VI. Ocular abnormalities require referral for medical evaluation. There are no hemorrhages noted in these photographs.

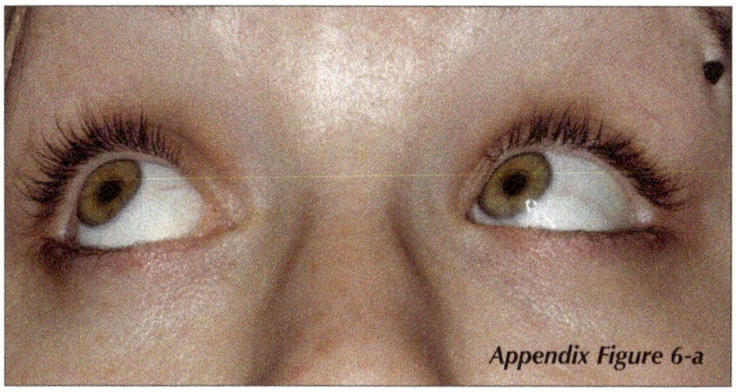

Appendix Figure 6-a

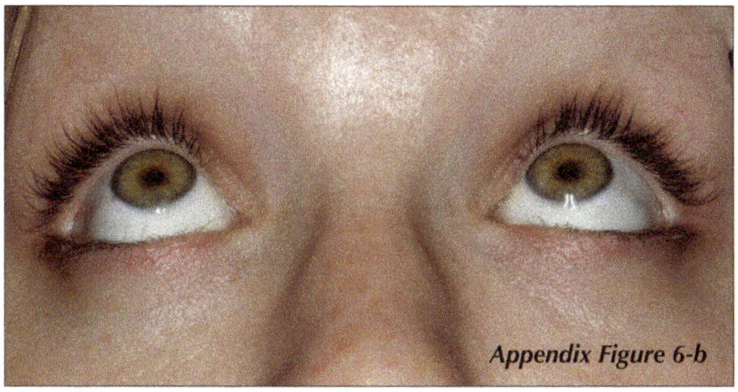

Appendix Figure 6-b

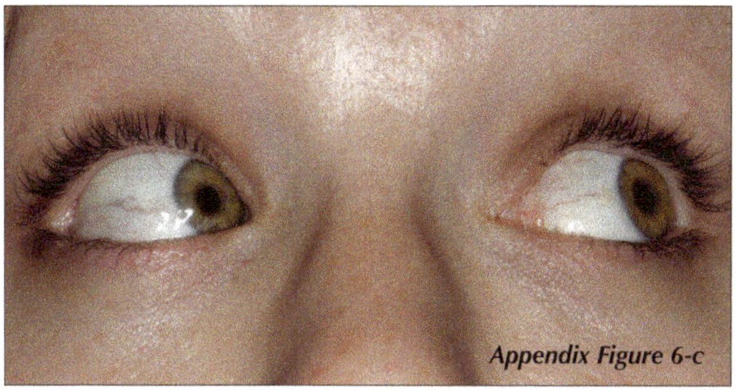

Appendix Figure 6-c

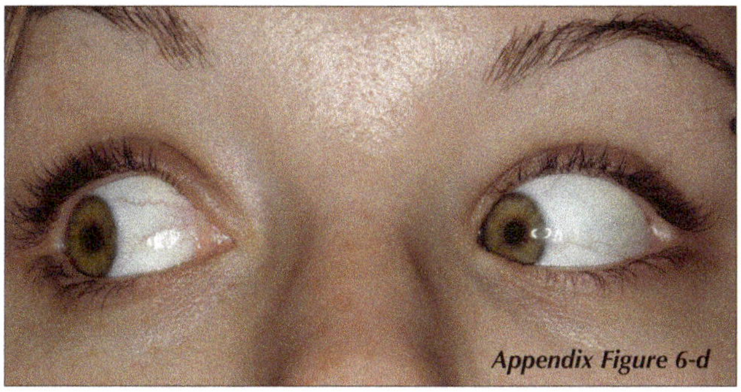

Appendix Figure 6-d

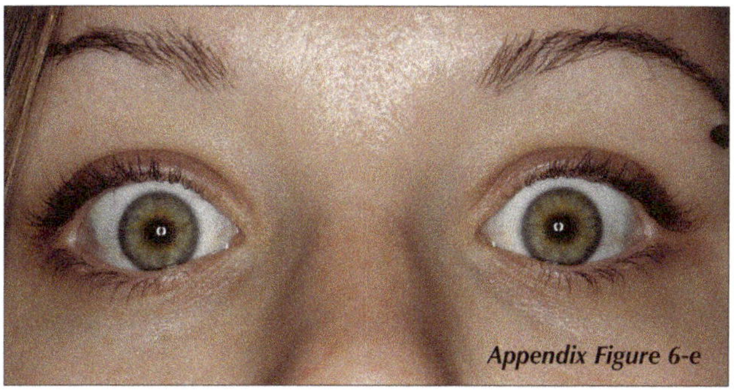

Appendix Figure 6-e

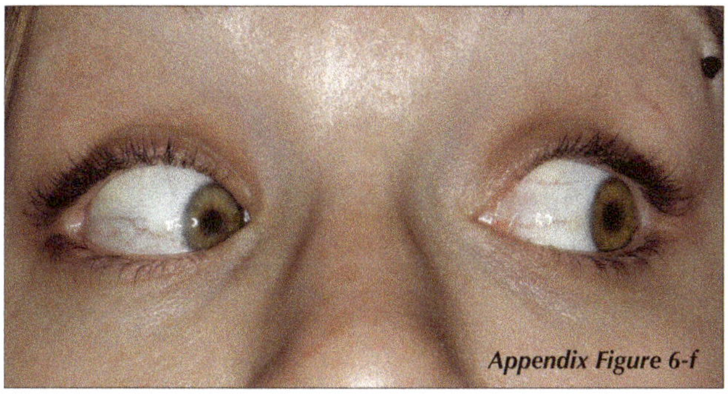

Appendix Figure 6-f

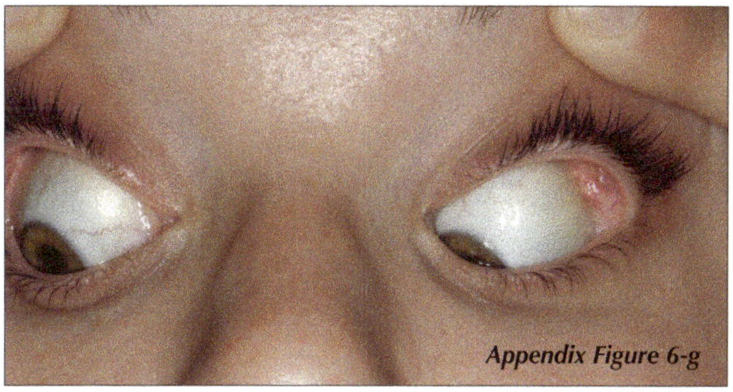

Appendix Figure 6-g

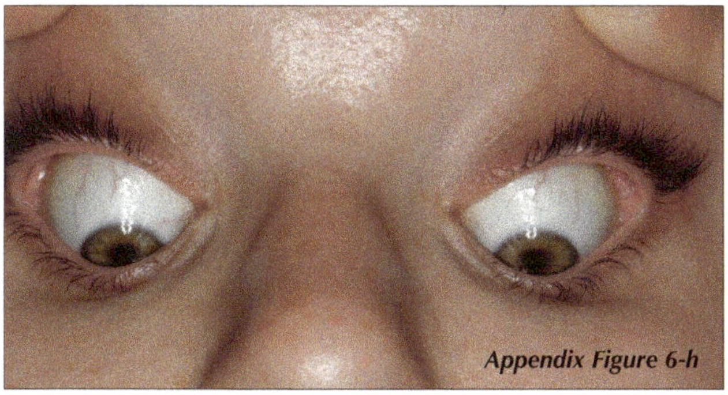

Appendix Figure 6-h

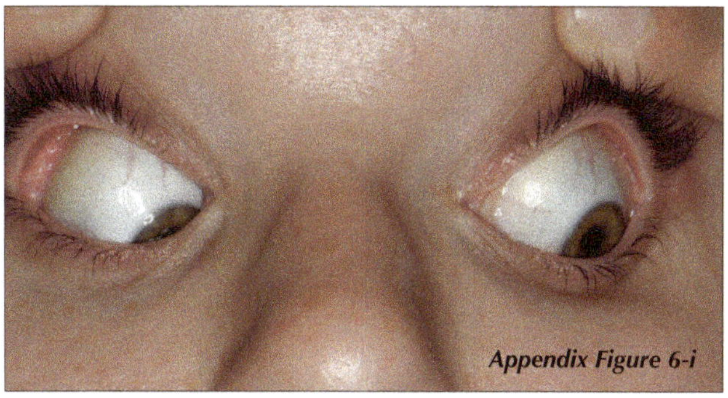

Appendix Figure 6-i

Appendix Figure 6-a through i. *Eye positions.*

7. Capture a series of close-up photos of each eye using the eye inversion technique. Apply pressure medially and laterally on the lower lids to expose the entire surface. This step exposes the back of the upper and lower eyelids where the examiner looks for petechiae, hemorrhaging, and other trauma.

   To achieve this on the upper lid, grasp the lid using the fingers of a gloved hand by the middle eyelashes, pull it downward and forward, and then pull it back over a cotton applicator placed at the upper margin of the tarsus while the patient looks downward.

   For the lower lid, place the cotton applicator on the lower margin of the tarsus and depress laterally while the patient looks upward. Capture a series of close-up photos of each eye using the inversion technique. Apply pressure medially and laterally on the lower lids to expose the entire surface. Use the same gaze positions as used in step 6 (**Appendix Figure 7-a** through **d**).

> ***Clinical Pearl:***
> *Expect drying of the ocular surface, which increases size of capillaries and is demonstrated in* ***Appendix Figure 7-a*** *through* ***d****. Drying may cause excessive tearing.*

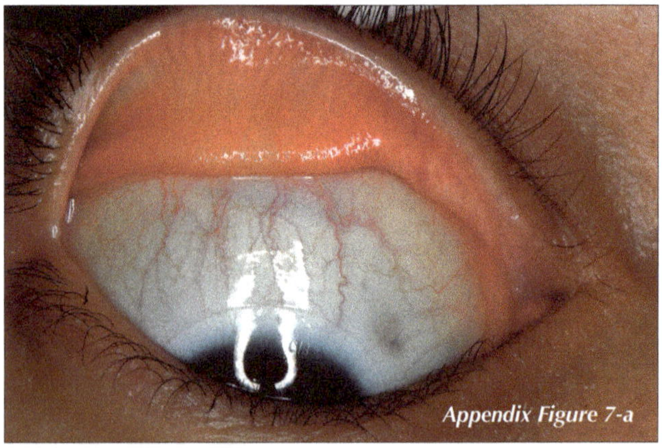

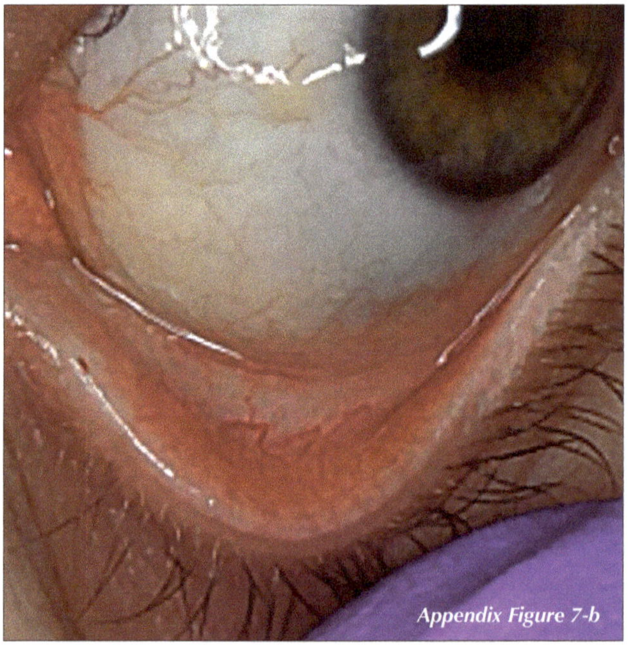

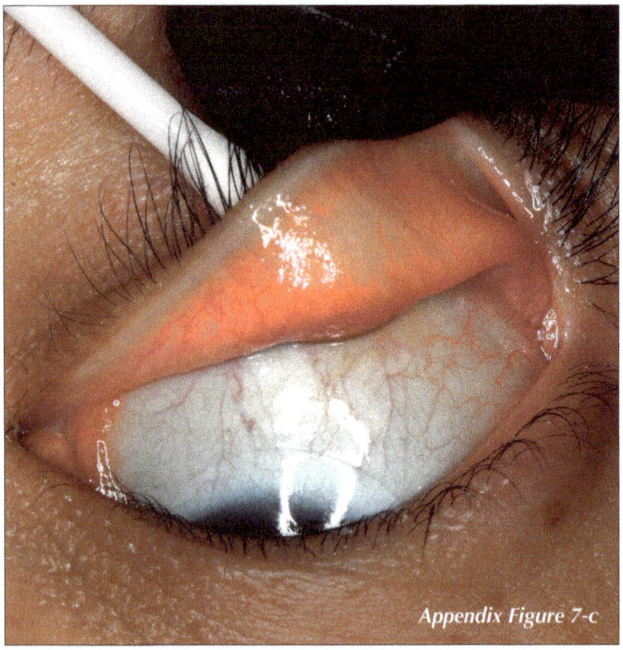

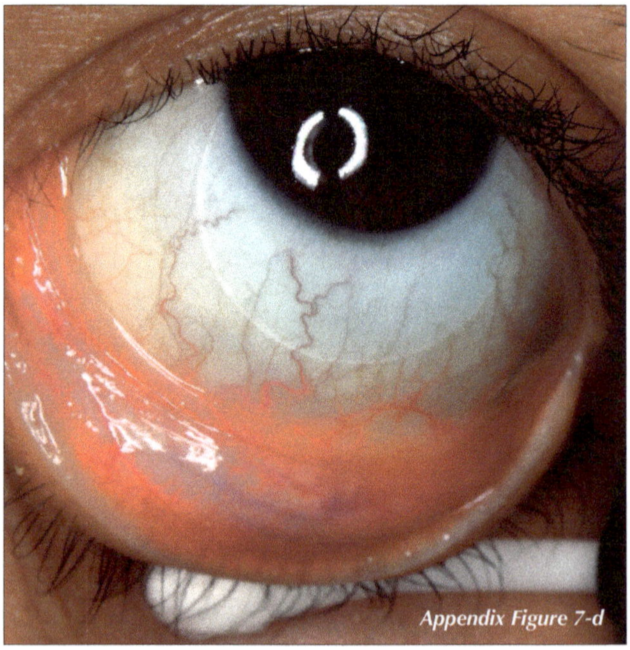

Appendix Figure 7-a and b. Right upper and lower eyelids.

Appendix Figure 7-c and d. Left upper and lower eyelids.

8. Capture a close-up photo of the upper and lower lips. If you see or suspect bruising, hemorrhaging, or detect any other area of interest, capture photos with a measurement scale first and then without a scale (**Appendix Figure 8-a** and **b**).

9. Capture a series of close-up photos of the oral cavity. The examiner assesses the soft palate, hard palate, uvula, and oropharynx (**Appendix Figure 9-a**).

   Next, capture a series of pictures of the frenula of the upper and lower lips (**Appendix Figure 9-b** and **c**). If you see or suspect bruising, hemorrhaging, or see any other areas of interest, capture additional close-up photos of the finding.

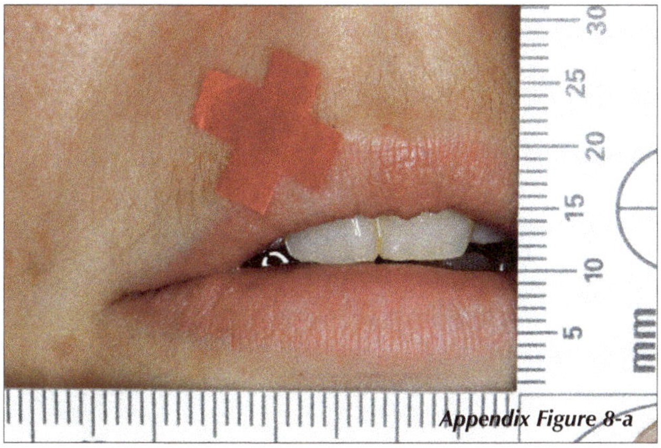

Appendix Figure 8-a

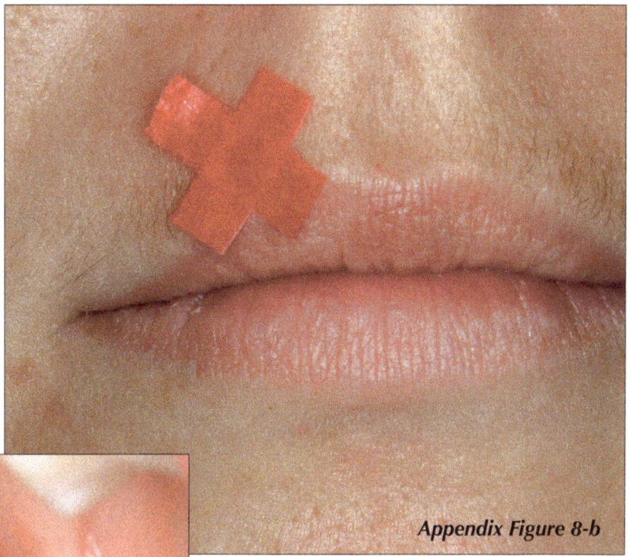

Appendix Figure 8-b

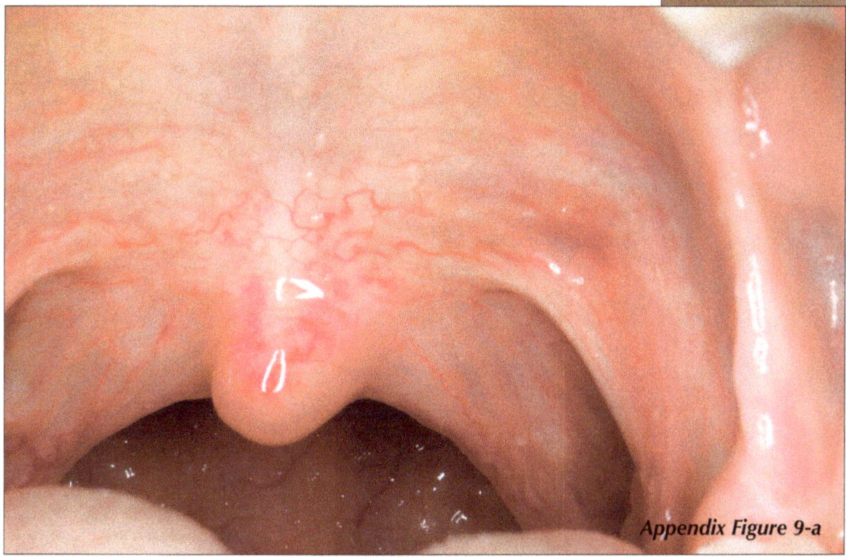

Appendix Figure 9-a

Appendix Figure 8-a and b. *Lips with and without a measurement scale.*

Appendix Figure 9-a. *Oral cavity.*

Appendix Figure 9-b and c. *Frenula of the upper and lower lips.*

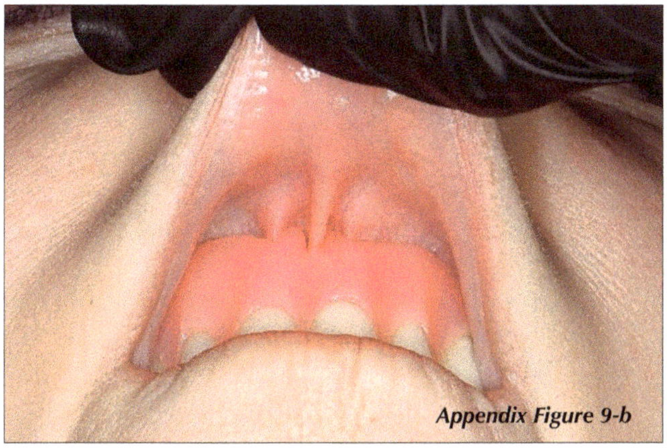

Appendix Figure 9-b

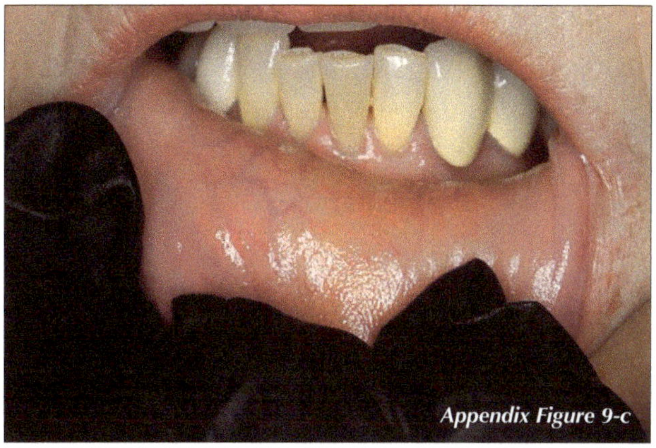

Appendix Figure 9-c

10. Capture a series of close-up photos of both hands showing the dorsal and palmar sides separately using the SDFI Hand Map. If you see or suspect bruising or see any other area of interest, capture additional photos with a measurement scale first, then without a scale (**Appendix Figure 10-a** and **b**).

11. Capture close-up photos of the fingertips and fingernails from both hands. If you see or suspect bruising or detect any area of interest, capture additional photos with a measurement scale first then without a scale (**Appendix Figure 11-a** and **b**).

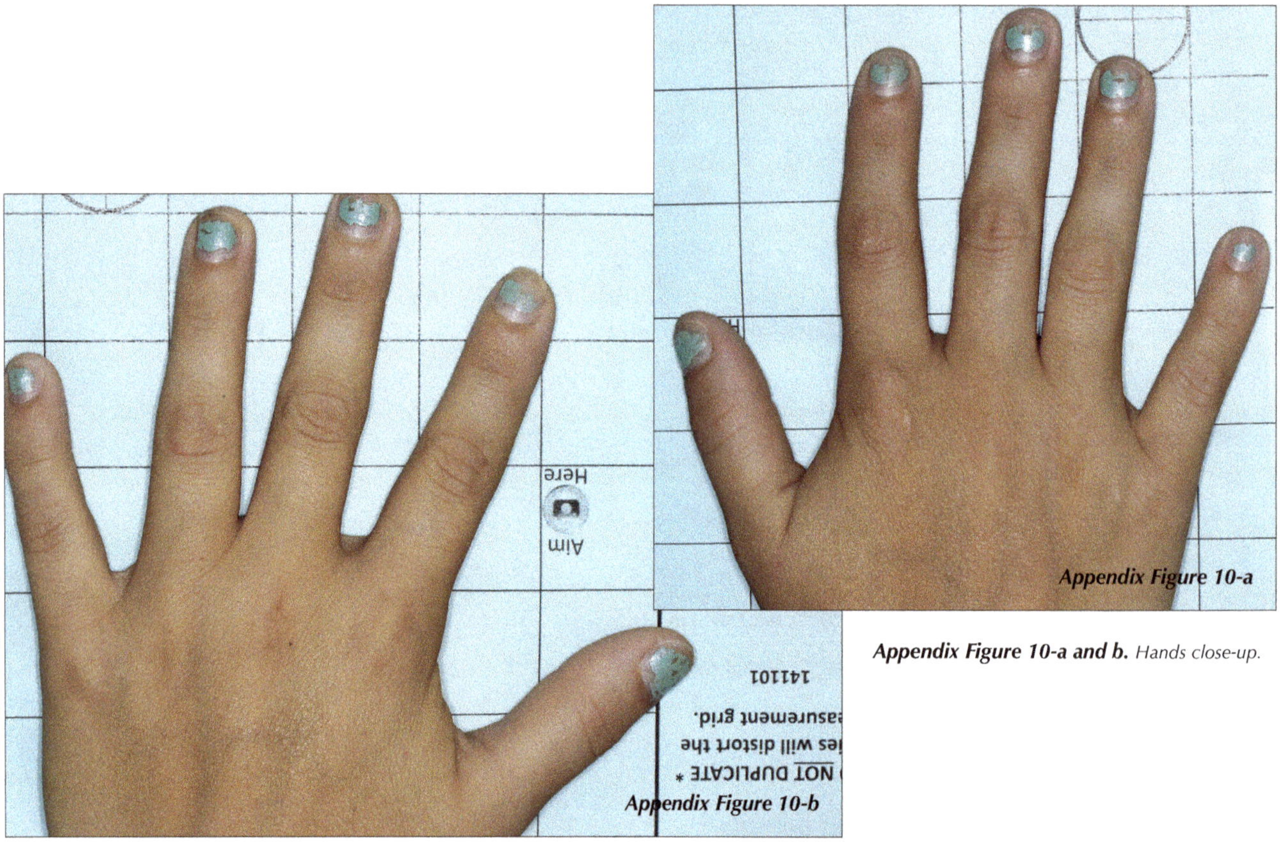

Appendix Figure 10-a and b. *Hands close-up.*

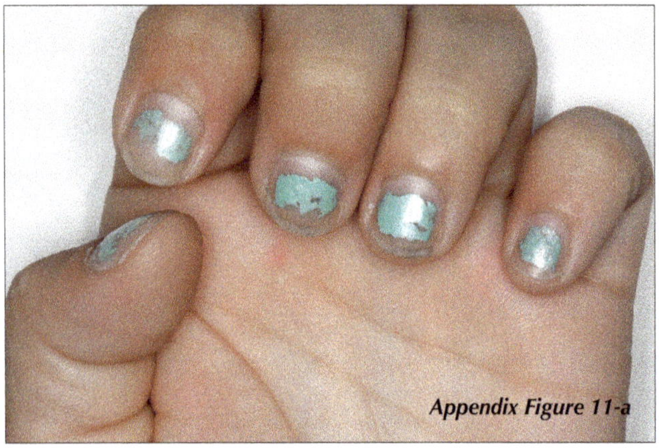

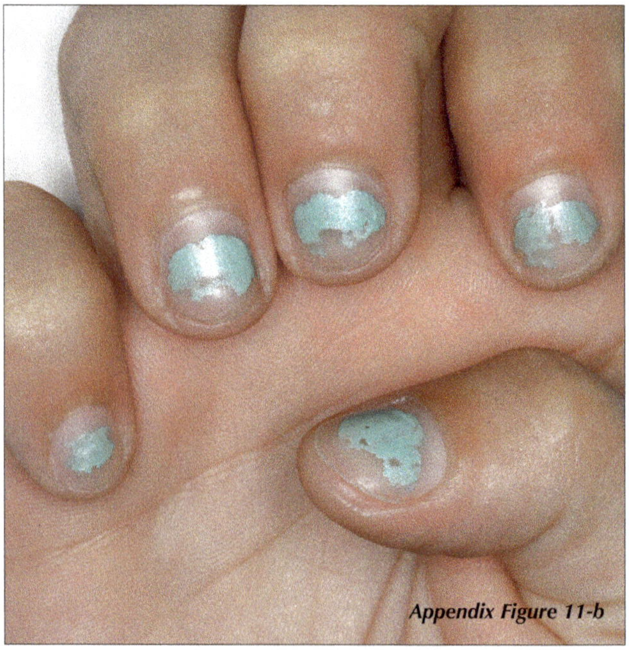

Appendix Figure 11-a and b. *Nails close-up.*

12. Use of a mannequin can be effective in understanding the dynamics of a nonfatal strangulation assault and how the patient and perpetrator were physically placed in relation to the event. This tool can also show the physical positions of the patient and the perpetrator at the time of the assault. In **Appendix Figure 12-a** through **c**, the patient is photographed demonstrating the way the perpetrator carried out the strangulation using the model Styrofoam head. This is a recreation of a traumatic event and is treated seriously; therefore, do not use a toy or stuffed animal. Do not apply pressure to the neck, as this may cause additional physical trauma or trigger the patient and result in psychological reactions. Before bringing the mannequin head out, be sure to inform the patient about demonstrating what happened during the assault. Be prepared for a wide range of reactions, from disbelief to violence, because the patient may react very strongly. Always use trauma-informed and patient-centered care principles, and let the patient accept or decline the recreation portion of the examination.

Appendix Figure 12-a through 12-c.
Mannequin demonstrations.

If a mannequin or Styrofoam head is available, take a middistance photo of the patient demonstrating the placement of the accused's hands. The recreation is a fluid exchange, necessitating the nursing process of continual assessments and interventions because the recreation may trigger the patient or increase understanding of the lethality of the act. The trigger could result in a personal crisis, necessitating the implementation of evidence-based interventions supporting the patient's choices in a trauma-informed environment. This includes explaining to the patient what they are experiencing, that it is a normal response to the stimulus, and they may choose differently at any point in the demonstration if it is uncomfortable, from waiting until feelings pass to stopping the demonstration altogether.

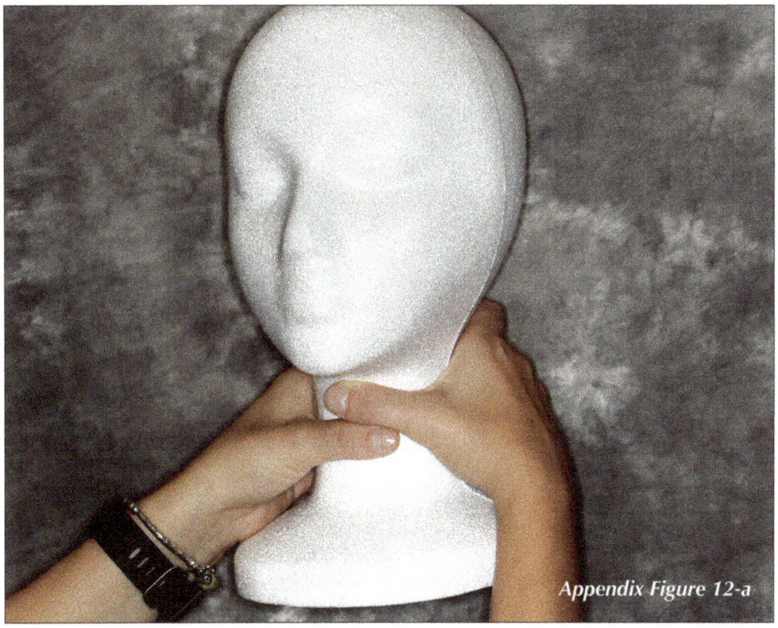

Appendix Figure 12-a

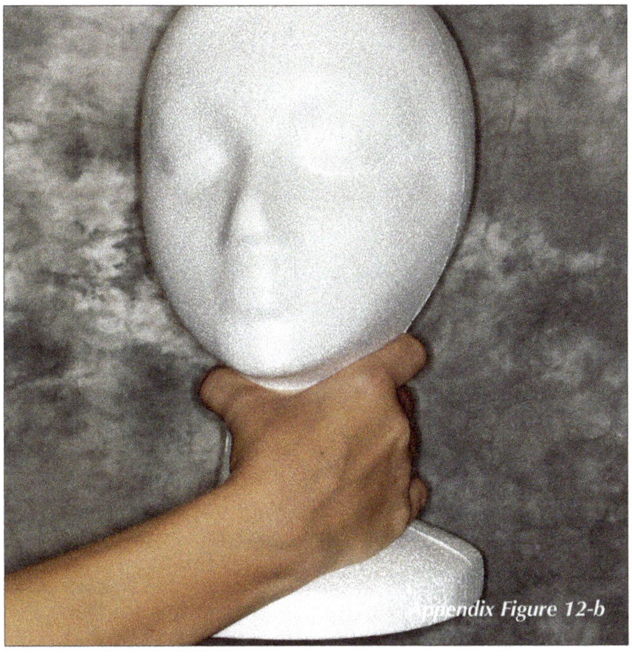

Appendix Figure 12-b

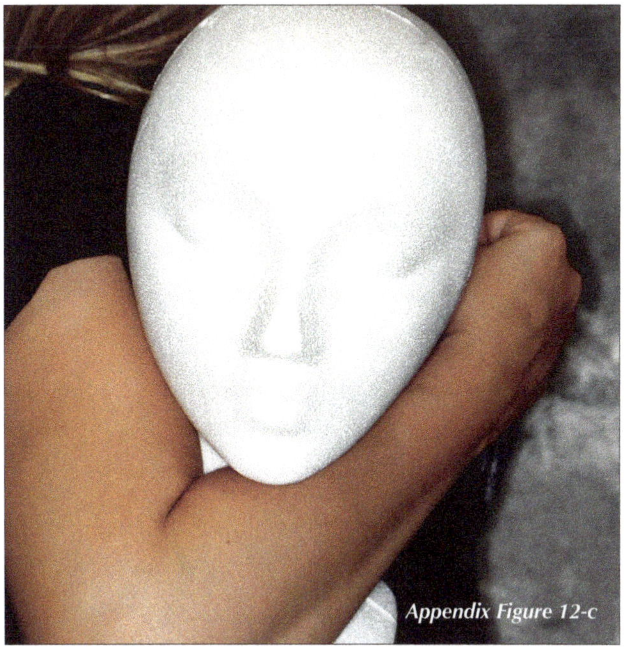

Appendix Figure 12-c

13. In the event the person being cared for is unable or unwilling to demonstrate the strangulation using a mannequin or model, the examiner may ask permission to use the Nonfatal Manual Strangulation Chart (**Appendix Figure 13-a**). The chart shows 8 different depictions of manual strangulation, also known as ***The 8 Pack.*** As a trauma-informed approach to a triggered reaction to the mannequins, the examiner can offer the patient an alternate approach to telling their experience. The chart allows patients to pick representations of their nonfatal strangulation experience among the numbered pictures, identifying which position is similar to what happened to them. A photograph can be taken with the patient's finger pointing to the picture or pictures that depict what happened (**Appendix Figure 13-b**). Another option is to have the patient circle and initial the correct hand position or positions.

14. The bookend card is a photo of a printed label and is the last picture the examiner will take for the examination. Again, it will include the case number, patient's name (eg, the patient's ID wristband), date, and the name and role of the examiner. This will mark the conclusion of the photodocumentation portion of the examination.

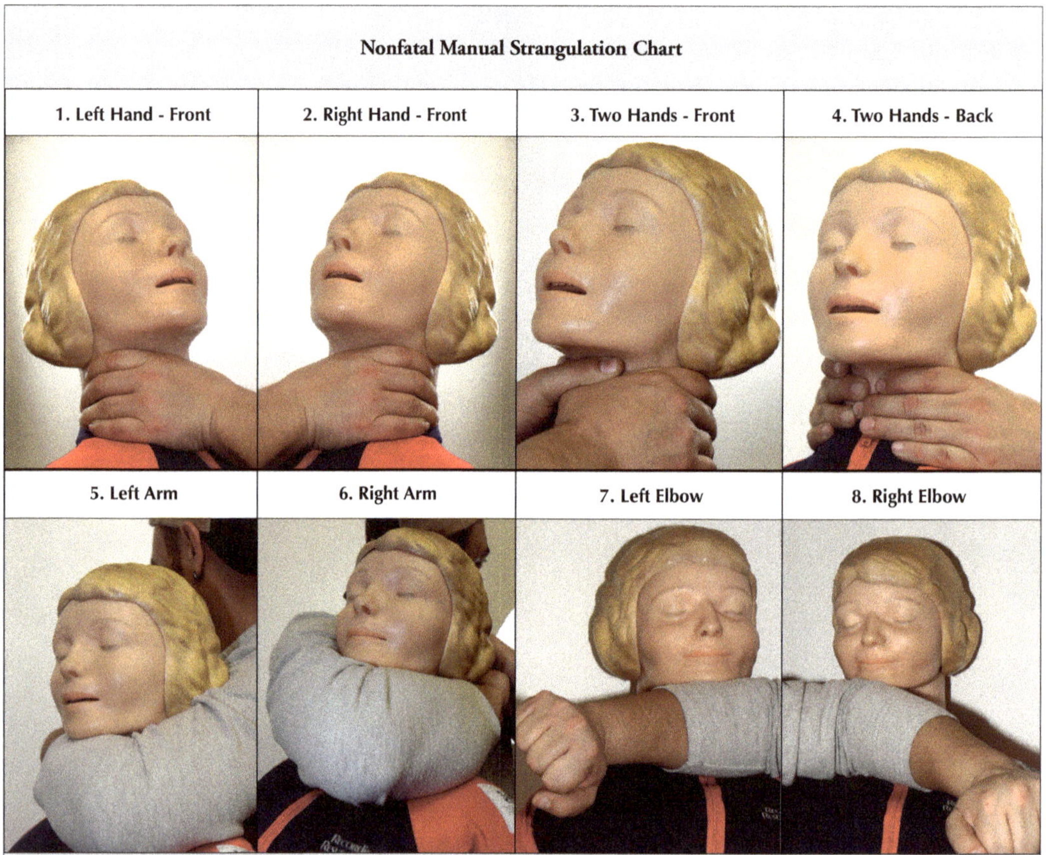

Examiner's Notes: ______________________________

Appendix Figure 13-a. Nonfatal Manual Strangulation Chart (8 positions of strangulation).

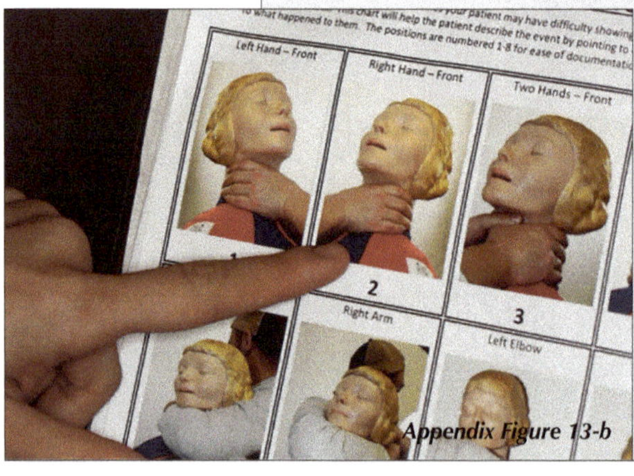

Appendix Figure 13-b. Patient pointing to the picture that depicts what happened.

Appendix Figure 13-b

Appendix Figure 13-a

Appendix 2. Academy of Forensic Nursing (AFN) Evidence Table*

— The purpose of evidence tables is to critically analyze and synthesize studies of importance to the forensic nursing community. Evidence tables discuss the strength of studies guiding practice through the critical appraisal process. The AFN Journal Club discusses all pertinent publications and completes the Evidence Tables. AFN Evidence Tables are made available to AFN members annually.

— To keep the table succinct, descriptions are brief and abbreviations have been used. Column 9 reflects Melnyk's levels of evidence.

— ***Level 1:*** Systematic review and meta-analysis of randomized controlled trials; clinical guidelines based on systematic reviews or meta-analyses

— ***Level 2:*** One or more randomized controlled trials

— ***Level 3:*** Controlled trial (no randomization)

— ***Level 4:*** Case-control or cohort study

— ***Level 5:*** Systematic review of descriptive and qualitative studies

— ***Level 6:*** Single descriptive or qualitative study

— ***Level 7:*** Expert opinion (commentary from subject matter expert)

There is no level for print media or media that promote individual thinking or opinion (eg, newspapers, TV, electronic communication). However, in articles you may see these items referenced to justify a need for the study. The information included in the table is as follows:

— ***Column 1:*** Complete citation in APA 6th edition format.

— ***Column 2:*** Conceptual framework/theoretical basis/purpose for study.

— ***Column 3:*** Design/method: Is the study quantitative or qualitative? Briefly describe what was done in the study.

— ***Column 4:*** Sample/setting: Sample/participant/study numbers, characteristics of the population, attrition rate and what causes the attrition.

— ***Column 5:*** Variables: define the independent variables and dependent variables studied (there may be more than one of each).

— ***Column 6:*** Measurement: What scales/tools/measures were used to measure the outcome variables?

— ***Column 7:*** Data analysis: What statistical tests were used to answer the clinical questions?

— ***Column 8:*** Study findings: Statistical or qualitative findings.

— ***Column 9:*** Strength of evidence, appraisal, worth to practice: Using Melnyk's levels of evidence as above, report study quality to include strengths, weaknesses, limitations, risks of harm if implemented, feasibility for use in real-life practice. Levels of evidence + quality of evidence = strength of evidence and confidence to inform practices, regardless of undergraduate or graduate preparation.

**Modified from Speck, 2006 Evidence Table*

Appendix 2. AFN Evidence Table *(continued)*

Appendix Table 1. AFN Evidence Table: Asphyxiation: Intentional Nonfatal Strangulation

Column 1	Column 2	Column 3	Column 4
Citation	Conceptual Framework/Theoretical Basis/Purpose	Design/Method/ Fidelity	Sample/Setting
Patch, M., Anderson, J. C., & Campbell, J. C. (2018). Injuries of women surviving intimate partner strangulation and subsequent emergency health care seeking: An integrative evidence review. *Journal of Emergency Nursing, 44*(4), 384-393. doi:10.1016/ j.jen.2017.12.001	N/A, evidence review	Followed PRISMA guidelines; 5 electronic databases searched; articles restricted to 2000 to 2015; resulted in 13 articles included: 5 quantitative, 2 qualitative, 1 mixed method, 5 case reports	Half of the included articles used convenience sampling from varied locations: DV shelters, police or legal settings, and medical centers; sample sizes ranged from 1 to 3 in case reports, 62 to 300 in qualitative studies, 14 to 17 in quantitative studies
Zuberi, O., Dixon, T., Richardson, A., Gandhe, A., Hadi, M., Joshi, J. (2019). CT angiograms of the neck in strangulation victims: Incidence of positive findings at a level one trauma center over a 7-Year period. *Emergency Radiology, 26*(5), 485-492. doi: 10.1007/ s10140-019-01690-3	Determine incidence of BCVI diagnosed by CTA of the neck in patients presenting with strangulation injury	Retrospective study of all patients that had undergone a CTA of the neck after being strangled at a Level 1 Trauma Center	142 patients included from Jan 1 2009 to April 30, 2016; 91.7% female and 18.3% male; average age 33 female, average age 30.9 male; manual strangulation in 83.8% of cases, followed by ligature, hanging, and, least common, mechanical strangulation
Matusz, E., Schaffer, J., Bachmeier, B., Kirschner, J., Musey, P., Roumpf, S., Strachan, C., Hunter, B. (2019). Evaluation of nonfatal strangulation in alert adults. *Annals of Emergency Medicine, 75*(3), 329-338. doi: 10.1016/j. annemergmed.2019.07.018	Define rate of serious injuries in alert strangled patients and determine which sx, if any, predict such injuries	Retrospective analysis of charts of alert, strangled patients treated in Level 1 trauma ED; aged 16 years and older, excluded transfers from outside hospitals, GCS less than 13, and no documented strangulation MOI	349 included patients from 2014 to 2018, 328 manually strangled and 21 near hanging; median age 30; 314 female; race not included
Shields, L., Corey, T., Weakley-Jones, B., Stewart, D. (2010). Living victims of strangulation: A 10-year review of case in metropolitan community. *American Journal of Forensic Pathology, 31*(4), 320-325.	N/A, case review	Retrospective chart reviews; living patients included over 10 years from 1998 to 2007; 2 outliers removed	102 victims; each chart included race, age, sex, location and manner of strangulation, relationship to perp, presence of others, S/S post NFS, previous DV; ages ranged from 17 to 68; all but one were female

(continued)

Appendix 2. AFN Evidence Table (continued)

Appendix Table 1. AFN Evidence Table: Asphyxiation: Intentional Nonfatal Strangulation *(continued)*

Column 5	Column 6	Column 7	Column 8	Column 9*
Dependent and Independent Variables	Measurement Tool	Data Analysis Results	Study Findings	Strength of Evidence/ Appraisal/Worth to Practice
N/A	N/A	N/A	Visualization improved with ALS especially for darker skin tones; acute and long term mental health symptoms described; pain, voice changes, difficulty breathing or swallowing prevalent S/S; less than half sought care after NFS; injury documentation by medical staff was noted to be considerably more robust than police	Level 5; provides a beginning framework to support current practice; good implications for nursing practice; observational and descriptive qualitative studies were retrospective and so concerns for recall bias; low rate of health care seeking behavior implies only severe cases of NFS are captured
Patient S/S categorized for potential associations with clinical injuries; each CTA reviewed by neuroradiologist for accuracy of original reading	Demographics, MOI, and ROS reported as percentages of total cases	21 acute injuries identified: 16 soft tissue injuries and 6 vascular injuries; after review by neuroradiologists, final prevalence for vascular injuries was 3/142; ROS = 51.4% neck pain, 47.2% LOC, 21.8% headache but predictive value of ROS and vascular injury was weak (4.1%, 4.5%, and 3.2% respectively)	Positive vascular injury could not be clinically predicted by history and physical examination; BCVIs can be initially asymptomatic; of 3/142 with vascular injury, none had neurologic sx	Level 4; none of the patients had f/u studies so unclear if some were anatomic variants versus vascular injury; only focused on vascular injury findings so other MOI in strangulation such as hypoxia not evaluated; CTA of neck post strangulation rarely identifies BCVI, so limited diagnostic yield
Patient S/S categorized for potential associations with clinical injuries	Results were measured as a % of total cases; results included basic demographics, S/S, and type of advanced imaging completed (if any)	6/349 found to have injuries diagnosed radiographically, 2 of which were clinically important (cervical artery dissections); among manually strangled patients, most common findings include neck pain (595), anterior neck bruising (43%), anterior neck tenderness (38%), and dysphagia (29%)	Both patients with clinically important injuries and all 4 patients with neck injury had GCS less than 15 or dysphagia; small number of injuries precludes association between patient S/S and injuries diagnosed radiographically; strangulation often occurs in conjunction with additional trauma	Level 4; most patients women, manually strangled, and GCS greater than or equal to 13 so not widely applicable results; not all patients had imaging so injuries could have been missed; authors proposed that patients with normal GCS and no dysphagia, dysphonia, or tenderness do not need advanced imaging based on findings
N/A	Results were measured as a % of total cases	N/A	Subjective: 40% difficulty breathing, 38% LOC, 25% difficulty swallowing; objective: 54% contusions, 40% abrasions, 23% redness	Level 5; cognitive/recall bias and omission inherent in patient history; subjective should guide objective; lack of evidence is not indication that NFS did not occur; rarely NFS from stranger; 7% lied to HCP about mechanism

(continued)

Appendix 2. AFN Evidence Table *(continued)*

Appendix Table 1. AFN Evidence Table: Asphyxiation: Intentional Nonfatal Strangulation ***(continued)***

Column 1	Column 2	Column 3	Column 4
Citation	Conceptual Framework/Theoretical Basis/Purpose	Design/Method/ Fidelity	Sample/Setting
Pinheiro, J., Cascallana, J. L., Lopez de Abajo, B., Otero, J. L., & Rodriguez-Calvo, M. S. (2018). Laryngeal anatomical variants and their impact on the diagnosis of mechanical asphyxias by neck pressure. *Forensic Science International, 290,* 1-10. doi:10.1016/j.forsciint.2018.06.019	Anatomic variants can affect dissection interpretation and make it difficult to diagnose larynx fractures	Samples obtained from 207 consecutive autopsies performed in Spain; 38 were asphyxia victims by compression of the neck, and 159 samples were deaths from other causes	Population-based study including only autopsies performed in the Institute of Legal Medicine in Galicia, Spain; 149 males and 57 females ranging in ages from 1 to 97 years
Sorenson, S. B., Manisha, J., & Sivitiz, E. (2014). A systematic review of the epidemiology of nonfatal strangulation, a human rights and health concern. *American Journal of Public Health, 104*(11), e54-e61.	N/A	Systematic review; used PRISMA guidelines; cross sectional studies and serial text word searches; limited to English from 1960 to 2014	23 articles based on 11 cross sectional nationally representative surveys of community-residing adults
Messing, J. T., Patch, M., Wilson, J. S., Kelen, G. D., & Campbell, J. (2018). Differentiating among attempted, completed, and multiple nonfatal strangulation in women experiencing intimate partner violence. *Women's Health Issues, 28*(1), 104-111. doi:10.1016/j.whi.2017.10.002.	IPV identification is low in health care settings; support and understanding of recognition of IPV-NFS is crucial	Trained researchers conducted semi-structured phone interviews with survivors of IPV; referred by police	1008 female survivors from 2009 to 2013; survivors were asked by police who responded to reports of IPV if they were willing to be contacted by the researchers; 7 jurisdictions in Oklahoma included
Faugno, D., Waszak, D., Strack, G., Brooks, M, & Gwinn, C. (2013). Strangulation forensic examination: Best practice for health care providers. *Advanced Emergency Nursing Journal, 35*(4), 314-327. doi:10.1097/TME.0b013e3182aa05d3.	N/A, clinical practice G=guideline	N/A	N/A
Holbrook, D., & Jackson, C. (2013). Use of an alternative light source to assess strangulation victims. *Journal of Forensic Nursing, 9*(3), 140-145. doi:10.1097/JFN.0b013e31829beb1e.	ALS may reveal soft tissue injuries not visible to naked eye	Retroactive review of 172 acute NFS patients >13 years old evaluated with a "SPEX" ALS	Over 2 years from an urban FNE program, 69% African American, only 1 male
Armstrong, M. & Strack, G. (2016). Recognition and documentation of strangulation crimes: A review. JAMA Otolaryngology--Head & Neck Surgery, 142(9), 891-897. doi:10.1001/jamaoto.2016.0293.	Review prompted after an otolaryngologist was called as an expert for strangulation but could not find anything described in the otolaryngology literature	N/A, review	29 references; mix of qualitative and quantitative studies, case reports, expert opinions, and health care related websites

(continued)

Appendix 2. AFN Evidence Table (continued)

Appendix Table 1. AFN Evidence Table: Asphyxiation: Intentional Nonfatal Strangulation *(continued)*

Column 5 Dependent and Independent Variables	Column 6 Measurement Tool	Column 7 Data Analysis Results	Column 8 Study Findings	Column 9* Strength of Evidence/ Appraisal/ Worth to Practice
N/A, not RCT	Descriptive analysis carried out and comparison between groups analyzed using Student t-test, Chi-Squared test, or Fisher's exact test; ANOVA used for testing 3 or more groups	Known anatomic variants were identified, such as triticeal cartilage and agenesis of thyroid horns, but 3 new anatomic variants were discovered: terminal segmentation of thyroid horns, ectopic superior thyroid horns, and lateral thyrohyoid ossification (author's terms proposal)	Probability of misdiagnosis of laryngeal fracture because of presence of anatomic variant was high at 71.5%; likelihood is greater if thyroid cartilage was affected; higher frequency of thyroid fractures with the prevalence and location of triticeal cartilage on lower third of the lateral thyrohyoid ligament are main reasons	Level 4; anatomic variants of larynx should always be considered when making diagnosis of hyoid or thyroid fractures in autopsy, with particular attention paid to triticeal cartilage; dissection technique is crucial; critical evaluation of anatomic variants in cases whereby there is fatal pressure on the neck is essential in avoiding misinterpretation, which has serious medicolegal consequences
N/A, not RCT	N/A, no specific measurement tool used; used own criteria	N/A	NFS is large enough to be a human rights violation; women report higher strangulation when structurally/socially vulnerable; NFS common globally	Level 5; not a true systematic review; search retrieval and data included; differences in definitions so unable to do proper SR; limited practice value; pilot study
Prevalence and correlates of NFS were examined; victim and relationship characteristics collected during the interviews constitute independent variables	Multinomial logistic regression used to examine strength of association between the independent variables and the types of NFS: attempted, completed, and multiple	Risk ratios were calculated to describe association between injury, risk factors for homicide, and other forms of IPV with each type of NFS; association looked at between multiple episodes of NFS and LOC	79.6% of women interviewed has experienced NFS as either attempted (11.7%), completed (30.16%), and multiple (37.8%); each type of NFS was independently significantly associated with sexual violence; multiple NFS associated with more IPV injury; LOC resulted in greater likelihood to seek medical attention	Level 6; large sample but not representative and limited to IPV survivors that reported to police, measurement of types of NFS are limited to survivor reports; able to support need to screen all patients for IPV and NFS to treat injury and enhance patient safety; significant association was identified with multiple episodes of NFS and known homicide risk factors
N/A	N/A	N/A	NFS prevalent in IPV; underreported; often missed by HCP because of lack of visible injury; recommend screening directly; complete MFE for all and disclosures	Level 7; key points, pearls of wisdom, and case successes provided to support expert opinions; summary of best practice
N/A	Light absorption under the ALS as seen by the reviewer(s)	93% nothing visible to unaided eye, 98% positive "intradermal indications" under the ALS	ALS can aid in NFS examination and tx, need to use a variety of wavelengths and goggle colors; no clinical relevance in relation to age or skin color	Level 6; findings notable to inform practice but additional education about ALS practice and interpretation needed; no other studies known that have duplicated these findings
N/A	N/A	N/A	In one study of 300 victims of NFS, 67% reported no symptoms and only 15% had visible photographable injuries; in other studies, 4 patients had not recognized injuries after assault, but all eventually required an emergency tracheotomy; in 1 study, children witnessed 41% of assaults	Level 5; treatment and assessment recommendations as well as review of A&P provided, specifically to otolaryngologists, but useful for all health care disciplines

Legend: N/A=Not available; IPV=Intimate partner violence; HCP= Health care provider; MFE= Medical forensic examination; NFS= Nonfatal strangulation; BCVI= Blunt cerebral vascular injury; CTA= Computed tomography angiography; MOI= Mechanism of injury; ROS= Review of systems; sx= symptoms; GCS= Glasgow Coma Scale; ALS= Alternative light source, S/S= Signs and symptoms; tx= Treatment; DV=Domestic violence; ANOVA= Analysis of variance; A&P= Anatomy and physiology; LOC= Loss of consciousness; ED = Emergency Department

Speck, 2010. Last revised 2018. Used by AFN with permission, based on Fineout-Overholt et al, 2010.

Fineout-Overholt E, Melnyk BM, Stillwell SB, Williamson KM. Evidence-based practice step by step: critical appraisal of the evidence: part I. Am J Nurs. 2010:110(7):47-52.

Appendix 3. Danger Assessment

DANGER ASSESSMENT*

Several risk factors have been associated with increased risk of homicide of women and men in violent relationships. We cannot predict what will happen in your case, but we would like you to be aware of the danger of homicide in situations of abuse and for you to see how any of the risk factors apply to your situation.

Using the calendar, please mark the approximate dates during the past year when you were abused by your partner or ex-partner. Write on that date how bad the incident was according to the following scale:

_______ 1. Slapping, pushing; no injuries and/or lasting pain

_______ 2. Punching, kicking; bruises, cuts, and/or continuing pain

_______ 3. "Beating up;" severe contusions, burns, broken bones

_______ 4. Threat to use weapon; head injury, internal injury, permanent injury, miscarriage, or choking (mark a © on the date to indicate choking/strangulation/cut off your breathing)

_______ 5. Use of weapon; wounds from weapon

(If any of the descriptions for the higher number apply, use the higher number.)

Mark **Yes** or **No** for each of the following questions. *("He" refers to your husband, partner, ex-husband, ex-partner, or whoever is currently physically hurting you.)*

_______ 1. Has the physical violence increased in frequency or severity over the past year?

_______ 2. Does he own a gun?

_______ 3. Have you left him after living together during the past year?

3a. If you have *never* lived with him, check here: _______

_______ 4. Is he unemployed?

_______ 5. Has he ever used a weapon against you or threatened you with a lethal weapon?

5a. If yes, was the weapon a gun? Check here: _______

_______ 6. Does he threaten to kill you?

_______ 7. Has he avoided being arrested for domestic violence?

_______ 8. Do you have a child that is not his?

_______ 9. Has he ever forced you to have sex when you did not wish to do so?

_______ 10. Does he ever try to choke/strangle you or cut off your breathing?

10a. If yes, has he done it more than once, or did it make you pass out, black out, or make you dizzy? Check here: _______

_______ 11. Does he use illegal drugs? By drugs, I mean "uppers" or amphetamines, "meth," speed, angel dust, cocaine, "crack," street drugs, or mixtures.

_______ 12. Is he an alcoholic or problem drinker?

_______ 13. Does he control most or all of your daily activities? For instance, does he tell you who you can be friends with, when you can see your family, how much money you can use, or when you can take the car?

13a. If he tries, but you do not let him, check here: _______

_______ 14. Is he violently and constantly jealous of you? (For instance, does he say: "If I can't have you, no one can.")

_______ 15. Have you ever been beaten by him while you were pregnant?

15a. If you have never been pregnant by him, check here: _______

_______ 16. Has he ever threatened or tried to commit suicide?

_______ 17. Does he threaten to harm your children?

_______ 18. Do you believe he is capable of killing you?

_______ 19. Does he follow or spy on you, leave threatening notes or messages, destroy your property, or call you when you don't want him to?

_______ 20. Have you ever threatened or tried to commit suicide?

_______ **Total "Yes" Answers**

Thank you. Please talk to your nurse, advocate, or counselor about what the Danger Assessment means in your situation.

Appendix 4. Danger Assessment for Clinicians (DA-5)

DANGER ASSESSMENT FOR CLINICIANS (DA- 5)

This brief risk assessment identifies women who are at high risk for homicide or severe injury by an intimate partner or former intimate partner.[1,2]

Mark **Yes** or **No** for each of the following questions.

_______ 1. Has the physical violence increased in frequency or severity over the past year?

_______ 2. Has your partner (or ex) ever used a weapon against you or threatened you with a weapon?

_______ 3. Do you believe your partner (or ex) is capable of killing you?

_______ 4. Has your partner (or ex) ever tried to choke (strangle) you?

_______ 4a. If yes, did he ever choke you?

_______ 4b. About how long ago?

_______ 4c. Did it happen more than once?

_______ 4d. Did you ever lose consciousness or think you may have?

_______ 5. Is your partner (or ex) violently and constantly jealous of you?

[1] *This is a brief adaptation of the Danger Assessment (2003). It is designed for use by a health care provider after a positive screen for intimate partner violence. The full Danger Assessment with weighted scoring provides the most accurate assessment of risk.*

[2] *Snider C, Webster D, O'Sullivan CS, Campbell J. Intimate partner violence: development of a brief risk assessment for the emergency department.* Acad Emerg Med. *2009;16(11):1208–1216.*

Protocol suggestions for use of DANGER ASSESSMENT-5

Use the 5-item version in the emergency department and other health care settings or at protective order hearings or child custody hearings once intimate partner violence has been identified.

— **If there are 4 or 5 yes responses,** tell the victim s/he is in danger, allow the victim to choose reporting to the police or to domestic violence advocacy program or confidential hotline (eg, 800-799-7233). Follow through by calling the number with the victim or with an in-person hand-off to a knowledgeable advocate.

— **If there are 3 of 5 yes responses,** do full a Danger Assessment (DA) with the calendar and weighted scoring if the victim is a woman. Inform the victim of the level of danger, and do safety planning based on the DA or refer to someone certified in administrating the DA and proceed based on results and best practices.

— **If there are 2 of 5 yes responses,** tell the victim there are 2 of 5 risk factors for serious injury/assault/homicide present and recommend further advocacy. If the victim agrees, follow through with a referral and (preferably in-person) hand-off to a knowledgeable advocate.

— **If there are 0 to 1 of 5 yes responses,** proceed with normal referral/procedural processes for domestic violence.

Brief Strangulation Protocol

If the patient answers "yes" to 4a and if the strangulation was a week ago or less, examine the inside of the throat and the neck, face, and scalp for physical signs of strangulation. See the strangulation assessment and radiographic evaluation information at *www.strangulationtraininginstitute.com*. Proceed with emergency medical care for strangulation, especially if there was a loss of consciousness or possible loss of consciousness. Victims are often unsure, but if they lost consciousness they will have become incontinent. You can ask the patient if they wet themselves. If the victim reports more than one strangulation, conduct a neurologic examination for brain injury or refer for examination and inform her of increased risk of homicide. Notify police and/or prosecutors if the victim wants this action (know state/local law on strangulation and mandatory reporting so that victim can be informed).

Appendix 5. HELPS Brain Injury Screening Tool

Consumer Information: ____________________

____

____

Agency/Screener's Information: ____________________

____

H Have you ever **H**it your **H**ead or been **H**it on the **H**ead? ☐ Yes ☐ No

Note: Prompt client to think about all incidents that may have occurred at any age, even those that did not seem serious: vehicle accidents, falls, assault, abuse, sports, etc. Screen for domestic violence and child abuse, and also for service related injuries. A TBI can also occur from violent shaking of the head, such as being shaken as a baby or child.

E Were you ever seen in the **E**mergency room, hospital, or by a doctor because of an injury to your head? ☐ Yes ☐ No

Note: Many people are seen for treatment. However, there are those who cannot afford treatment, or who do not think they require medical attention.

L Did you ever **L**ose consciousness or experience a period of being dazed and confused because of an injury to your head? ☐ Yes ☐ No

Note: People with TBI may not lose consciousness but experience an "alteration of consciousness." This may include feeling dazed, confused, or disoriented at the time of the injury, or being unable to remember the events surrounding the injury.

P Do you experience any of these **P**roblems in your daily life since you hit your head? ☐ Yes ☐ No

Note: Ask your client if s/he experiences any of the following problems, and ask when the problem presented. You are looking for a combination of two or more problems that were not present prior to the injury.

- ☐ headaches
- ☐ dizziness
- ☐ anxiety
- ☐ depression
- ☐ difficulty concentrating
- ☐ difficulty remembering
- ☐ difficulty reading, writing, calculating
- ☐ poor problem solving
- ☐ difficulty performing your job/school work
- ☐ change in relationships with others
- ☐ poor judgment (being fired from job, arrests, fights)

S Any significant **S**icknesses? ☐ Yes ☐ No

Note: Traumatic brain injury implies a physical blow to the head, but acquired brain injury may also be caused by medical conditions, such as: brain tumor, meningitis, West Nile virus, stroke, seizures. Also screen for instances of oxygen deprivation such as following a heart attack, carbon monoxide poisoning, near drowning, or near suffocation.

Scoring the HELPS Screening Tool

A HELPS screening is considered positive for a *possible* TBI when the following 3 items are identified:

1.) An event that could have caused a brain injury (yes to H, E **or** S), **and**

2.) A period of loss of consciousness or altered consciousness after the injury or another indication that the injury was severe (yes to L or E), **and**

3.) The presence of two or more chronic problems listed under P that were not present before the injury.

Note:

- A positive screening is **not sufficient to diagnose TBI** as the reason for current symptoms and difficulties - other possible causes may need to be ruled out
- **Some individuals could present exceptions** to the screening results, such as people who have TBI-related problems but answered "no" to some questions
- Consider positive responses within the context of the person's self-report and documentation of altered behavioral and/or cognitive functioning

---

The original HELPS TBI screening tool was developed by M. Picard, D. Scarisbrick, R. Paluck, 9/91, International Center for the Disabled, TBI-NET, U.S. Department of Education, Rehabilitation Services Administration, Grant #H128A00022. The Helps Tool was updated by project personnel to reflect recent recommendations by the CDC on the diagnosis of TBI. See http://www.cdc.gov/ncipc/pub-res/tbi_toolkit/physicians/mtbi/diagnosis.htm.

This document was supported in part by Grant 6 H21 MC 00039-03-01 from the Department of Health and Human Services (DHHS) Health Resources and Services Administration, Maternal and Child Bureau to the Michigan Department of Community Health. The contents are the sole responsibility of the authors and do not necessarily represent the official views of DHHS.

Appendix 6. Lethality Assessment

Physical and sexual violence are a public health crisis. More than 10 million women and men in the United States are assaulted by a former or current partner every year.[1] Medical practitioners are often the first or only professional to come in contact with someone in an abusive situation, so they are in a unique position to intervene. It is important for health care providers to know not only how to identify domestic violence, but also how to properly respond both medically, psychologically, and socially.

Patients should always be treated with dignity and respect, having voice and choice in a trauma-informed approach to their lifetime experience and current health status. Health care providers need to be aware that leaving an abusive relationship is often a long and gradual process. Providers engage patients in the health care system to support them through the long-term and stepwise process of decision making toward attaining greater safety. A top priority is the safety of the patient and their children. When children are in danger, child protection mandates reporting.

Domestic violence is common enough to warrant routine screening. Early recognition and intervention significantly reduce morbidity and mortality associated with domestic violence. Screening should be done in a safe environment, away from anyone who accompanied the patient. If this cannot be done, postpone the screening for domestic violence. Screening questions should be direct and specific, as well as nonjudgmental and nonthreatening.

A positive screening for domestic violence necessitates further questioning to determine if the patient is in immediate danger for lethality. Often, victims of domestic abuse do not believe that their partner would ever take it that far. It is important for health care providers to screen for lethality in order to help the patient get to safety as soon as possible. Indicators of escalating danger can include an increase in the frequency or severity of the assault, threats to any children in the home, a firearm in the home, and new threats of homicide or suicide.

The health care provider should be supportive of the patient's decisions and assure and empower them. Statements such as "No one deserves abuse," "You are not alone," and "It must be difficult for you to leave. We are here to help whenever you are ready" can help the patient feel safe and supported. If the patient is responding emotionally, do not say "It is not your fault" to make yourself feel better. While you do not want to blame the victim, you also do not know the situation or complicit activities, (eg, drug use, which is best addressed in cognitive behavioral therapy when the patient is ready). With any motivational method, ask the patient questions to determine their state of mind towards possible change, such as "What type of assistance would you like?" "Have you thought about what you need to make the change?" and "What steps are you ready to take toward those goals?" Always assess for depression and suicide[2-4] by asking directly, "Are you having any suicidal thoughts?" or "Have you made plans to die?" Any affirmative answer requires the provider to follow up with referrals to the hospital for protection and resources designed to coordinate in a community response to the issue.

An expanded assessment should be given, which may need to be continued at a follow-up visit. The health care provider should assess the patient's general view toward the abuse, the degree of control the abuser has over the patient, the medical and psychological effects the abuse has had on the patient, and the effects of the abuse on any children in the home, as well as further assessment for suicide or homicide. Many states have mandatory reporting legislation when children are exposed to domestic violence, so know your laws, and report if you determine children are present during the violence.

Always remember that screening for domestic abuse is ongoing. A patient may not express concerns the first time the health care provider inquiries about their relationship, but over time, as patient-provider trust builds or the intimate relationship evolves, signs and symptoms of abuse may become evident, and disclosure becomes likely.

Appendix 7. Recommendations for the Medical/Radiographic Evaluation of Acute Adult, Non-Fatal Strangulation

TRAINING INSTITUTE on STRANGULATION PREVENTION

RECOMMENDATIONS for the MEDICAL/RADIOGRAPHIC EVALUATION of ACUTE ADULT, NON-FATAL STRANGULATION

Prepared by **Bill Smock, MD** and **Sally Sturgeon, DNP, SANE-A**
Office of the Police Surgeon, Louisville Metro Police Department
Endorsed by the **National Medical Advisory Committee**: Bill Smock, MD, Chair; Cathy Baldwin, MD; William Green, MD; Dean Hawley, MD; Ralph Riviello, MD; Heather Rozzi, MD; Steve Stapczynski, MD; Ellen Tailiaferro, MD; Michael Weaver, MD

POLICE LOUISVILLE METRO

GOALS:
1. Evaluate carotid and vertebral arteries for injuries
2. Evaluate bony/cartilaginous and soft tissue neck structures
3. Evaluate brain for anoxic injury

Strangulation patient presents to the Emergency Department

History of and/or physical exam with ANY of the following:

- **Loss of Consciousness** (anoxic brain injury)
- **Visual changes**: "spots", "flashing light", "tunnel vision"
- **Facial, intra-oral or conjunctival petechial hemorrhage**
- **Ligature mark or** neck **contusions**
- **Soft tissue neck injury/swelling of the neck/carotid tenderness**
- **Incontinence** (bladder and/or bowel from anoxic injury)
- **Neurological signs or symptoms** (LOC, seizures, mental status changes, amnesia, visual changes, cortical blindness, movement disorders, stroke-like symptoms.)
- **Dysphonia/Aphonia** (hematoma, laryngeal fracture, soft tissue swelling, recurrent laryngeal nerve injury)
- **Dyspnea** (hematoma, laryngeal fractures, soft tissue swelling, phrenic nerve injury)
- **Subcutaneous emphysema** (tracheal/laryngeal rupture)

↓

Consider administration of one 325mg aspirin if there is any delay in obtaining a radiographic study

↓

Recommended Radiographic Studies to Rule Out Life-Threatening Injuries*
(including delayed presentations of up to 1 year)

- **CT Angio of carotid/vertebral arteries** (*GOLD STANDARD* for evaluation of vessels and bony/cartilaginous structures, less sensitive for soft tissue trauma) ***or***
- **CT neck with contrast** (less sensitive than CT Angio for vessels, good for bony/cartilaginous structures) ***or***
- **MRA of neck** (less sensitive than CT Angio for vessels, best for soft tissue trauma) ***or***
- **MRI of neck** (less sensitive than CT Angio for vessels and bony/cartilaginous structures, best study for soft tissue trauma) ***or***
- **MRI/MRA of brain** (most sensitive for anoxic brain injury, stroke symptoms and inter-cerebral petechial hemorrhage)
- **Carotid Doppler Ultrasound** (*NOT RECOMMENDED:* least sensitive study, unable to adequately evaluate vertebral arteries or proximal internal carotid)

**References on page 2*

(-) → Continued ED/Hospital Observation (based on severity of symptoms and reliable home monitoring)

(+) →
- Consult Neurology Neurosurgery/Trauma Surgery for admission
- Consider ENT consult for laryngeal trauma with dysphonia
- Perform a lethality assessment per institutional policy

History of and/or physical exam with:

- **No LOC** (anoxic brain injury)
- **No visual changes**: "spots", "flashing light", "tunnel vision"
- **No petechial hemorrhage**
- **No soft tissue trauma to the neck**
- **No dyspnea, dysphonia or odynophagia**
- **No neurological signs or symptoms** (i.e. LOC, seizures, mental status changes, amnesia, visual changes, cortical blindness, movement disorder, stroke-like symptoms)
- And **reliable home monitoring**

↓

Discharge home with detailed instructions, including a lethality assessment, and to return to ED if: neurological signs/symptoms, dyspnea, dysphonia or odynophagia develops or worsens

Brochure Design by Yesenia Aceves — StrangulationTrainingInstitute.com — Version 4.8.19

Reprinted with permission from Training Institute on Strangulation Prevention.

Appendix 7. Recommendations for the Medical/Radiographic Evaluation of Acute Adult, Non-Fatal Strangulation *(continued)*

REFERENCES

(Recommendations based upon case reports, case studies, and cited medical literature)
Click below for hyperlinks, please note that some sources may require purchase or subscription.

1. Christe A, Thoeny H, Ross S, et al. Life-threatening versus non-life-threatening manual strangulation: are there appropriate criteria for MR imaging of the neck?. Eur Radiol 2009;19: 1882-1889

2. Christe A, Oesterhelweg L, Ross S, et al. Can MRI of the Neck Compete with Clinical Findings in Assessing Danger to Life for Survivors of Manual Strangulation? A Statistical Analysis, Legal Med 2010;12:228-232

3. Yen K, Thali MJ, Aghayev E, et al. Strangulation Signs: Initial Correlation of MRI, MSCT, and Forensic Neck Findings, J Magn Reson Imaging 2005;22:501-510

4. Stapczynski JS, Strangulation Injuries, Emergency Medicine Reports 2010;31(17):193-203

5. Yen K, Vock P, Christe A, et al. Clinical Forensic Radiology in Strangulation Victims: Forensic expertise based on magnetic resonance imaging (MRI) findings, Int J Legal Med 2007;121:115-123

6. Malek AM, Higashida RT, Halback VV, et al. Patient Presentation Angiographic Features and Treatment of Strangulation-Induced Bilateral Dissection of the Cervical Carotid Artery: Report of three cases, J Neurosurg 2000;92(3):481-487

7. Di Paolo M, Guidi B, Bruschini L, et al. Unexpected delayed death after manual strangulation: need for care examination in the emergency room, Monaldi Arch Chest Dis 2009;Sep;71(3):132-4

8. Dayapala A, Samarasekera A and Jayasena A, An Uncommon Delayed Sequela After Pressure on the Neck: An autopsy case report, Am J Forensic Med Pathol 2012;33:80-82

9. Hori A, Hirose G, Kataoka, et al. Delayed Postanoxic Encephalopathy After Strangulation, Arch Neurol 1991;48:871-874

10. Iacovou E, Nayar M, Fleming J, Lew-Gor S, A pain in the neck: a rare case of isolated hyoid bone trauma, JSCR 2011;7(3)

11. Oh JH, Min HS, Park TU, Sang JL, Kim SE, Isolated Cricoid Fracture Associated with Blunt Neck Trauma; Emerg Med J 2007;24:505-506

12. Gill JR, Cavalli DP, Ely SF, Stahl-Herz J, Homicidal Neck Compression of Females: Autopsy and Sexual Assault Findings, Acad Forensic Path 2013;3(4):454-457

13. Sethi PK, Sethi NK, Torgovnick J, Arsura E, Delayed Left Anterior and Middle Cerebral Artery Hemorrhagic Infarctions After Attempted Strangulation, A case report; Am J Forensic Med Pathol 2012;33:105-106

14. Clarot F, Vaz E, Papin F, Proust B, Fatal and Non-fatal Bilateral Delayed Carotid Artery Dissection after Manual Strangulation, Forensic Sci Int 2005;149:143-150

15. Molack J, Baxa J, Ferda J, Treska V, Bilateral Post-Traumatic Carotid Dissection as a Result of a Strangulation Injury, Ann Vasc Surg 2010;24:1133e9-1133e11

16. Plattner T, Bollinger S, Zollinger U, Forensic Assessment of Survived Strangulation, Forensic Sci Int 2005;153:202-207

17. Miao J, Su C, Wang W, et al. Delayed Parkinsonism with Selective Symmetric Basal Ganglia Lesion after Manual Strangulation, J Clin Neurosci 2009;16:573-575

18. Purvin V, Unilateral Headache and Ptosis in a 30-Year-Old Woman, Surv Ophthalmol 1997;42(2):163-168

19. Nazzal M, Herial NA, MacNealy MW: Diagnostic Imaging in Carotid Artery Dissection: A case report and review of current modalities; Ann Vasc Surg 2014;28;739.e5-739.e9

20. Chokyu TT, Miyamoto T, Yamaga H, Terada T, Itakura T: Traumatic Bilateral Common Carotid Artery Dissection Due to Strangulation: A case report; Interventional Neuroradiology;12:149-154, 2006

This project is supported all or in part by Grant No. 2016-TA-AX-K067 awarded by the Office on Violence Against Women, U.S. Department of Justice. The opinions, findings, conclusions, and recommendations expressed in this publication/program/exhibition are those of the author(s) and do not necessarily reflect the views of the Department of Justice, Office on Violence Against Women.

Appendix 8. Recommendations for the Medical/Radiographic Evaluation of the Pregnant Adult Patient with Nonfatal Strangulation

TRAINING INSTITUTE on STRANGULATION PREVENTION

RECOMMENDATIONS for the MEDICAL/RADIOGRAPHIC EVALUATION of the PREGNANT ADULT PATIENT WITH NON-FATAL STRANGULATION

Prepared by Michael Weaver, MD and Barbra Bachmeier, JD, MSN, NP-C

Endorsed by the **National Medical Advisory Committee**: Bll Smock, MD, Chair; Cathy Baldwin-Johnson, MD; William Green, MD; Dean Hawley, MD; Sally Henin, MD; Ralph Riviello, MD; Heather Rozzi, MD; Steve Stapczynski, MD; Ellen Tailiaferro, MD

GOALS:

1. Evaluate carotid and vertebral arteries for injuries
2. Evaluate bony/cartilaginous and soft tissue neck structures
3. Evaluate brain for anoxic injury
4. Evaluate/Monitor the fetus

Pregnant Strangulation patient presents to the Emergency Department

↓

Evaluate per institution Trauma Pregnancy Protocol/ OB Consultation

History of and/or physical exam with ANY of the following:

- **Loss of consciousness** (anoxic brain injury)
- **Visual changes**: "spots", "flashing light", "tunnel vision"
- **Facial, intraoral or conjunctival petechial hemorrhage**
- **Ligature mark or neck contusions**
- **Soft tissue neck injury/swelling of the neck/cartoid tenderness**
- **Incontinence** (bladder and/or bowel from anoxic injury)
- **Neurological signs or symptoms** (LOC, seizures, mental status changes, amnesia, visual changes, cortical blindness, movement disorders, stroke-like symtoms, unilateral headache, and bruit)
- **Dysphonia/Aphonia** (hematoma, laryngeal fracture, soft tissue swelling, recurrent laryngeal nerve injury)
- **Dyspnea** (hematoma, laryngeal fractures, soft tissue swelling, phrenic nerve injury)
- **Subcutaneous emphysema** (tracheal/laryngeal rupture)

↓

Recommended Radiographic Studies to Rule Out Life-Threatening Injuries*
(including rare delayed presentations of up to 2 years)

- **CT Angio of carotid/vertebral arteries** - (***GOLD STANDARD*** for evaluation of vessels and bony/cartilaginous structures, less sensitive for soft tissue trauma. Safe for all stages of pregnancy and/or lactating patients.) ***or***
- **CT neck with contrast** - (less sensitive than CT Angio for vessels, good for bony/ cartilaginous structures. Safe for all stages of pregnancy and/or lactating patients.) ***or***
- **MRIs without gadolinium**:
  - **MRA of neck** (less sensitive than CT Angio for vessels) ***or***
  - **MRI of neck** (less sensitive than CT Angio for vessels and bony/cartilaginous structures, best study for soft tissue trauma) ***or***
  - **MRI/MRA of brain** (most sensitive for anoxic brain injury, stroke symptoms and intercerebral petechial hemorrhage)

  Safe to perform during all trimesters for pregnant and/or lactating patients.
- **MRIs with gadolinium** (***NOT RECOMMENDED:*** Use should be limited to situations in which the benefits clearly outweigh possible risks.)
- **Carotid Doppler Ultrasound** (***NOT RECOMMENDED:*** Least sensitive study, unable to adequately evaluate vertebral arteries or proximal internal carotid.)

(−) → Continued ED/ Hospital Observation (based on severity of symptoms, reliable home monitoring, and a lethality assessment discussion)

(+) →
- Consult Neurology Neurosurgery/ Trauma Surgery/ OB for admission
- Consider ENT consult for laryngeal trauma with dysphonia

**References on page 2*

History of and/or physical exam with:

- **No LOC** (anoxic brain injury)
- **No visual changes**: "spots", "flashing light", "tunnel vision"
- **No petechial hemorrhage**
- **No soft tissue trauma to the neck**
- **No dyspnea, dysphonia or odynophagia**
- **No neurological signs or symptoms** (i.e. LOC, seizures, mental status changes, amnesia, visual changes, cortical blindness, movement disorder, stroke-like symtoms)
- And **reliable home monitoring**

↓

Discharge home with detailed instructions including a lethality assessment, per institution Trauma Pregnancy Protocol/OB Consultation to return to ED if: neurological signs/symptoms, dyspnea, dysphonia or odynophagia develops or worsens

Brochure Design by Yesenia Aceves

StrangulationTrainingInstitute.com

Version 4.1 5/18

Reprinted with permission from Training Institute on Strangulation Prevention.

Appendix 8. Recommendations for the Medical/Radiographic Evaluation of the Pregnant Adult Patient with Nonfatal Strangulation *(continued)*

TRAINING INSTITUTE on STRANGULATION PREVENTION

RECOMMENDATIONS for the MEDICAL/RADIOGRAPHIC EVALUATION of the PREGNANT ADULT PATIENT WITH NON-FATAL STRANGULATION

PREGNANCY REFERENCES

(Recommendations based upon expert consensus, case reports, and cited medical literature)

1. Copel J, El-Sayed Y, Heine RP, et al. Guidelines for Diagnostic Imaging During Pregnancy and Lactation. Obst Gyn2017; 130(4): e210-e216 *This document is endorced by the American College of Radiologoy and the American Institute of Ultrasound in Medicine.*

2. Ray JG, Vermeulen MJ, Bharatha A, et al. Association Between MRI Exposure During Pregnancy and Fetal and Childhood Outcomes. J Ameri Med Assoc 2016; 316(9): 952-961

3. Limanovich DE, Tack D, Lee KD, et al. Cardiothoracic Imaging in the Pregnant Patient. J Thor Imag 2014; 29(1): 38-49

4. Bekiesinka-Figatowska M, Romaniuk-Doroszewska A, Szkudlinska-Pawlak S, et al. Diagnostic Imaging on Pregnant Women: The Role of Magnetic Resonance Imaging. Polish J Radio 2017; 82: 220-226

5. Prola-Netto J, Woods M, Roberts VHJ, et al. Gadolinium Chelate Safety in Pregnancy: Barely Detectable Gadolinium Levels in the Juvenile Nonhuman Primate After in Utero Exposure. Radio 2018; 286(1): 122-128

6. Oh KY, Roberts VHJ, Schabel MC, et al. Gadolinium Chelate Contrast Material in Pregnancy: Fetal Biodistribution in the Nonhuman Primate. Radio 2015; 276(1): 110-118

7. Wieseler KM, Bhargava P, Kanal KM, et al. Imaging in Pregnant Patients: Examination Appropriateness. RadioGraphics 2010; 30: 1215-1233

8. Wang PI, Chong ST, Kielar AZ, et al. Imaging of Pregnancy and Lactating Patients: Part 1, Evidence-Based Review and Recommendations. Ameri J Radio 2012; 198: 778-785

9. Wang PI, Chong ST, Kielar AZ, et al. Imaging of Pregnancy and Lactating Patients: Part 2, Evidence-Based Review and Recommendations. Ameri J Radio 2012; 198: 785-792

10. Patel SJ, Reede DL, Katz DS, et al. Imaging for the Pregnancy Patient for Nonobstetric Conditions: Algorithms and Radiation Dose Considerations. RadioGraphics 2007; 27(6): 1705-1723

11. Wagner LK and Applegate KE. More Cautions on Imaging of Pregnant Patient. RadioGraphics 2011; 31(3): 891-895

GENERAL STRANGULATION REFERENCES

1. Christe A, Thoeny H, Ross S, et al. Life-threatening versus non-life-threatening manual strangulation: are there appropriate criteria for MR imaging of the neck?. Eur Radiol 2009;19: 1882-1889

2. Christe A, Oesterhelweg L, Ross S, et al. Can MRI of the Neck Compete with Clinical Findings in Assessing Danger to Life for Survivors of Manual Strangulation? A Statistical Analysis, Legal Med 2010;12:228-232

3. Yen K, Thali MJ, Aghayev E, et al. Strangulation Signs: Initial Correlation of MRI, MSCT, and Forensic Neck Findings, J Magn Reson Imaging 2005;22:501-510

4. Stapczynski JS, Strangulation Injuries, Emergency Medicine Reports 2010;31(17):193-203

5. Yen K, Vock P, Christe A, et al. Clinical Forensic Radiology in Strangulation Victims: Forensic expertise based on magnetic resonance imaging (MRI) findings, Int J Legal Med 2007;121:115-123

6. Malek AM, Higashida RT, Halback VV, et al. Patient Presentation Angiographic Features and Treatment of Strangulation-Induced Bilateral Dissection of the Cervical Carotid Artery: Report of three cases, J Neurosurg 2000;92(3):481-487

7. Di Paolo M, Guidi B, Bruschini L, et al. Unexpected delayed death after manual strangulation: need for care examination in the emergency room, Monaldi Arch Chest Dis 2009;Sep;71(3):132-4

8. Dayapala A, Samarasekera A and Jayasena A, An Uncommon Delayed Sequela After Pressure on the Neck: An autopsy case report, Am J Forensic Med Pathol 2012;33:80-82

9. Hori A, Hirose G, Kataoka, et al. Delayed Postanoxic Encephalopathy After Strangulation, Arch Neurol 1991;48:871-874

10. Iacovou E, Nayar M, Fleming J, Lew-Gor S, A pain in the neck: a rare case of isolated hyoid bone trauma, JSCR 2011;7(3)

11. Oh JH, Min HS, Park TU, Sang JL, Kim SE, Isolated Cricoid Fracture Associated with Blunt Neck Trauma; Emerg Med J 2007;24:505

12. Gill JR, Cavalli DP, Ely SF, Stahl-Herz J, Homicidal Neck Compression of Females: Autopsy and Sexual Assault Findings, Acad Forensic Path 2013;3(4):454-457

13. Sethi PK, Sethi NK, Torgovnick J, Arsura E, Delayed Left Anterior and Middle Cerebral Artery Hemorrhagic Infarctions After Attempted Strangulation, A case report; Am J Forensic Med Pathol 2012;33:105-106

14. Clarot F, Vaz E, Papin F, Proust B, Fatal and Non-fatal Bilateral Delayed Carotid Artery Dissection after Manual Strangulation, Forensic Sci Int 2005;149:143-150

15. Molack J, Baxa J, Ferda J, Treska V, Bilateral Post-Traumatic Carotid Dissection as a Result of a Strangulation Injury, Ann Vasc Surg 2010;24:1133e9-1133e11

16. Plattner T, Bollinger S, Zollinger U, Forensic Assessment of Survived Strangulation, Forensic Sci Int 2005;153:202-207

17. Miao J, Su C, Wang W, et al. Delayed Parkinsonism with Selective Symmetric Basal Ganglia Lesion after Manual Strangulation, J Clin Neurosci 2009;16:573-575

18. Purvin V, Unilateral Headache and Ptosis in a 30-Year-Old Woman, Surv Ophthalmol 1997;42(2):163-168

19. Nazzal M, Herial NA, MacNealy MW: Diagnostic Imaging in Carotid Artery Dissection: A case report and review of current modalities; Ann Vasc Surg 2014;28;739.e5-739.e9

20. Chokyu TT, Miyamoto T, Yamaga H, Terada T, Itakura T: Traumatic Bilateral Common Carotid Artery Dissection Due to Strangulation: A case report; Interventional Neuroradiology;12:149-154, 2006

Brochure Design by Yesenia Aceves

StrangulationTrainingInstitute.com

Version 4.1 5/18

Appendix 9. Strangulation Discharge Instructions

Because you have reported being "choked" or strangled, we are providing you with the following instructions:

Please report to the nearest ED or call 911 immediately if you notice:

— Difficulty breathing or shortness of breath

— Loss of consciousness or "passing out"

— Changes in your voice or difficulty speaking

— Difficulty swallowing, lump in throat, or muscle spasms in throat or neck

— Tongue swelling

— Behavioral changes or memory loss

— Thoughts of harming self or others

— Swelling to throat or neck

— Persistent cough or coughing up blood

— Persistent vomiting or vomiting up blood

— Left- or right-sided weakness, numbness, or tingling to extremities or face

— Headache not relieved by pain medication (Tylenol or Motrin as directed on bottle)

— Seizures

It is important that the above symptoms be evaluated by a health care provider (HCP).

After evaluation, keep a log of any changes in symptoms for your HCP and law enforcement. If symptoms worsen, call your HCP, or go to the nearest ED. We recommend you follow-up with law enforcement regarding symptom changes.

It is important that you have a follow-up medical evaluation in 72 hours at the ED or clinic where you were initially examined or the HCP of your choice. Make sure to bring your discharge instructions with you.

I have been made aware of and understand the importance of following the above outlined instructions.

______________________________________ ____________________
Patient or Authorized Representative Signature Date/Time

______________________________________ ____________________
Forensic Nurse Examiner Signature Date/Time

Appendix 10. Sturgeon's SAVEcD Tool - Strangulation Assessment for Victims With Evidence Collection and Documentation

Victim Name ____________________ Date of Birth _________ Case #______ Report # ________________

Left Eye - Outer Eyelid/Upper and Lower Conjunctiva/Sclera

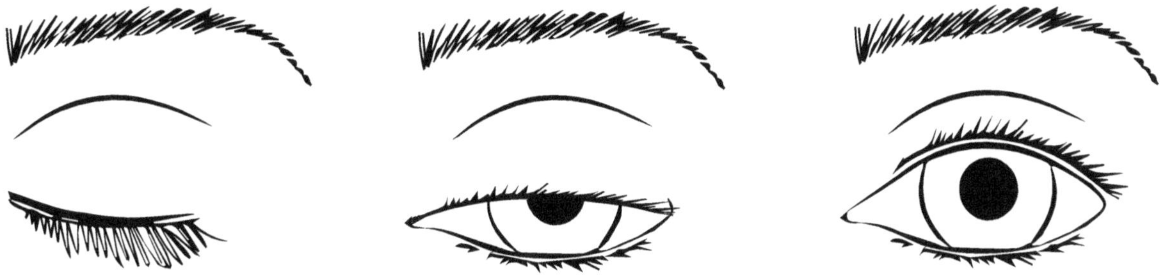

Right Eye - Sclera/Upper and Lower Conjunctiva/Outer Lid

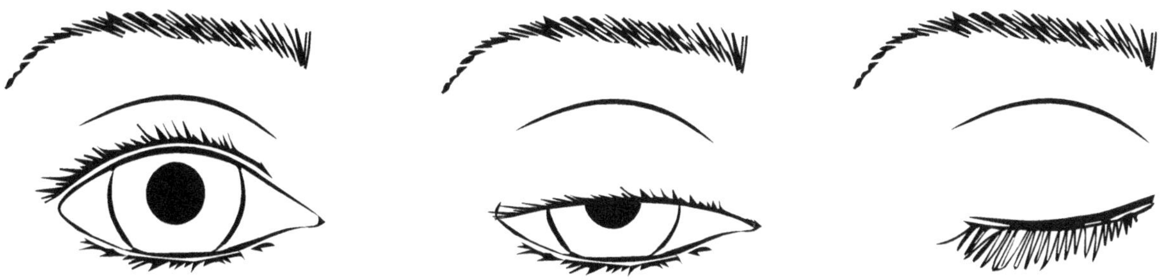

Mouth - Palate/Tongue/Frenulums/Inner and Outer Lips

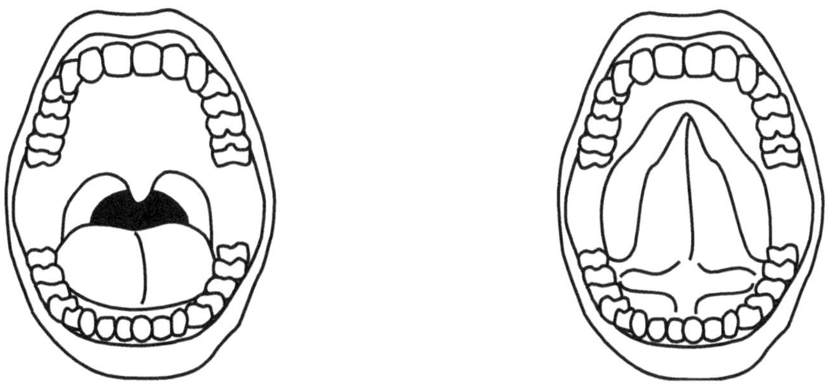

Forensic Nurse Examiner Name/Signature ________________________________

Courtesy of Sally Sturgeon, DNP, RN, SANE-A, AFN-BC.

Appendix 11. Signs and Symptoms of Strangulation

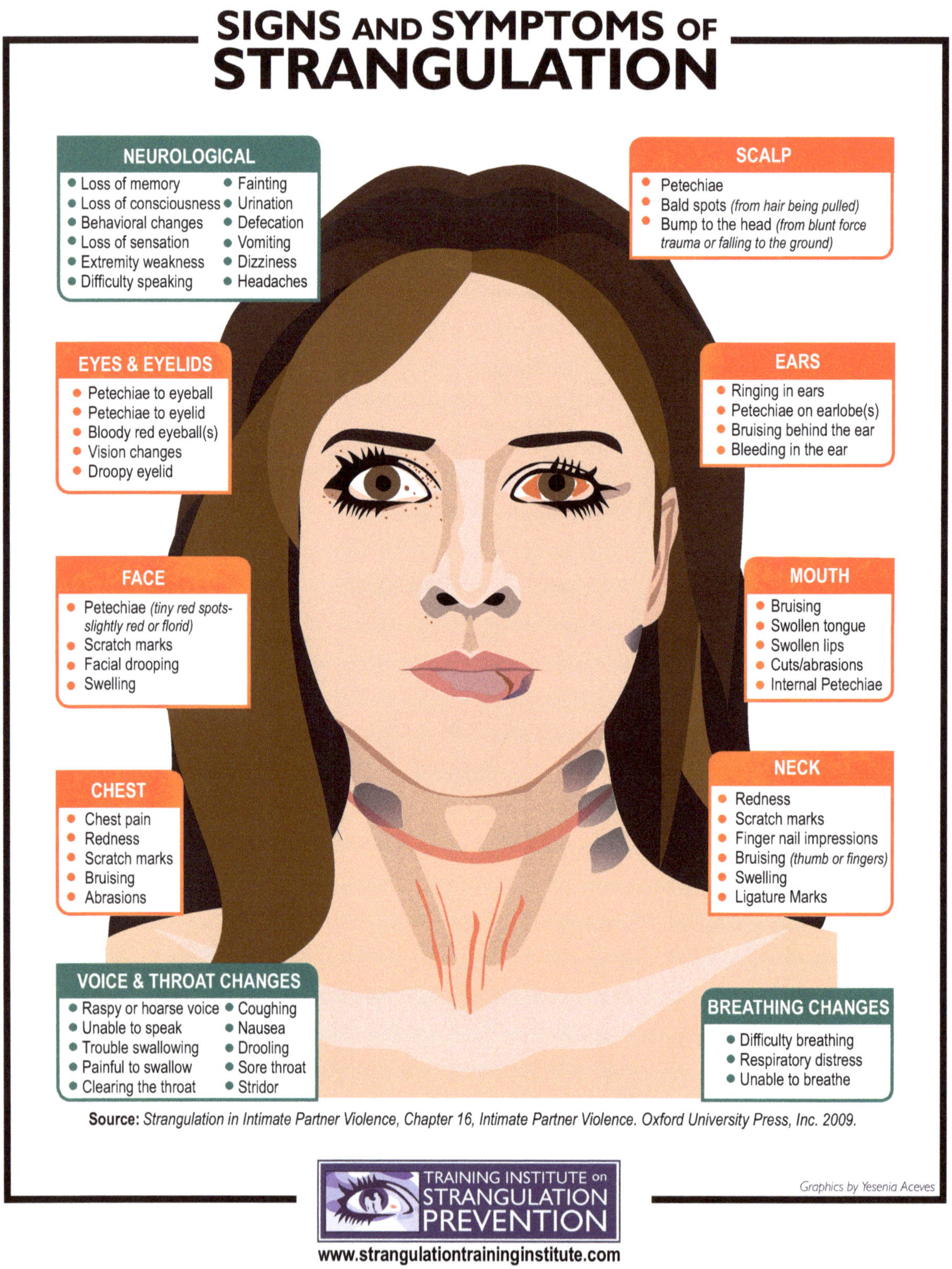

Reprinted with permission from Training Institute on Strangulation Prevention.

Appendix 12. Strangulation Injuries

Appendix Table 2. Strangulation Injuries

Signs and Symptoms		Location and Type	
Breathing	**Behavioral**	**Face**	**Under chin**
— Difficulty breathing	— Restlessness	— Red, flushed	— Redness
— Hyperventilation	— Agitation	— Petechiae	— Bruising
— Coughing	— Combativeness	— Abrasions	— Abrasions
— Unable to breathe	— Memory loss	— Bloody nose	**Ear**
Voice	— Hallucinations	**Mouth**	— Petechiae
— Unable to speak	— Acute posttraumatic stress syndrome	— Bruising	— Ruptured ear drum
— Raspy voice	**Other**	— Swelling of tongue/lips	— Bruising behind ear
— Hoarseness	— Dizziness	— Petechiae	**Head**
— Pain with speaking	— Headaches	**Neck**	— Petechiae
Swallowing	— Loss of consciousness	— Redness	— Pulled hair
— Difficulty swallowing	— Incontinence of urine	— Bruising	— Swelling
— Pain with swallowing	— Incontinence of stool	— Abrasions	**Chest/Shoulders**
— Neck pain	— Nausea/vomiting	— Swelling	— Redness
		— Ligature mark	— Bruising
		Eyes/Eyelids	— Abrasions
		— Petechiae	
		— Blood-red eyes	

Courtesy of Ruth Downing, MSN, RN, CNP, SANE-A and Forensic Healthcare Consulting; Delaware, Ohio.

Appendix 13. Nonfatal Strangulation in the "Walking and Talking" Patient

Nonfatal Strangulation in the "Walking and Talking" Patient

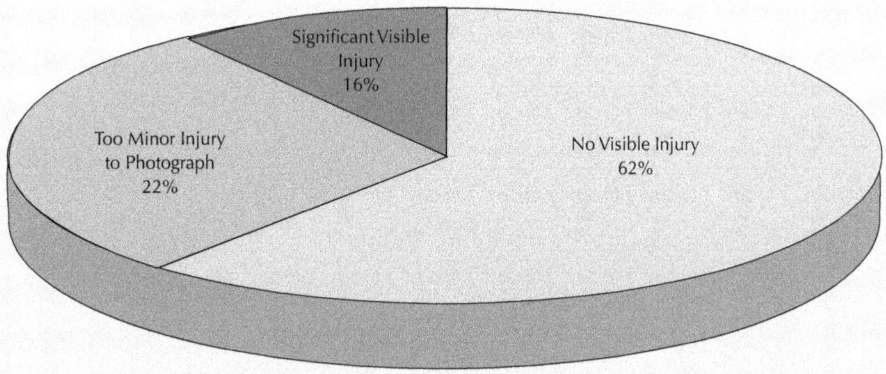

Adapted from Strack GB, McClane GE, 1990.

Appendix 14. Physiological Consequences of Strangulation Occlusion of Arterial Blood Flow: Seconds to Minutes Timeline

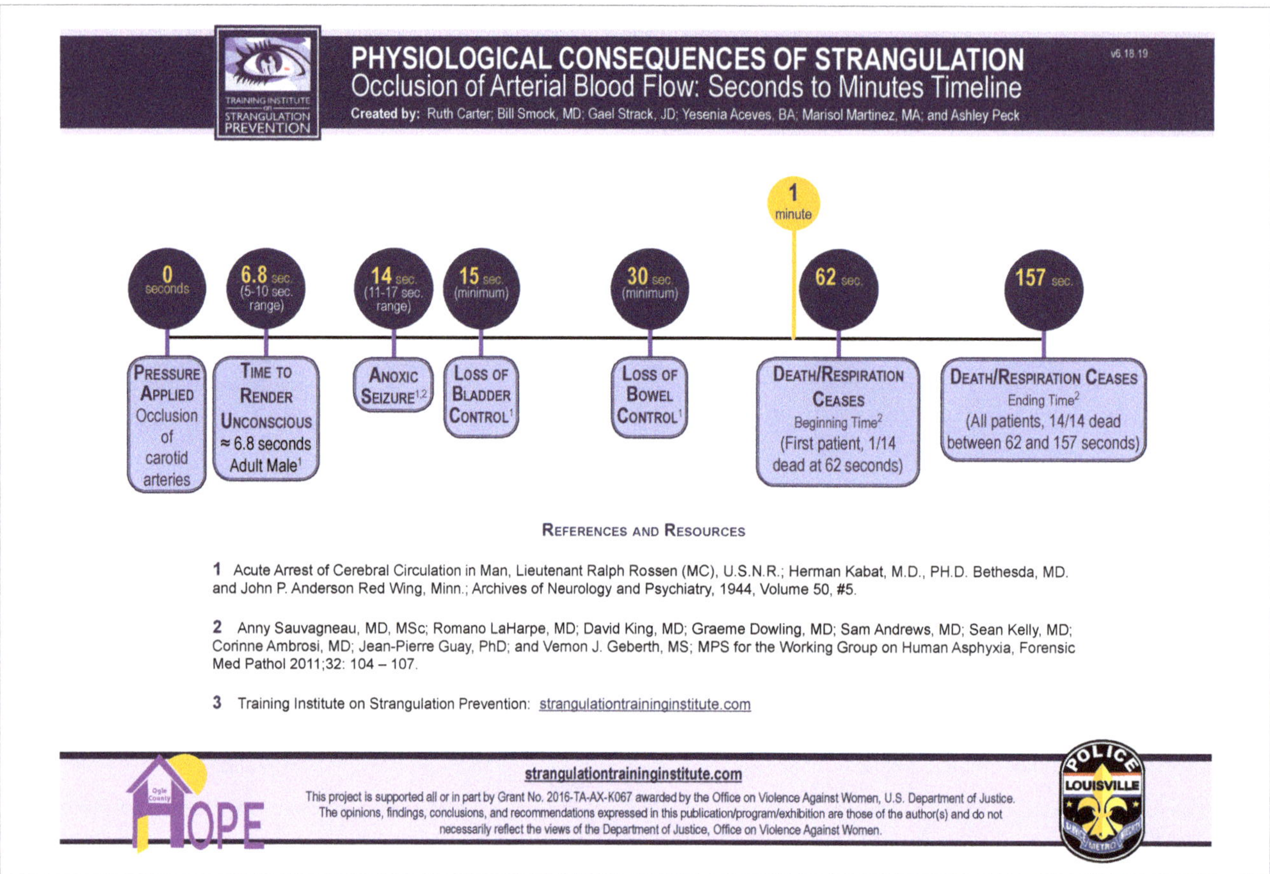

Appendix 15. Common Procedural Technology (CPT) Codes

Appendix Table 3. CPT Codes

Code	Description
R05	Cough
R06	Abnormality of breathing
R07	Pain in throat/chest
R51	Headache
R52	Generalized pain
R55	Syncope
R60.0	Localized edema
R64.84	Jaw pain
S00-09	Injury to head
S10-19	Injury to neck
T74	Codes must be confirmed — Assault/strangulation/abuses
T71	Asphyxiation, unspecified — A-initial — D-repeat visit — S-subsequent visits
T71.9	Strangulation — A/D/S

Appendix 16. Petechial Hemorrhage Challenge

The pathophysiology and forensic science of petechial hemorrhage development can be difficult to understand and even more difficult to explain to a jury. This "challenge" exercise goes deep into the science, medicine, and physiology of petechial hemorrhages in an effort to assist you in explaining how petechial hemorrhages are created, how someone can be fatally or nonfatally strangled and have no petechial hemorrhages, and how blood flows into and out of the head and neck.

Are You Ready for the "Petechial Hemorrhage Court Challenge?

(Answer these questions as if you were on the stand. Remember that responding "I don't know" is perfectly appropriate. Do not render an opinion unless you are confident of the medicine and science behind your opinion.)

1. What are petechial hemorrhages?
2. What part of the circulatory system is involved in the development of petechial hemorrhages?
3. What are the 2 physiologic events required to create petechial hemorrhages?
4. How often are petechial hemorrhages documented in nonfatal strangulation?
5. What are your medical references?
6. Describe the arterial blood flow to the head/brain.
7. Describe the venous blood flow from the head/brain.
8. What percentage of blood flow to the head/brain is contributed by the carotid arteries?
9. What percentage of blood flow to the head/brain is contributed by the vertebral arteries?
10. How much pressure (PSI) is required to occlude a jugular vein?
11. What is your medical reference?
12. How much pressure (PSI) is required to occlude a carotid artery?
13. What is your medical reference?
14. How much pressure (PSI) is required to occlude a vertebral artery?
15. What is your medical reference?
16. How much time is required to create facial petechial hemorrhage associated with strangulation?
17. Can you be strangled unconscious and have no petechial hemorrhages?
18. If yes, please explain under what circumstances you can be strangled unconscious and have no petechial hemorrhages.
19. How much time is required for external petechial hemorrhages to resolve?
20. Is the pathophysiology of petechial hemorrhage development different in a strangulation versus a hanging?
21. What is a "complete" hanging?

22. What is an "incomplete" hanging?

23. What is positional asphyxia?

24. In a case of positional asphyxia, where on the body can you see petechial hemorrhages?

25. What is the pathophysiology of how petechiae are created in positional asphyxia?

26. Would you expect to see more or less facial petechial hemorrhages in a complete hanging versus an incomplete hanging?

27. Explain why the incidence of petechial hemorrhages increases or decreases with complete hangings.

28. What is a "pale" hanging?

29. What percentage of hangings are pale hangings?

30. What are your medical references?

31. What are Tardieu spots?

32. Can Tardieu spots be present in deaths not associated with hanging or strangulation?

33. What are some causes of petechiae, other than strangulation?

34. Can petechial hemorrhages be associated with CPR?

35. What does the medical literature say with regard to the maximum number of petechial hemorrhages associated with CPR?

36. What is meant by "florid" facial petechial hemorrhage?

37. What is the pathophysiology of florid petechial hemorrhage in nonfatal or fatal strangulation?

38. When you observe florid petechial hemorrhages, what can you say regarding the circumstances of their development?

39. What are visceral petechial hemorrhages?

40. If petechial hemorrhages are present externally, are petechial hemorrhages always present internally?

41. Do vertebral arteries provide "significant" blood flow to the brain?

42. What parts of the brain are primarily supplied by the vertebral arteries?

43. If sufficient anterior lateral pressure (>11 pounds) is applied to the neck, sufficient to occlude the carotid arteries, will the jugular veins also be occluded?

44. Please explain your answer.

45. Can the vertebral arteries be occluded from the application of external pressure?

46. If yes, describe the anatomic location(s) where external pressure can occlude blood flow to the brain via the vertebral arteries.

47. If both the carotid and vertebral arteries were occluded, would you expect to see the development of petechial hemorrhages in the face?

48. Please explain your answer.

49. Define collateral arterial circulation within the brain.

50. Is there collateral circulation within the brain between the carotid and vertebral arteries?

51. Which arteries provide collateral circulation within the brain?

52. Would there be increased blood flow to the brain, via the vertebral arteries, if the carotid arteries were completely occluded?

53. Please explain your answer.

54. What is the name of the syndrome involving collateral circulation of the upper extremity via the vertebral arteries in order to perfuse the arm?

55. Can you describe the collateral blood circulation associated with this syndrome?

56. Would you expect petechial hemorrhages to develop if the carotid arteries and jugular veins are completely occluded bilaterally (30+ seconds) and the vertebral arteries are open?

57. Please explain your answer.

58. Would you expect petechial hemorrhages to develop if only 1 carotid artery was occluded?

59. Please explain your answer.

60. Are petechial hemorrhages required to prove that either fatal or nonfatal strangulation has occurred?

61. Please explain your answer.

Developed and researched by:

MaKayla Campbell, BS
University of Louisville School of Medicine
Louisville, Kentucky

Shelby Easley, BS
University of Kentucky College of Medicine
Lexington, Kentucky

Bill Smock, MD
Police Surgeon
Louisville Metro Police Department
Louisville, Kentucky

Beth Fitzgerald-Weekley, RN, BSN, SANE-A
Professional Forensic Services, LLC
Salt Lake City, Utah

Petechial Hemorrhage Challenge Answer Key

1. *What are petechial hemorrhages?*

   Petechial hemorrhages are ruptured capillaries from increased venous pressure. Petechial hemorrhages are nonblanching and nonpalpable.

2. *What part of the circulatory system is involved in the development of petechial hemorrhages?*

   Capillaries

3. *What are the 2 physiologic events required to create petechial hemorrhages?*

   Increased venous pressure from obstructed venous outflow with continued arterial inflow

4. *How often are petechial hemorrhages documented in nonfatal strangulation?*

   22% to 25% of cases

5. *What are your medical references?*

   Johnson J. Non-fatal strangulation: client presentation without physical injury. Maryville University, 2017.

   Shields LBE, Corey TS, Weakley-Jones B, Stewart D. Living victims of strangulation: a 10-year review of cases in a metropolitan community. *Am J Forensic Med Pathol.* 2010;31(4):320-325.

6. *Describe the arterial blood flow to the head/brain.*

   There are 2 sets of arteries that supply blood to the brain: common carotid arteries (70% to 80% of blood flow to the brain) and vertebral arteries (20% to 30% of blood flow to the brain). The common carotid arteries begin at the aorta. The right common carotid is a branch from the brachiocephalic artery attached to the aorta, and the left common carotid is directly attached to the aorta. The common carotids on each side run into the neck, then bifurcate at the superior edge of the laryngeal cartilage and into the internal and external carotid arteries. The internal carotid arteries supply the anterior and medial aspects of the brain, and the vertebral arteries supply the posterior cortex. The vertebral arteries arise from the subclavian arteries that run superiorly through the transverse processes of the C6-C1, ultimately coming together to form the basilar artery.[5,6]

7. *Describe the venous blood flow from the head/brain.*

   The 2 sets of veins responsible for most of the venous blood flow from the head/brain are the internal and external jugular veins. The internal jugular veins run on the lateral aspects of the neck alongside the common carotid arteries, while the smaller external jugular veins run superficial to the sternocleidomastoid muscle.

8. *What percentage of blood flow to the head/brain is contributed by the carotid arteries?*

   70% to 80%[7]

9. *What percentage of blood flow to the head/brain is contributed by the vertebral arteries?*

   20% to 30%[7]

10. *How much pressure (PSI) is required to occlude a jugular vein?*

    4.4 PSI

11. *What is your medical reference?*

    Brouardel P. *La Pendaison, La Strangulation, La Suffocation, La Submersion.* Paris, France: Librairie JB Baillière et fils; 1897.

12. *How much pressure (PSI) is required to occlude a carotid artery?*

    11 to 13.2 PSI

13. *What is your medical reference?*

    Brouardel P. *La Pendaison, La Strangulation, La Suffocation, La Submersion.* Paris, France: Librairie JB Baillière et fils; 1897.

    Yamasaki S, Takase I, Takada N, Nishi K. Measurement of force to obstruct the cervical arteries and distribution of tension exerted on a ligature hanging. *Leg Med (Tokyo).* 2009;11(4):175-180.

14. *How much pressure (PSI) is required to occlude a vertebral artery?*

    15 to 66.1 PSI

15. *What is your medical reference?*

    DiPoce J, Guelfguat M, DiPoce J. Radiologic findings in cases of attempted suicide and other self-injurious behavior. *Radiographics.* 2012;32(7):2005-2024.

    Yamasaki S, Takase I, Takada N, Nishi K. Measurement of force to obstruct the cervical arteries and distribution of tension exerted on a ligature hanging. *Leg Med (Tokyo).* 2009;11(4):175-180.

16. *How much time is required to create facial petechial hemorrhage associated with strangulation?*

    Ten to 20 seconds of back pressure[8] or 10 to 30 seconds of back pressure.[9]

    Blunt force trauma, forceful vomiting, and forceful coughing can create petechial hemorrhage immediately. Petechial hemorrhages associated with strangulation are from a gradual buildup of venous pressure with continued arterial inflow.

17. *Can you be strangled unconscious and have no petechial hemorrhages?*

    Yes[10,11]

18. *If yes, please explain under what circumstances you can be strangled unconscious and have no petechial hemorrhages.*

    — Based on the 1943 Rossen et al[10] study, an adult male can be rendered unconscious in the range of 4 to 10 seconds (average 6.8 seconds) of obstructive pressure to the carotid and vertebral arteries. Therefore, you can be rendered unconscious before there was sufficient venous pressure to create petechial hemorrhages.

    — If 100% of the arterial inflow to the head is obstructed by compression of both the carotid and vertebral arteries, then there is no increased venous pressure because there is no arterial inflow and therefore no petechial hemorrhages.[11]

19. *How much time is required for external petechial hemorrhages to resolve?*

    Resolution depends on the concentration and anatomic location of the hemorrhages. According Plattner et al,[12] 1 day. Clinical experience indicates 48 to 72 hours in the skin or mouth and days to weeks in the sclera.

20. *Is the pathophysiology of petechial hemorrhage development different in a strangulation versus a hanging?*

    The pathophysiology is the same in strangulation and hanging. Both mechanisms involve blocking the venous return from the head/brain (most commonly the jugular vein) and continued arterial inflow to the head/brain.

21. *What is a "complete" hanging?*

    A hanging with the full body weight suspended by the ligature (ie, no part of the body is touching the ground)

22. *What is an "incomplete" hanging?*

    A hanging without the full body weight suspended by the ligature (ie, feet, legs, bottom touching the ground)

23. *What is positional asphyxia?*

    Positional asphyxia occurs when the body is immobilized in a certain position or when the application of external pressure to the chest, neck, and/or abdomen prevents adequate ventilation, resulting in death from hypoxia and hypercarbia.

24. *In a case of positional asphyxia, where on the body can you see petechial hemorrhages?*

    Petechial hemorrhages can be seen anywhere in the body depending on where and how the ability to respire was compromised. Pressure on the chest and abdomen can restrict blood return to the superior vena cava and cause petechial hemorrhages in the upper chest. Visceral petechial hemorrhages are common in positional asphyxia.

25. *What is the pathophysiology of how petechiae are created in positional asphyxia?*

    Increased venous pressure from blockage of venous return with continued arterial inflow results in capillary rupture. Petechial hemorrhages can be seen anywhere in the body depending on where and how the ability to respire was compromised. Pushing during childbirth results in increased intrathoracic and intra-abdominal pressure, which can cause petechiae in the chest, neck, or face.

26. *Would you expect to see more or less facial petechial hemorrhages in a complete hanging versus an incomplete hanging?*

    The incidence of petechial hemorrhages is much less with complete hangings (**Appendix Table 4**). Almost all pale hangings are complete hangings.[13-15]

Appendix Table 4. Partial Versus Full Suspension with Associated Findings

Category	Number (%)	Category	Number (%)
Partial suspensions	**191 (83.41)**	**Full suspensions**	**38 (16.59)**
Male adults	144 (75.39)	Male adults	28 (73.68)
Female adults	25 (13.09)	Female adults	5 (13.16)
Male children	16 (3.14)	Male children	4 (10.53)
Female children	6 (3.14)	Female children	1 (2.63)
Acute neck injury	32 (16.75)	Acute neck injury	0 (0.00)
Petechial hemorrhages	77 (40.31)	Petechial hemorrhages	6 (15.79)

27. *Explain why the incidence of petechial hemorrhages increases or decreases with complete hangings.*

    As weight, and therefore pressure, increases on the ligature, the probability of occluding both the carotid and vertebral arteries increases. In a complete hanging, the victim's entire body weight is suspended by the ligature. The pressure created by the full body weight would increase the likelihood of compressing both the carotid and vertebral arteries. If all blood flow is prevented from reaching the brain, intravascular venous pressure cannot increase. Therefore, complete hanging victims are less likely to show signs of venous congestion than incomplete hanging victims. In an incomplete hanging, the vertebral arteries are less likely to be compressed, which increases the probability of petechiae development.[11,13-15]

28. *What is a "pale" hanging?*

    A pale hanging is a hanging in which there is no venous congestion and no petechial hemorrhages. A pale hanging occurs when both the carotid and vertebral arteries are occluded, resulting in no arterial inflow into the head.[11]

    Petechiae are more common in partial hangings. In full suspension, usually both the arteries and veins are obstructed, and no blood flow goes in or out of the head. Petechiae are much less likely in such cases. Often, the face of the victim is pale. In our case review, there were more petechial hemorrhages in the partial suspension population, 77 out of 191 (40.31%), compared to 6 out of 38 (15.79%) in the full suspension population.[16]

29. *What percentage of hangings are pale hangings?*

    4% to 16%

30. *What are your medical references?*

    Dean DE, Kohler LJ, Sterbenz GCS, et al. Observed characteristics of suicidal hangings: an 11-year retrospective review. *J Forensic Sci.* 2012;57(5):1226-1230.

    Gill JR, Cavalli DP, Ely SF, Stahl-Herz J. Homicidal neck compression of females: autopsy and sexual assault findings. *Acad Forensic Pathol.* 2013;3(4):454-457.

31. *What are Tardieu spots?*

    Tardieu spots are purple to black capillary ruptures caused by increased pressure. They can occur in strangulation or from postmortem lividity throughout the body. They are also called Tardieu ecchymoses and Tardieu petechiae. They are named after the French forensic physician Auguste Tardieu (1818 to 1879), who incorrectly considered them pathognomonic for strangulation or suffocation.[11,17,18]

32. *Can Tardieu spots be present in deaths not associated with hanging or strangulation?*

    Yes, postmortem venous pooling, especially in the scalp, can create Tardieu spots.

33. *What are other causes of petechiae, other than strangulation?*

    Blunt force trauma, weightlifting, sneezing, forceful laughing, forceful vomiting, forceful coughing, Valsalva maneuver, seizures, childbirth, scuba diving, sky diving, and infections can also create petechial hemorrhage.[19]

34. *Can petechial hemorrhages be associated with CPR?*

    Yes

35. *What does the medical literature say with regard to the maximum number of petechial hemorrhages associated with CPR?*

    One to a maximum of 9 hemorrhages[20]

36. *What is meant by "florid" facial petechial hemorrhage?*

    This refers to massive petechial hemorrhages of the entire face.

37. *What is the pathophysiology of florid petechial hemorrhage in nonfatal or fatal strangulation?*

    The carotid arteries and jugular veins are blocked while blood in the vertebral arteries continues to flow into the head and brain. As collateral circulation allows blood to reach the small vessels throughout the face while venous pressure continues to build, these capillaries all over the face and neck will burst. Florid petechiae are found above the area where the pressure was applied.

38. *When you observe florid petechial hemorrhages, what can you say regarding the circumstances of their development?*

    Victims who demonstrate florid petechiae are either dead or have been rendered unconscious. The development of florid petechial hemorrhages requires a significant amount of venous back pressure from a prolonged period of neck pressure.

39. *What are visceral petechial hemorrhages?*

    Petechiae found on internal organs

40. *If petechial hemorrhages are present externally, are petechial hemorrhages always present internally?*

    No, the development of petechiae in any organ system depends on the duration of venous obstruction and the amount of arterial inflow.

41. *Do vertebral arteries provide "significant" blood flow to the brain?*

    Yes[21]

42. *What parts of the brain are primarily supplied by the vertebral arteries?*

    The vertebral arteries are the primary blood supply to the posterior circulation of the brain and supply the upper spinal cord, the brain stem, the midbrain, and the cerebellum. The vertebral arteries supply to multiple areas of the brain including the basilar artery, posterior inferior cerebellar artery (PICA), anterior inferior cerebellar artery (AICA), pontine branches, superior cerebellar artery (SCA), posterior cerebral artery (PCA), and the posterior communicating artery.[22]

43. *If sufficient anterior lateral pressure (>11 pounds) is applied to the neck, sufficient to occlude the carotid arteries, will the jugular veins also be occluded?*

    Yes, "Only 4.4 pounds of pressure is necessary to occlude the jugular veins, and they lie adjacent to the carotids, in virtually every case that the carotids are occluded, the jugular veins are also occluded."[11]

44. *Can you please explain your answer?*

    The internal jugular vein is immediately lateral to the carotid artery. When more than 11 pounds of pressure is applied to the lateral neck, both the jugular vein and the carotid artery will be blocked (**Appendix Figure 14**).[11]

45. *Can the vertebral arteries be occluded from the application of external pressure?*

    Yes

46. *If yes, describe the anatomic location(s) where external pressure can occlude blood flow to the brain via the vertebral arteries.*

    Subclavian Arteries: The apparatus created for the 1943 Rossen et al[10] study was designed to occlude both the carotid and vertebral arteries. The

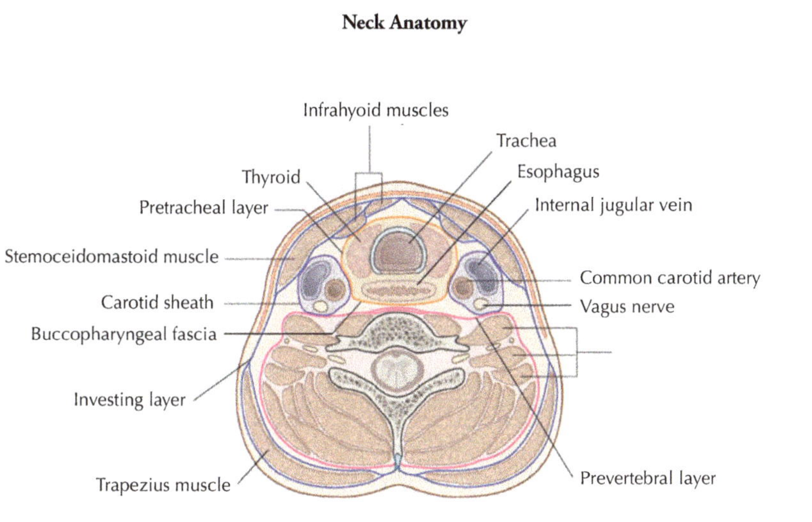

Appendix Figure 14

Appendix Figure 14. *The jugular veins are immediately lateral to the carotid artery. When more than 11 pounds of pressure are applied to the lateral neck, both the jugular vein and carotid artery will be occluded.*

apparatus applied pressure over the subclavian arteries, blocking blood flow into the subclavian and vertebral arteries. The physician in the Rossen study documented how blockage of the subclavian and carotid arteries prevented the development of venous congestion.

Vertebral Arteries: When a ligature applies lateral pressure on the neck, in between the transverse processes of the cervical spine, the ligature can occlude the vertebral arteries. This would create "pale hanging" or "pale strangulation." Application of a "rear naked choke" with pressure on the anterior and lateral aspect of the neck can also occlude 100% of blood flow to the brain from pressure on the carotid and vertebral arteries (**Appendix Figure 15-a** and **b**).

47. *If both the carotid and vertebral arteries were occluded, would you expect to see the development of petechial hemorrhages in the face?*

    No

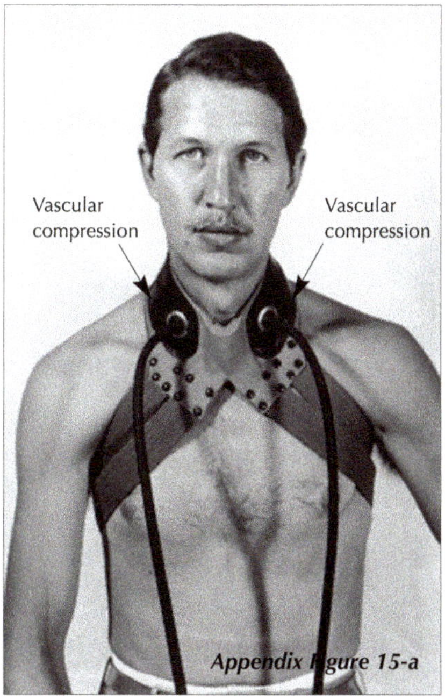

Appendix Figure 15-a

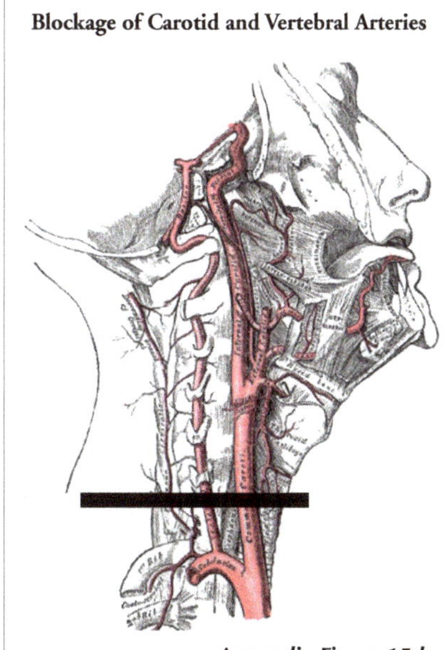

Appendix Figure 15-b

Appendix Figure 15-a. *Vascular compression occluding both carotid and vertebral arteries as demonstrated from the Rossen study.*

Appendix Figure 15-b. *Pressure at the base of the neck can result in bilateral blockage of both the carotid and vertebral arteries. Blockage of both arteries completely blocks blood flow to the brain.*

48. Please explain your answer.

Occlusion of both the carotid and vertebral arteries will result in a "pale hanging" or "pale strangulation" with no petechial hemorrhages.[11,23]

49. Define collateral arterial circulation within the brain.

Collateral arterial circulation is the alternative circulation around a blocked artery. Blood, like any fluid under pressure, always flows from high pressure to low pressure. In the brain, blood flows into the circle of Willis from the carotid and basilar arteries. When the carotid arteries are blocked the vertebral arteries will shunt blood via the Circle of Willis to the arteries in the face. This arterial blood flow, in concert with the occlusion of the jugular veins, meets the physiological requirements for the development of ocular and facial petechial hemorrhages. The communicating arteries in the circle of Willis will shunt blood to an area of low pressure (**Appendix Figure 16**).

Cerebral Artery Anatomy

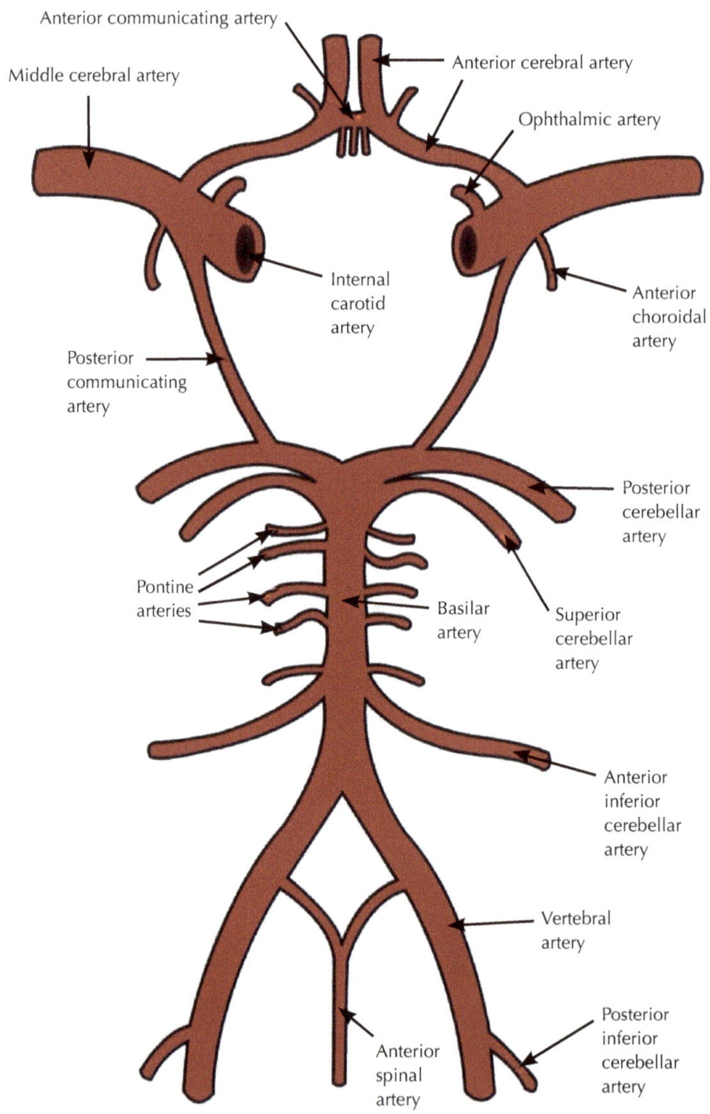

Appendix Figure 16

Appendix Figure 16. *Cerebral artery anatomy.*

50. *Is there collateral circulation within the brain between the carotid and vertebral arteries?*

Yes, if during strangulation the carotid arteries are blocked, the communicating arteries will shunt blood from the vertebral arteries to the face and ophthalmic arteries (**Appendix Figure 17**). This is the mechanism for the development of petechial hemorrhages. [24,25]

Blockage of Carotid Arteries

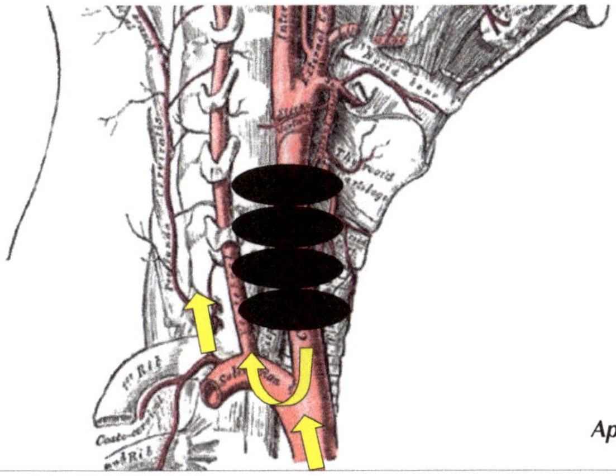

Appendix Figure 17

Appendix Figure 17. *Finger pressure blocking the carotid artery results in the shunting of blood via the vertebral arteries. This is also called "collateral circulation" of blood flow to the brain.*

51. *Which arteries provide collateral circulation within the brain?*

The arteries that form and contribute flow to the circle of Willis

52. *Would there be increased blood flow to the brain, via the vertebral arteries, if the carotid arteries were completely occluded?*

Yes

53. *Please explain your answer.*

The body's mean arterial pressure will not change with occlusion of the carotid arteries. Because of the pressure created by the heart, blood will be shunted via the vertebral arteries to the areas of the brain with low pressure (ie, the areas usually supplied by the carotids).

54. *What is the name of the syndrome involving collateral circulation of the upper extremity via the vertebral arteries in order to perfuse the arm?*

Subclavian steal syndrome (**Appendix Figure 18**)

55. *Can you describe the collateral blood circulation associated with this syndrome?*

In subclavian steal syndrome, the subclavian artery is occluded and blood is shunted via the vertebral artery to the low-pressure area in the subclavian artery.

56. *Would you expect petechial hemorrhages to develop if the carotid arteries and jugular veins are completely occluded bilaterally (30+ seconds) and the vertebral arteries are open?*

Yes

57. *Please explain your answer.*

Collateral circulation from the vertebral arteries to the basilar artery to the circle of Willis would provide the needed arterial inflow to increase the pressure within the capillary bed to create petechial hemorrhages on the face.

58. *Would you expect petechial hemorrhages to develop if only 1 carotid artery was occluded?*

No

Appendix Figure 18. *When the subclavian artery is blocked, blood flows to the arm via collateral flow in the vertebral arteries. Fluid under pressure will always flow from high pressure to low pressure.*

Subclavian Steal Syndrome

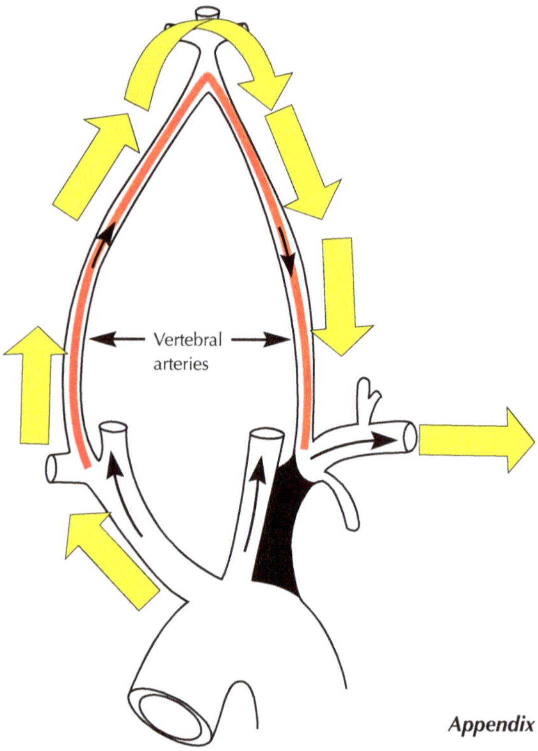

Appendix Figure 18

59. *Please explain your answer.*

    Collateral circulation from the open carotid and vertebral arteries and the jugular vein would provide relatively normal blood flow to the brain. This is the same anatomic and physiologic situation that occurs when someone has unilateral carotid stenosis.

60. *Are petechial hemorrhages required to prove that either fatal or nonfatal strangulation has occurred?*

    No

61. *Please explain your answer.*

    The definition of strangulation is the occlusion of air flow, blood flow, or both because of the application of external pressure on the neck. The development of petechial hemorrhages is dependent on a sufficient period of time of venous obstruction to create increased venous pressure in the capillaries from the compression of a vein, in the neck or the jugular, for the vessels to rupture. There must also be continued arterial inflow into the capillary beds to increase the pressure. The literature states somewhere between 10 and 30 seconds of increased venous back pressure is required. Based on the Rossen et al[10] study, an adult male can be rendered unconscious in less than 10 seconds of continual pressure. If more than 10 seconds is required, someone could be strangled and rendered unconscious and have had insufficient time to develop enough back pressure to create petechial hemorrhage. Pressure on the trachea can occlude the airway, without any vascular involvement, and there will never be petechial hemorrhage, yet the victim was clearly strangled. If 100% of the blood flow to the head via the carotid and vertebral arteries is blocked, pale fatal or nonfatal strangulation will occur. In summary, you can be fatally or nonfatally strangled and never develop a single petechial hemorrhage.

Appendix 17. Power and Control Wheel

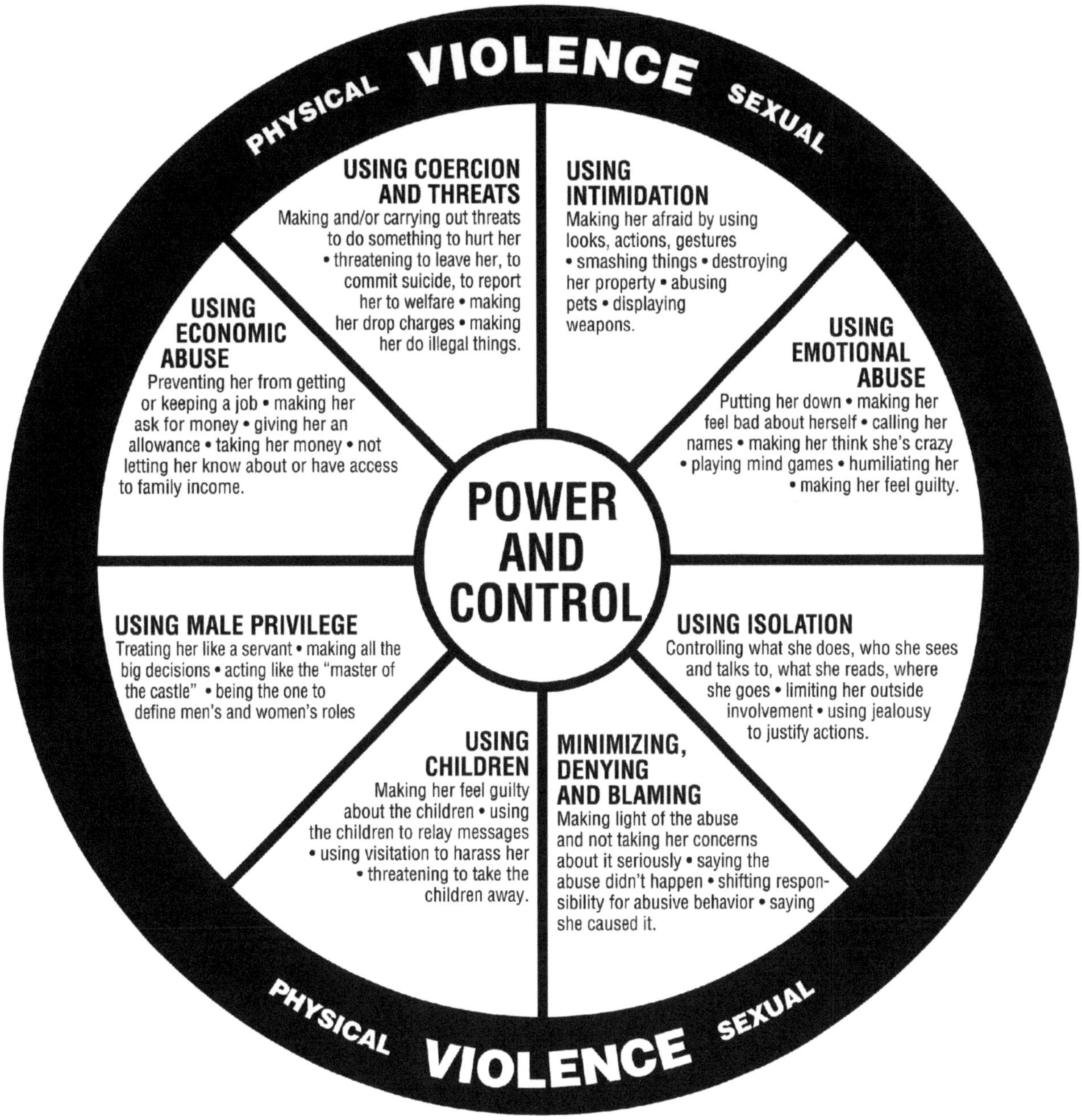
PHYSICAL
VIOLENCE
SEXUAL
USING COERCION AND THREATS
Making and/or carrying out threats to do something to hurt her • threatening to leave her, to commit suicide, to report her to welfare • making her drop charges • making her do illegal things.
USING INTIMIDATION
Making her afraid by using looks, actions, gestures • smashing things • destroying her property • abusing pets • displaying weapons.
USING ECONOMIC ABUSE
Preventing her from getting or keeping a job • making her ask for money • giving her an allowance • taking her money • not letting her know about or have access to family income.
USING EMOTIONAL ABUSE
Putting her down • making her feel bad about herself • calling her names • making her think she's crazy • playing mind games • humiliating her • making her feel guilty.
POWER AND CONTROL
USING MALE PRIVILEGE
Treating her like a servant • making all the big decisions • acting like the "master of the castle" • being the one to define men's and women's roles
USING ISOLATION
Controlling what she does, who she sees and talks to, what she reads, where she goes • limiting her outside involvement • using jealousy to justify actions.
USING CHILDREN
Making her feel guilty about the children • using the children to relay messages • using visitation to harass her • threatening to take the children away.
MINIMIZING, DENYING AND BLAMING
Making light of the abuse and not taking her concerns about it seriously • saying the abuse didn't happen • shifting responsibility for abusive behavior • saying she caused it.
PHYSICAL
VIOLENCE
SEXUAL

DOMESTIC ABUSE INTERVENTION PROGRAMS
202 East Superior Street
Duluth, Minnesota 55802
218-722-2781
www.theduluthmodel.org

Appendix 18. ICD-10 Codes

The World Health Organization (WHO) compiled a system of coding that is used internationally for filing health insurance claims in systems of care that depend on reimbursement and for tracking diseases, disorders, injuries, and morbidity/mortality statistics. ICD-10 stands for International Statistical Classification of Diseases and Related Health Problems and is currently in its eleventh revision.[26] ICD-10 is an alphanumeric coding system that uses as few as 3 to as many as 7 characters to represent an "objective story" about how and why a patient presents for health care. For more specifics about ICD-10 coding, a good reference is the WHO ICD-10 Training Tool.[27]

ICD-10 categories are separated into codes from A through Z[28]:

A00-B99: Certain infectious and parasitic diseases

C00-D49: Neoplasms

D50-D89: Diseases of the blood and blood-forming organs and certain disorders involving the immune mechanism

E00-E89: Endocrine, nutritional, and metabolic diseases

F01-F99: Mental, behavioral, and neurodevelopmental disorders

G00-G99: Diseases of the nervous system

H00-H59: Diseases of the eye and adnexa

H60-H95: Diseases of the ear and mastoid process

I00-I99: Diseases of the circulatory system

J00-J99: Diseases of the respiratory system

K00-K95: Diseases of the digestive system

L00-L99: Diseases of the skin and subcutaneous tissue

M00-M99: Diseases of the musculoskeletal system and connective tissue

N00-N99: Diseases of the genitourinary system

O00-O9A: Pregnancy, childbirth, and the puerperium

P00-P96: Certain conditions originating in the perinatal period

Q00-Q99: Congenital malformations, deformations, and chromosomal abnormalities

R00-R99: Symptoms, signs, and abnormal clinical and laboratory findings, not elsewhere classified

S00-T88: Injury, poisoning, and certain other consequences of external causes

V00-Y99: External causes of morbidity

Z00-Z99: Factors influencing health status and contact with health services

The first 3 characters represent disease, disorder, injury, infection, or symptomology. The additional 4 to 6 characters provide increasingly specific information about body site (eg, right breast, upper outer quadrant). A 3-character code can stand alone if additional specificity is not needed (**Appendix Table 5** Examples A and B).

Appendix Table 5. Examples of ICD-10 Codes

Category			Dot	Specificity			
Letter	Digit	Digit	Dot	Digit	Digit	Digit	Letter
Example A: Headache							
R	5	1					
Example B: Overnight Observation, Report of Strangulation							
Z	0	4					
Example C: Open Bite of Breast							
S	2	0	.	1	7		
Example D: Open Bite of Vulva, Initial Visit							
S	3	0	.	8	7	4	A
Example E: Retained Condom in Vagina, Initial Visit							
T	1	9	.	2	X	X	A
Example F: Open Bite of Vulva, Follow-Up Visit							
S	3	0	.	8	7	4	D
Example G: Open Bite of Vulva, Sequelae							
S	3	0	.	8	7	4	S

The seventh character provides information about initial versus subsequent visits and additional sequela.[26] This seventh character can only be used in the seventh position. If the initial codes are less than 6 characters, an "x" is used as a placeholder for each position that is not required for the initial code. This seventh code is primarily used to capture details in injuries, consequences of external causes, and pregnancy-related conditions[26] (**Appendix Table 5** Example C). An initial visit uses "A" for the seventh character (**Appendix Table 5** Example D and E); if this was an additional visit after the acute care period, "D" is used for the seventh character. (**Appendix Table 5** Example G).[26]

The website www.ICD10Data.com allows you to search by key terms and gives directions for increasing the specificity of certain situations. For example, the search term "sore throat" directs to R07.0, which is titled "pain in throat" but also gives additional options to consider, including acute versus chronic, difficulty swallowing, and neck pain.[28] (Use of online ICD-10 coding sites allows for keyword text search for assistance in appropriate coding.) If a patient reports strangulation with throat pain and a contusion, the following codes are available for use:

- — R07.0: Pain in throat
- — S10.0XXA: Contusion of throat
- — S10.14XA: External constriction of part of throat
- — Z04.71: Overnight observation for alleged physical abuse of adult to rule out possible sequelae of strangulation
- — Z65.4: Victim of crime
- — Z65.8: Specified problem related to psychosocial issues, domestic violence

Appendix Table 6 shows more examples of ICD-10 code listings.

Appendix Table 6. Examples of ICD-10 Code Listings for Forensic Patients (Not All Inclusive)

R00-R99: SYMPTOMS, SIGNS, AND ABNORMAL CLINICAL FINDINGS

R05: Cough
R06: Abnormality of breathing
R07: Pain in throat
R51: Headache
R55: Syncope
R60: Localized edema

S00-T88: INJURY TO BODY REGION(S) OR CONSEQUENCES OF EXTERNAL CAUSES

S00-S99: Injuries to specific body regions
T07-T14: Injuries in multiple body regions or unspecified regions
T20-T32: Burns
T36-T65: Poisoning: drugs, medications, biological substances, nonmedicinal substances
T71: Asphyxiation
T74-T76: Abuse, neglect, maltreatment (confirmed versus suspected); adult and/or child
T79: Complications of trauma, not otherwise classified

V00-X58: ENVIRONMENTAL EVENTS, ACCIDENTS, EXPOSURE

V00-V97: Transportation accidents
W00-W19: Slip, trip, stumble, falls
X71-X83: Intentional self-harm

X92-Y33: ASSAULT

X93-X95: Firearm related
X99-Y00: Assault by objects
Y04: Assault by bodily force (fight, bite, strike, other)
Y07: Perpetrator of assault, maltreatment, neglect
Y08-Y09: Assault by other means
Y21-Y33: Undetermined event: specific documentation that intent cannot be determined

Z CODES: REASONS FOR ENCOUNTERS OF HEALTH SERVICES

Z04: Examination/observation for other reasons
Z13: Screening for other disorders
Z18: Retained foreign body/fragments
Z20: Contact/suspected exposure to communicable disease
Z29.8: Encounter for other prophylactic measures (must specify in chart)
Z30.012: Encounter for prescription of emergency contraception
Z53: Encounter for procedure/treatment, not carried out (declined examination)
Z55-Z65: Hazards related to socioeconomic and psychosocial circumstances
Z69: Mental health services for victim or perpetrator of abuse
Z76.89: Encounter for health services in other specified circumstances (forensic examination)

ICD-10 coding is available to forensic health care providers (nurses, nurse practitioners, physician assistants, and physicians) when seeking reimbursement options. In addition, use of ICD-10 codes provide data to improve understanding about the scope of the problem in your community and seen in your facility or agency. Sexual assault programs are federally mandated to not charge victims for the medical forensic examination. ICD-10 coding also provides additional data for services, which enhances future planning for the program with advanced medical and nursing practices. Registered nurses cannot charge under the ICD-09 and ICD-10 coding for services. However, accurate coding provides improved data reflecting prevalence and incidence of physical assaults related to strangulation, in addition to reimbursement and planning for future fiscal needs for all forensic patients who are seen in hospitals, clinics, and agencies. A strategy to sustain forensic programs includes advanced medical and nursing practitioner administrators working with finance and billing offices to identify appropriate billing, coding, and charging structures. This will help in recognizing advanced medical forensic evaluation and planning services provided to the patients seeking services from their organization. In addition, the codes provide the foundation for specific services supporting victims of domestic violence, data for future funding and grants, and information necessary for quality and safety in evidence-based interventions, which are directed to improve outcomes for all traumatized patients.

Appendix 19. Five Myths About Strangulation

FIVE MYTHS ABOUT STRANGULATION

Prepared by Gerald Fineman, Assistant District Attorney, Riverside County, and Dr. William Green, Medical Director, California Clinical Forensic Medical Training Center/ CDAA

1

MYTH

STRANGULATION AND CHOKING ARE THE SAME THING

FACT

STRANGULATION is the external application of physical force that impedes either air or blood to or from the brain.

CHOKING is an internal obstruction of the airway by a foreign object.

SOLUTION

Use a diagram.

Compare to the flow of electrical current.

Compare to the flow of air/water through a closed system (fish tank).

2

MYTH

STRANGULATION ALWAYS LEAVES VISIBLE INJURIES

FACT

Studies show that over half the victims of strangulation lack visible external injury. A victim without visible external injury can still die from strangulation.

SOLUTION

Demonstrate cutting off blood flow to your fingertips by squeezing your wrist with your other hand. Upon release of the grip, you will likely have no identifiable marks. If you do, they will be very short in duration.

3

MYTH

IF THE VICTIM CAN SPEAK, SCREAM, OR BREATHE, THEY ARE NOT BEING STRANGLED

FACT

Since strangulation involves obstruction of blood flow, a person can have complete obstruction and continue breathing until the moment they die from lack of oxygenated blood flow to the brain.

SOLUTION

Again, grab your wrist and squeeze. You can still breathe, yet blood flow is obstructed to the fingertips. If this was the victim's neck, they could still have an open trachea (windpipe) but have lack of blood flow to the brain.

4

MYTH

STRANGULATION CANNOT BE HARMFUL BECAUSE MANY PEOPLE PRACTICE IT (MARTIAL ARTS, MILITARY, LAW ENFORCEMENT)

FACT

Martial arts are a form of combat. The military and law enforcement use strangulation as a lethal form of force.

RISK

There are numerous incidents of death resulting from strangulation. This can even occur during otherwise supervised events, such as sporting events, law enforcement training, etc.

5

MYTH

STRANGULATION VICTIMS SHOULD BE ABLE TO DETAIL THEIR ATTACK

FACT

Trauma impacts the brains ability to store memory. In addition, the hippocampus (part of the brain where memory is stored) is the most sensitive to oxygen deprivation.

When a victim is strangled, both factors can impact the ability to recall.

SOLUTION

Give the example of how limiting the flow of electricity to a digital recording device will prevent it from recording.

strangulationtraininginstitute.com | institute@allianceforhope.com | (888) 511-3522 | 101 West Broadway, Suite 1770, San Diego, CA 92101

This project is supported all or in part by Grant No. 2016-TA-AX-K067 awarded by the Office on Violence Against Women, U.S. Department of Justice. The opinions, findings, conclusions, and recommendations expressed in this publication/program/exhibition are those of the author(s) and do not necessarily reflect the views of the Department of Justice, Office on Violence Against Women.

References

1. National statistics. The National Coalition Against Domestic Violence Web site. https://ncadv.org/statistics#:~:text=On%20average%2C%20nearly%2020%20people,10%20million%20women%20and%20men. Accessed June 29, 2020.
2. Maurer DN, Darnall CR. Screening for depression. *Am Fam Physician*. 2012;85(2):139-144.
3. Suicide prevention. The Joint Commission Web site. https://www.jointcommission.org/resources/patient-safety-topics/suicide-prevention/. Updated July 1, 2019. Accessed June 29, 2020.
4. Suicide assessment five-step evaluation and triage. Substance Abuse and Mental Health Services Administration Web site. https://store.samhsa.gov/sites/default/files/d7/priv/sma09-4432.pdf. Accessed June 29, 2020.
5. Augustine GJ, Fitzpatrick D. The blood supply to the brain and spinal cord. In: Purves D, ed. *Neuroscience*. 2nd ed. Oxford, England: Oxford University Press; 2001.
6. Blood vessels of the brain. The Internet Stroke Center Web site. http://www.strokecenter.org/professionals/brain-anatomy/blood-vessels-of-the-brain/. Accessed June 5, 2020.
7. Zarrinkoob L, Ambarki K, Wåhlin A, Birgander R, Eklund A, Malm J. Blood flow distribution in cerebral arteries. *J Cereb Blood Flow Metab*. 2015;35(4):648-654.
8. Bschor F. Diangosis of congestive hemorrhage in the region of the head in strangulation and other causes of death [Article in German]. *Beitr Gerichtl Med*. 1969;25:146-152.
9. Payne-James J, Jones R, Karch SB, Manlove J. *Simpson's Forensic Medicine*. 13th ed. Boca Raton, FL: CRC Press; 2011.
10. Rossen R, Kabat H, Anderson JP. Acute arrest of cerebral circulation in man. *Arch Neur Psych*. 1943;50(5):510-528.
11. DiMaio VJM, Dana SE. *Handbook for Forensic Pathology*. 2nd ed. Boca Raton, FL: CRC Press; 2006.
12. Plattner T, Bolliger S, Zollinger S. Forensic assessment of survived strangulation. *Forensic Sci Int*. 2005;153(2-3):202-207.
13. Ambade VN, Kolpe D, Tumram N, Meshram S, Pawar M, Kukde H. Characteristic features of hanging: a study in rural district of central India. *J Forensic Sci*. 2015;60(5):1216-1223.
14. Kurtulus A, Yonguc GN, Boz B, Acar K. Anatomopathological findings in hangings: a retrospective autopsy study. *Med Sci Law*. 2013;53(2):80-84.
15. Samarasekera A, Cooke C. The pathology of hanging deaths in western Australia. *Pathology*. 1996;28(4):334-338.
16. Dean DE, Kohler LJ, Sterbenz GCS, et al. Observed characteristics of suicidal hangings: an 11-year retrospective review. *J Forensic Sci*. 2012;57(5):1226-1230.
17. Ely SF, Hirsch CS. Asphyxial deaths and petechiae: a review. *J Forensic Sci*. 2000;45(6):1274-1277.
18. Geserick G, Krocker K, Wirth I. Tardieu's spots and asphyxia—a literature study [Article in German]. *Arch Kriminol*. 2010;226(5-6):145-160.
19. Rao VJ, Wetli CV. The forensic significance of conjunctival petechiae. *Am J Forensic Med Pathol*. 1988;9(1):32-34.
20. Schröder AS, Müller F, Gehl A, Sehner S, Anders S. Post-mortem development of conjunctival petechiae following temporary prone position. *Forensic Sci Int*. 2012;223(1-3):e53-e55.
21. Nagashima C, Iwama K, Sakata E, Miki Y. Effects of temporary occlusion of a vertebral artery on the human vestibular system. *J Neurosurg*. 1970;33(4):388-394.
22. Stopford JSB. The arteries of the pons and medulla oblongata. *J Anat Physiol*. 1916;50(pt 2):131-164.
23. Clément R, Guay JP, Redpath M, Sauvageau A. Petechiae in hanging: a retrospective study of contributing variables. *Am J Forensic Med Pathol*. 2011;32(4):378-382.
24. Moore WS, Yee JM, Hall AD. Collateral cerebral blood pressure. An index of tolerance to temporary carotid occlusion. *Arch Surg*. 1973;106(4):521-513.
25. Webb WG, Adler RK. *Neurology for the Speech-Language Pathologist*. 6th ed. St. Louis, MO: Mosby; 2016.
26. Andrus B, Bohnett C. Understanding the ICD-10 code structure. WebPT Web site. https://www.webpt.com/blog/post/understanding-icd-10-code-structure. Published October 29, 2013. Accessed October 1, 2019.
27. ICD-10 training tool. World Health Organization Web site. http://apps.who.int/classifications/apps/icd/icd10training/ICD-10%20training/Start/index.html. Accessed December 4, 2019.
28. The web's free 2019 ICD-10-CM/PCS medical coding reference. ICD10Data Web site. https://www.icd10data.com/. Accessed December 4, 2019.

Recommended Reading

Altmann AE, Ozanne-Smith J. Non-fatal asphyxiation and foreign body ingestion in children 0-14 years. *Inj Prev.* 1997;3(3):176-182.

Anscombe AM, Knight BH. Case report. Delayed death after pressure on the neck: possible causal mechanisms and implications for mode of death in manual strangulation discussed. *Forensic Sci Int.* 1996;78(3):193-197.

Baker RB, Sommers MS. Physical injury from intimate partner violence: measurement strategies and challenges. *J Obstet Gynecol Neonatal Nurs.* 2008;37(2):228-233.

Bergin A, Berkowitz R. Domestic violence in military families: non-fatal strangulation. *Md Med.* 2012;13(3):19-29.

Black MC, Basile KC, Breiding MJ, et al. *The National Intimate Partner and Sexual Violence Survey (NISVS): 2010 summary report.* Atlanta, GA: National Center for Injury Prevention and Control; 2011.

Butz RO Jr. Length and cross-section growth patterns in the human trachea. *Pediatrics.* 1968;42(2):336-341.

Campbell JC. *Assessing Dangerousness.* Newbury Park, CA: Sage Publications; 1995.

Campbell JC, Anderson JC, McFadgion A, et al. The effects of intimate partner violence and probably traumatic brain injury on central nervous system symptoms. *J Womens Health (Larchmt).* 2018;27(6):761-767.

Campbell JC, Glass N, Sharps PW, Laughon K, Bloom T. Intimate partner homicide: review and implications of research and policy. *Trauma Violence Abuse.* 2007;8(3):246-269.

Campbell JC. Nursing assessment for risk of homicide with battered women. *ANS Adv Nurs Sci.* 1986;8(4):36-51.

Campbell JC, Webster D, Koziol-McLain J, et al. Risk factors for femicide in abusive relationships: results from a multisite case control study. *Am J Public Health.* 2003;93(7):1089-1097.

Christe A, Oesterhelweg L, Ross S, et al. Can MRI of the neck compete with clinical findings in assessing danger to life for survivors of manual strangulation? A statistical analysis. *Leg Med (Tokyo).* 2010;12(5):228-232.

Christe A, Thoeny H, Ross S, et al. Life-threatening versus non-life-threatening manual strangulation: are there appropriate criteria for MR imaging of the neck? *Eur Radiol.* 2009;19(8):1882-1889.

Clarot F, Vaz E, Papin F, Proust B. Fatal and non-fatal bilateral delayed carotid artery dissection after manual strangulation. *Forensic Sci Int.* 2005;149(2-3):143-150.

Dayapala A, Samarasekera A, Jayasena A. An uncommon delayed sequela after pressure on the neck: an autopsy case report. *Am J Forensic Med Pathol.* 2012;33(1):80-82.

Di Paolo M, Guidi B, Bruschini L, Vessio G, Domenici R, Ambrosino N. Unexpected delayed death after manual strangulation: need for careful examination in the emergency room. *Monaldi Arch Chest Dis.* 2009;71(3):132-134.

Ely SF, Hirsch CS. Asphyxial deaths and petechiae: a review. *J Forensic Sci.* 2000;45(6):1274-1277.

Faugno DK, Copeland RA, Crum JL, Speck PM. *Advanced-Level Adolescent and Adult Sexual Assault Assessment: SANE/SAFE Forensic Learning Series*. Saint Louis, MO: STM Learning, Inc; 2012.

Faugno D, Waszak D, Strack GB, Brooks MA, Gwinn CG. Strangulation forensic examination: best practice for health care providers. *Adv Emerg Nurs J.* 2013;35(4):314-327.

Funk M, Schuppel J. Strangulation injuries. *WMJ.* 2003;102(3):41-45.

Gill JR, Cavalli DP, Ely SF, Stahl-Herz J. Homicidal neck compression of females: autopsy and sexual assault findings. *Acad Forensic Path.* 2013;3(4):454-457.

Glass N, Laughon K, Campbell J, et al. Non-fatal strangulation is an important risk factor for homicide of women. *J Emerg Med.* 2008;35(3):329-335.

Härm T, Rajs J. Types of injuries and interrelated conditions of victims and assailants in attempted homicidal strangulation. *Forensic Sci Int.* 1981;18(2):101-123.

Hawley DA. Death by strangulation. Paper presented at: How to Improve Your Investigation and Prosecution of Domestic Violence and Strangulation Cases; June 2002; Delaware, OH.

Hawley DA. Death by strangulation and suffocation. In: Training Institute on Strangulation Prevention, California District Attorneys Association, eds. *The Investigation and Prosecution of Strangulation Cases*. San Diego, CA: Training Institute on Strangulation Prevention; 2013:63-76.

Hawley DA, McClane GE, Strack GB. A review of 300 attempted strangulation cases part III: injuries in fatal cases. *J Emerg Med.* 2001;21(3):317-322.

Hawton K, Bergen H, Casey D, Simkin S. General hospital presentations of non-fatal hanging over a 28-year period: case-control study. *Br J Psychiatry.* 2008;193(6):503-504.

Hettrick H, Hill C, Hardigan P. Early detection of pressure injury using a forensic alternate light source. *Wounds.* 2017;29(8):222-228.

Iacovou E, Nayar M, Fleming J, Lew-Gor S. A pain in the neck: a rare case of isolated hyoid bone trauma. *J Surg Case Rep.* 2011;2011(7):3.

Iserson KV. Strangulation: a review of ligature, manual, and postural neck compression injuries. *Ann Emerg Med.* 1984;13(3):179-185.

Iverson KM, Pogoda TK. Traumatic brain injury among women veterans: an invisible wound of intimate partner violence. *Med Care.* 2015;53(4 suppl 1):S112-S119.

Khokhlov VD. Pressure on the neck calculated for any point along the ligature. *Forensic Sci Int.* 2001;123(2-3):178-181.

Klevens J. An overview of intimate partner violence among Latinos. *Violence Against Women.* 2007;13(2):111-122.

Laughon K, Glass N, Worrell C. Review and analysis of laws related to strangulation in 50 states. *Eval Rev.* 2009;33(4):358-369.

Le Blanc-Louvry I, Papin F, Vaz E, Proust B. Cervical arterial injury after strangulation—different types of arterial lesions. *J Forensic Sci.* 2013;58(6):1640-1643.

Maguire SA, Watts PO, Shaw AD, et al. Retinal haemorrhages and related findings in abusive and non-abusive head trauma: a systematic review. *Eye (Lond).* 2013;26(1):28-36.

Malek AM, Higashida RT, Halbach VV, et al. Patient presentation, angiographic features, and treatment of strangulation-induced bilateral dissection of the cervical internal carotid artery. *J Neurosurg.* 2000;92(3):481-487.

Marieb EN, Hoehn K. *Human Anatomy and Physiology.* 9th ed. Glenview, IL: Pearson; 2013.

McClane GE, Strack GB, Hawley D. A review of 300 attempted strangulation cases part II: clinical evaluation of the surviving victim. *J Emerg Med.* 2001;21(3):311-315.

McKenzia K, Scott DA, Campbell MA, McClure RJ. The use of narrative text for injury surveillance research: a systematic review. *Accid Anal Prev.* 2010;42(2):354-363.

Miao J, Su C, Wang W, et al. Delayed parkinsonism with selective symmetric basal ganglia lesion after manual strangulation. *J Clin Neurosci.* 2009;16(4):573-575.

Molacek J, Baxa J, Houdek K, Ferda J, Treska V. Bilateral post-traumatic carotid dissection as a result of a strangulation injury. *Ann Vasc Surg.* 2010;24(8):1133e9-1133e11.

Oh JH, Min HS, Park TU, Lee SJ, Kim SE. Isolated cricoid fracture associated with blunt neck trauma. *Emerg Med J.* 2007;24(7):505-506.

Plattner T, Bolliger S, Zollinger U. Forensic assessment of survived strangulation. *Forensic Sci Int.* 2005;153(2-3):202-207.

Pollitt EN, Anderson JC, Scafide KN, Holbrook D, D'Silva G, Sheridan DJ. Alternate light source findings of common topical products. *J Forensic Nurs.* 2016;12(3):97-103.

Pritchard AJ, Reckdenwald A, Nordham C. Nonfatal strangulation as part of domestic violence: a review of research. *Trauma Violence Abuse.* 2017;18(4):407-424.

Ramchand T, Choudhry OJ, Shukla PA, Tomovic S, Kuperan AB, Eloy JA. Management of hyoid bone fractures: a systematic review. *Otolaryngol Head Neck Surg.* 2012;147(2):204-208.

Sauvageau A, Boghossian E. Classification of asphyxia: the need for standardization. *J Forensic Sci.* 2010;55(5):1259-1267.

Scafide KN, Sharma S, Tripp NE, Hayat MJ. Bruise detection and visibility under alternate light during the first three days post-trauma. *J Forensic Leg Med.* 2020;69:101893.

Scafide KN, Sheridan DJ, Downing NR, Hayat MJ. Detection of inflicted bruises by alternate light: results of a randomized controlled trial. *J Forensic Sci.* 2020:doi: 10.1111/1556-4029.14294.

Sethi PK, Sethi NK, Torgovnick J, Arsura E. Delayed left anterior and middle cerebral artery hemorrhagic infarctions after attempted strangulation: a case report. *Am J Forensic Med Pathol.* 2012;33(1):105-106.

Sheridan DJ. Forensic documentation of battered women. *J Nurse Midwifery.* 1996;41(6):467-472.

Shields LBE, Corey TS, Weakley-Jones B, Stewart D. Living victims of strangulation: a 10-year review of cases in a metropolitan community. *Am J Forensic Med Pathol.* 2010;31(4):320-325.

Smith DJ, Mills T, Taliaferro E. Frequency and relationship of reported symptomology in victims of intimate partner violence: the role of multiple strangulation attacks. *J Emerg Med.* 2001;21(3):323-329.

Sorenson SB, Joshi M, Sivitz E. A systematic review of the epidemiology of nonfatal strangulation, a human rights and health concern. *Am J Public Health.* 2014;104(11):e54-e61.

Stapczynski JS. Strangulation injuries. *Emerg Med Rep*. 2010;31(17):193-203.

Strack GB, McClane GE, Hawley D. A review of 300 attempted strangulation cases part I: criminal legal issues. *J Emerg Med*. 2001;21(3):303-309.

Stuart EP. Campbell JC. Assessment of patterns of dangerousness with battered women. *Issues Ment Health Nurs*. 1989;10(3-4):245-260.

Taliaferro E, Hawley D, McClane D, Strack G. Strangulation in intimate partner violence. In: Mitchell C, Anglin D, eds. *Intimate Partner Violence: A Health-Based Perspective*. Oxford, England: Oxford University Press; 2009.

Wilbur L, Higley M, Hatfield J, et al. Survey results of women who have been strangled while in an abusive relationship. *J Emerg Med*. 2001;21(3):297-302.

Yen K, Thali MJ, Aghayev E, et al. Strangulation signs: initial correlation of MRI, MSCT, and forensic neck findings. *J Magn Reson Imaging*. 2005;22(4):501-510.

Yen K, Vock P, Christe A, et al. Clinical forensic radiology in strangulation victims: forensic expertise based on magnetic resonance imaging (MRI) findings. *Int J Legal Med*. 2007;121(2):115-123.

Zilkens RR, Phillips MA, Kelly MC, Mukhtar SA, Semmens JB, Smith DA. Non-fatal strangulation in sexual assault: a study of clinical and assault characteristics highlighting the role of intimate partner violence. *J Forensic Leg Med*. 2016;43:1-7.

Answer Key

Note to Students

Community standards and agency protocols for evidence collection, prophylactic treatment, patient referrals, and follow-up vary across the United States and internationally. It is the student's responsibility to know his or her community standards, agency protocols, and the rationale surrounding any variations where national or international standards or recommendations exist.

When documenting findings in the medical forensic record, documentation should include approximate length, width, shape, and color of injuries. This level of documentation is not possible when reviewing photodocumentation as presented in these case studies. Limitations to assessment of injury via photodocumentation are related to several variables, including scale, angle, lighting, equipment settings, picture quality, and provider technique (eg, separation, traction).

The case studies in this book are brief summaries of complex patient encounters. The figures provided with each case study represent a sample of the photodocumentation collected during the medical forensic examination. Please note that detail and extent of evidence collection, prophylactic treatment, patient referrals, and recommended follow-up are based on these brief summaries, not on the additional details that would be available during an actual patient encounter. Additionally, the authors purposefully created the answer key for a broad audience to reflect the diversity and scope of practice of individuals completing this book. In doing so, it is recognized that the answer key may often reflect those roles that have a more limited scope of practice (eg, registered nurse [RN] versus advanced practice registered nurse [APRN] or physician).

Chapter 1: 32-Year-Old Female Strangulation Patient with Hyoid Bone Fracture and Suicidal Ideation

Anatomic Skills 1-1

A. Greater horns

B. Lesser horns

C. Body

D. Thyroid cartilage

E. Trachea

Activity 1-1. Injury Identification

F. Red, curve-shaped area, approximately 1.5 to 2 cm in length and 4 mm wide

G. Faint discoloration of lighter, egg-shaped area on jawline that measures approximately 4 cm in length

H. Round, yellowish-brown contusion measuring 2.5 cm x 3.5 cm on inner aspect of right arm with irregular lower edge

Activity 1-2. Assessment

— Use patient-friendly, nonmedical language when evaluating the patient (eg, difficulty breathing, swallowing, or talking).

— What was the method of strangulation (eg, 1 hand, 2 hands, ligature)?

— What were the symptoms of strangulation (eg, loss of consciousness, light-headedness, other neurologic symptoms)?

— Is there any neck pain (now or after strangulation)?

— Is there any difficulty breathing (now or after strangulation)?

— Are there any changes in the patient's voice (now or after strangulation)?

— Are there any changes in vision (now or after strangulation)?

— Does the patient have any difficulty swallowing (now or after strangulation)?

— Does the patient have any pain or bleeding (now or after strangulation)?

— Was there any incontinence of the bowel or bladder? Did the patient change clothes before coming in?

— What are notable characteristics of the patient's behavior and demeanor (eg, flat affect, looking away) and short-term memory?

— How long did the strangulation last (best estimate by patient)? What was the pressure on a scale of 0 to 10?

Activity 1-3. Physical Assessment

— Neurologic checks (eg, full cranial nerve assessment, cervical nerves in upper body, strength)

— Skin assessment for petechial hemorrhages (eg, conjunctiva, retinal splinter hemorrhages, scalp, ears)

— Speech assessment (eg, for clarity, slurring, hoarseness)

— Memory assessment (eg, orientation, sensory memory, recent and remote memory questions)

— Strength assessment and balance (eg, hands, jaws, squint)

— Assessment of oral cavity for tears to frenulum, bruising to buccal mucosa, petechiae, tongue, uvula midline, symmetrical smile, and other injuries

— Assessment for previous head injury

— Danger Assessment (eg, previous physical assaults, suicidal ideation and attempts, previous strangulation)

— Pulse oximetry reading

— Head-to-toe assessment, including checking and palpating abdomen

— Peripheral vision test and 6 cardinal fields of gaze

Activity 1-4. Evidence Collection

— Use evidence collection kit for *strangulation and sexual assault*, as stated by the patient or implied by the history. Kit should include a reference standard of the patient's DNA from the uninjured buccal area (if injury is present, consider drawing blood for DNA). Swab skin over contusions, fingernails, oral cavity, sides of face, and ears.

— Document the history given by the patient, using quotation marks for the patient's exact words.

— Assess and inspect specific anatomic locations for visible injury and pain on palpation.

— Photograph and measure, documenting all injuries, bruises, and areas the patient notes as painful. All photographs should be taken with and without an American Board of Forensic Odontology (ABFO) ruler.

— Photograph the 9 diagnostic positions of gaze of the eyes, including the inner aspects of the upper and lower lids.

— Take multiple photographs at 90-degree angles, 360 degrees around the neck.

— Inspect and photograph the oral cavity, including the hard palate, soft palate, uvula, and oropharynx, for petechiae or other injury.

— Inspect and photograph the ears, including anterior and posterior. Initial injury, unless it involves dermal capillary injury, may not be visible but over time may surface, allowing for reassessment and documentation.

— For reference (a baseline), measure and mark the neck at present and at follow-up in 72 hours to 14 days.

— Some programs use an alternate light source (ALS) light to scan the neck for substances and to highlight injury. At this time, research does not support that ALS light identifies bruising; however, invert filters may identify bruises. More research is necessary to determine the usefulness of both methods. An ALS light can be used to identify substances.

— Photograph the hands using the size mat available on the Secure Digital Forensic Imaging (SDFI) website, taking note of the fingernails and any injuries. The advantage of using a size mat is to measure the size and angle of the photographs.

Activity 1-5. Treatment and Care

— The results of the physical examination are consistent with the history of the assault provided by the patient.

— Apply ice indirectly to the neck (eg, cloth or towel barrier between ice and skin) to reduce swelling as tolerated.

— Prepare the patient for radiographic studies.

— Discuss safety planning with the patient.

— Recommend medical observation for 12 to 23 hours, with continuous monitoring of pulse oximetry and vital signs as needed.

— Assess if the patient has a safe place to go after examination and discharge, and if not, involve the advocate or social services as necessary.

— The forensic nurse refers the patient to a community partner (eg, advocate, YWCA, other locally identified agencies) for shelter and victim of crime application.

— Victim advocate offers to assist in obtaining or referring for restraining order protection, if needed. The forensic nurse provides information to the patient and supports their decision about the order of protection.

— Provide a Danger Assessment and discuss the results with the patient, being transparent about the evidence-based risk assessment (eg, "The results reflect a population of persons and may not apply to you as an individual. However, these results can inform your decision about your situation.").

— Depending on jurisdictional mandated reporting laws, report to police or notify the agency within the jurisdiction if the patient requests law enforcement involvement. (Failure to report when mandatory may result in legal action against the nurse and/or health care provider.)

— Discuss findings with the patient and provide patient-specific strangulation discharge information, such as detailed instructions to return to the emergency department (ED) if neurologic signs or symptoms, dyspnea, dysphonia, odynophagia, or seizures develop or worsen. Provide written instructions if the patient feels comfortable taking them with her. Discuss the possibility of a lifetime increased risk of neurologic consequences.

— Schedule follow-up forensic examination for 72 hours to 14 days after assault for additional medical forensic evaluation if possible within the framework of your program.

— Assess patient access to primary provider care or clinic care for follow-up in 14 days.

Activity 1-6 Lethality Assessment

Indicators of escalating danger include the following:

— Increase in frequency or severity of the assaults

— Increase of new threats of homicide or suicide

— Threats to children present in the home

— Presence of a firearm or deadly weapon in the home

Questions to assess immediate risk of violence include the following. Patients who answer "yes" to at least 3 of the following questions may be at especially high immediate risk of violence.

— Has the physical violence happened more often or gotten worse over the past 6 months?

— Has your partner ever used a weapon or threatened you with a weapon?

— Has your partner ever tried to strangle you?

— Do you believe your partner could kill you?

— Has your partner ever beaten you while you were pregnant?

— Is your partner violently and constantly jealous of you?

— Do you feel unsafe in your home?

Chapter 2: 21-Year-Old Male Patient Assaulted by an Acquaintance

Anatomic Skills 2-1

A. Back of the neck

B. Right front of the neck

C. Right upper eyelid

Activity 2-1. Injury Identification

A. Linear bruising that circles the neck

B. Linear red bruising cluster on the left side of neck with a red linear patterned bruise around the neck

C. Right upper eyelid and side of the face with multiple flat, red petechial hemorrhages

D. Left upper eyelid and side of the face with multiple flat, red petechial hemorrhages

Activity 2-2. Assessment

— Use patient-friendly, nonmedical language when evaluating the patient (eg, difficulty breathing, swallowing, or talking).

— What was the method of strangulation (eg, 1 hand, 2 hands, ligature)?

— What were the symptoms of strangulation (eg, loss of consciousness, light-headedness, other neurologic symptoms)?

— Is there any neck pain (now or after strangulation)?

— Is there any difficulty breathing (now or after strangulation)?

— Are there any changes in the patient's voice (now or after strangulation)?

— Are there any changes in vision (now or after strangulation)?

— Does the patient have any difficulty swallowing (now or after strangulation)?

— Does the patient have any pain or bleeding (now or after strangulation)?

— Was there any incontinence of the bowel or bladder? Did the patient change clothes?

— What are notable characteristics of the patient's demeanor and behavior and demeanor (eg, flat affect, looking away) and short-term memory? Does the patient have any suicidal or homicidal ideation?

— How long did the strangulation last (best estimate by patient)? What was the pressure on a scale of 0 to 10?

Activity 2-3. Physical Assessment

— Neurologic checks (eg, full cranial nerve assessment, cervical nerves in upper body, strength)

— Skin assessment for petechial hemorrhages (eg, conjunctiva, retinal hemorrhages, scalp, ears)

— Speech assessment (eg, for clarity, slurring, hoarseness)

— Memory assessment (eg, orientation, sensory memory, recent and remote memory questions)

— Strength assessment and balance (eg, hands, jaws, squint)

— Assessment of oral cavity for tears to frenulum, bruising to buccal mucosa, petechiae, tongue, uvula midline, symmetrical smile, and other injuries

— Assessment for previous head injury

— Danger Assessment (eg, previous physical assaults, suicidal ideation and attempts, previous strangulation)

— Pulse oximetry reading

— Head-to-toe assessment, including checking and palpating abdomen

— Peripheral vision test and 6 cardinal fields of gaze

Activity 2-4. Evidence Collection

— Use evidence collection kit for *strangulation and sexual assault*, as stated by the patient or implied by the history. Kit should include a reference standard of the patient's DNA from the uninjured buccal area (if injury is present, consider drawing blood for DNA). Swab skin over contusions, fingernails, oral cavity, sides of face, and ears.

— Document the history given by the patient, using quotation marks around the patient's exact words.

— Assess and inspect specific anatomic locations for visible injury and pain on palpation.

— Photograph and measure, documenting all injuries, bruises, and areas the patient notes as painful. All photographs should be taken with and without an ABFO ruler.

— Photograph the 9 diagnostic positions of gaze of the eyes, including the inner aspects of the upper and lower lids.

— Take photographs at 90-degree angles, 360 degrees around the neck.

— Inspect and photograph the oral cavity, including the hard palate, soft palate, uvula, and oropharynx, for petechiae or other injury.

— Inspect and photograph the ears, including anterior and posterior. Initial injury, unless it involves dermal capillary injury, may not be visible but over time may surface, allowing for reassessment and documentation.

— For reference (a baseline), measure and mark the neck at present and at follow-up in 72 hours to 14 days.

— Some programs use an ALS light to scan the neck for substances and to highlight injury. At this time, research does not support that ALS light identifies bruising; however, invert filters may identify bruises. More research is necessary to determine the usefulness of both methods. An ALS light can be used to identify substances.

— Photograph the hands using the size mat available on the SDFI website, taking note of the fingernails and any injuries. The advantage of using a size mat is to measure the size and angle of the photographs.

Activity 2-5. Treatment and Care

— The results of the physical examination are consistent with the history of the assault provided by the patient.

— Apply ice indirectly to the neck (eg, cloth or towel barrier between ice and skin) to reduce swelling as tolerated.

— Prepare the patient for radiographic studies.

— Discuss safety planning with the patient.

— Recommend medical observation for 12 to 23 hours, with continuous monitoring of pulse oximetry and vital signs as needed.

— Assess if the patient has a safe place to go after examination and discharge, and if not, involve the advocate or social services as necessary.

— The forensic nurse refers the patient to a community partner (eg, advocate, YWCA, other locally identified agencies) for shelter and victim of crime application.

— Victim advocate offers to assist in obtaining or referring for restraining order protection, if needed. The forensic nurse provides information to the patient and supports their decision about the order of protection.

— Provide a Danger Assessment and discuss the results with the patient, being transparent about the evidence-based risk assessment (eg, "The results reflect a population of persons and may not apply to you as an individual. However, these results can inform your decision about your situation.").

— Depending on jurisdictional mandated reporting laws, report to police or notify the agency within the jurisdiction if the patient requests law enforcement involvement. (Failure to report when mandatory may result in legal action against the nurse or health care provider.)

— Discuss findings with the patient and provide patient-specific strangulation discharge information, such as detailed instructions to return to the ED if neurologic signs or symptoms, dyspnea, dysphonia, odynophagia, or seizures develop or worsen. Discuss the possibility of a lifetime increased risk of neurologic consequences.

— Schedule follow-up forensic examination for 72 hours to 14 days after assault for additional medical forensic evaluation if possible within the framework of your program.

— Assess patient access to primary provider care or clinic care for follow-up in 14 days.

Chapter 3: 66-Year-Old Female Patient Assaulted by Her Son

Anatomic Skills 3-1

A. Chin

B. Right neck

C. Left neck

D. Anterior mid-neck

Anatomic Skills 3-2

E. Chin

F. Right neck

G. Left neck

H. Anterior mid-neck

Activity 3-1. Injury Identification

I. Abrasion left neck, submandibular area

J. Abrasion, left neck/clavicle area

K. Ecchymosis and abrasions, lateral and inferior tongue

L. Circular purple bruise, 2 cm, right mandible

M. Black-brown bruise, 1.5 cm x 1.5 cm, overlying the metacarpophalangeal joint of the first finger of the right hand

Activity 3-2. Assessment

— Use patient-friendly, nonmedical language when evaluating the patient (eg, difficulty breathing, swallowing, or talking).

— What was the method of strangulation (eg, 1 hand, 2 hands, ligature)?

— What were the symptoms of strangulation (eg, loss of consciousness, light-headedness, other neurologic symptoms)?

— Is there any neck pain (now or after strangulation)?

— Is there any difficulty breathing (now or after strangulation)?

— Are there any changes in the patient's voice (now or after strangulation)?

— Are there any changes in vision (now or after strangulation)?

— Does the patient have any difficulty swallowing (now or after strangulation)?

— Does the patient have any pain or bleeding (now or after strangulation)?

— Was there any incontinence of the bowel or bladder? Did the patient change clothes before coming in?

— What are notable characteristics of the patient's behavior and demeanor (eg, flat affect, looking away) and short-term memory?

— How long did the strangulation last (best estimate by patient)? What was the pressure on a scale of 0 to 10?

Activity 3-3. Physical Head to Toe Assessment

— Neurologic checks (eg, full cranial nerve assessment, cervical nerves in upper body, strength)

— Skin assessment for petechial hemorrhages (eg, conjunctiva, retinal splinter hemorrhages, scalp, ears)

— Speech assessment (eg, for clarity, slurring, hoarseness)

— Memory assessment (eg, orientation, sensory memory, recent and remote memory questions)

— Strength assessment and balance (eg, hands equal strength bilaterally, jaws, squint)

— Assessment of oral cavity for tears to frenulum, bruising to buccal mucosa, petechiae, tongue, uvula midline, symmetrical smile, and other injuries

— Assessment for previous head injury

— Danger Assessment (eg, previous physical assaults, suicidal ideation and attempts, previous strangulation)

— Pulse oximetry reading

— Head-to-toe assessment, including checking and palpating abdomen

— Peripheral vision test and 6 cardinal fields of gaze

Activity 3-4. Evidence Collection

— Use evidence collection kit for *strangulation*, as stated by the patient or implied by the history. Kit should include a reference standard of the patient's DNA from the uninjured buccal area (if injury is present, consider drawing blood for DNA). Swab skin over contusions, fingernails, oral cavity, sides of face, and ears.

— Document the history given by the patient, using quotation marks for the patient's exact words.

— Assess and inspect specific anatomic locations for visible injury and pain on palpation.

— Photograph and measure, documenting all injuries, bruises, and areas the patient notes as painful. All photographs should be taken with and without an ABFO ruler.

— Photograph the 9 diagnostic positions of gaze of the eyes, including the inner aspects of the upper and lower lids.

— Take multiple photographs at 90-degree angles, 360 degrees around the neck.

— Inspect and photograph the oral cavity, including the hard palate, soft palate, uvula, and oropharynx, for petechiae or other injury.

— Inspect and photograph the ears, including anterior and posterior. Initial injury, unless it involves dermal capillary injury, may not be visible but over time may surface, allowing for reassessment and documentation.

— For reference (a baseline), measure and mark the neck at present and at follow-up in 72 hours to 14 days.

— Some programs use an ALS light to scan the neck for substances and to highlight injury. At this time, research does not support that ALS light identifies bruising; however, invert filters may identify bruises. More research is necessary to determine the usefulness of both methods. An ALS light can be used to identify substances.

— Photograph the hands using the size mat available on the SDFI website, taking note of the fingernails and any injuries. The advantage of using a size mat is to measure the size and angle of the photographs.

Activity 3-5. Treatment and Care

— The results of the physical examination are consistent with the history of the assault provided by the patient.

— Apply ice indirectly to the neck (eg, cloth or towel barrier between ice and skin) to reduce swelling as tolerated.

— Prepare the patient for radiographic studies.

— Discuss safety planning with the patient.

— Recommend medical observation for 12 to 23 hours, with continuous monitoring of pulse oximetry and vital signs as needed.

— Assess if the patient has a safe place to go after examination and discharge, and if not, involve the advocate or social services as necessary.

— The forensic nurse refers the patient to a community partner (eg, advocate, YWCA, other locally identified agencies) for shelter and victim of crime application.

— Victim advocate offers to assist in obtaining or referring for restraining order protection, if needed. The forensic nurse provides information to the patient and supports their decision about orders of protection.

— Provide a Danger Assessment and discuss the results with the patient, being transparent about the evidence-based risk assessment (eg, "The results reflect a population of persons and may not apply to you as an individual. However, these results can inform your decision about your situation.").

— Depending on jurisdictional mandated reporting laws, report to police or notify the agency within the jurisdiction if the patient requests law enforcement involvement. (Failure to report when mandatory may result in legal action against the nurse and/or health care provider.)

— Discuss findings with the patient and provide patient-specific strangulation discharge information, such as detailed instructions to return to the ED if neurologic signs or symptoms, dyspnea, dysphonia, odynophagia, or seizures develop or worsen. Provide written instructions if the patient feels comfortable taking them with her. Discuss the possibility of a lifetime increased risk of neurologic consequences.

— Schedule follow-up forensic examination for 72 hours to 14 days after assault for additional medical forensic evaluation if possible within the framework of your program.

— Assess patient access to primary provider care or clinic care for follow-up in 14 days.

Activity 3-6 Lethality Assessment

Indicators of escalating danger include the following:

— Increase in frequency or severity of the assaults

— Increase of new threats of homicide or suicide

— Threats to children present in the home

— Presence of a firearm or deadly weapon in the home

Questions to assess immediate risk of violence include the following. Patients who answer "yes" to at least 3 of the following questions may be at especially high immediate risk of violence.

— Has the physical violence happened more often or gotten worse over the past 6 months?

— Has your son ever used a weapon or threatened you with a weapon?

— Has your son ever tried to strangle you?

— Do you believe your son could kill you?

— Do you feel unsafe in your home?

Chapter 4: 17-Year-Old Female Patient Assaulted by a Nonintimate Acquaintance Stalker

Anatomic Skills 4-1

A. Left periorbital area

B. Left ear

C. Left cheek

Activity 4-1. Injury Identification

D. Petechiae to left upper eyelid

E. Petechiae to left temple

F. Petechiae to left cheek

G. Ecchymosis to left periorbital area, purple/blue, about 1 cm × 2 cm area

H. Multiple linear red abrasion marks on wrist, 1 cm around the wrist

I. Punctate abrasion

Activity 4-2. Assessment

— Use patient-friendly, nonmedical language when evaluating the patient (eg, difficulty breathing, swallowing, or talking).

— What was the method of strangulation (eg, 1 hand, 2 hands, ligature)?

— What were the symptoms of strangulation (eg, loss of consciousness, light-headedness, other neurologic symptoms)?

— Is there any neck pain (now or after strangulation)?

— Is there any difficulty breathing (now or after strangulation)?

— Are there any changes in the patient's voice (now or after strangulation)?

— Are there any changes in vision (now or after strangulation)?

— Does the patient have any difficulty swallowing (now or after strangulation)?

— Does the patient have any pain or bleeding (now or after strangulation)?

— Was there any incontinence of the bowel or bladder? Did the patient change clothes before coming in?

— What are notable characteristics of the patient's behavior and demeanor (eg, flat affect, looking away) and short-term memory?

— How long did the strangulation last (best estimate by patient)? What was the pressure on a scale of 0 to 10?

Activity 4-3. Physical Assessment

— Neurologic checks (eg, cranial nerves I-XII, cervical nerves C1-C8 in upper body)

  — Cranial nerves (CN I-XII, equal bilaterally)

  — Cervical nerves (ROM and strength: head and neck, diaphragm, deltoids, biceps, wrist extenders, triceps, hand)

— Skin assessment for petechial hemorrhages (eg, conjunctiva, retinal splinter hemorrhages, scalp, ears) and demarcation from ligature; palpate for tenderness, lumps, and bumps

— Speech assessment (eg, for clarity, slurring, hoarseness)

— Memory assessment (eg, orientation, sensory memory, recent and remote memory questions)

— Strength assessment and balance (eg, gait, hands, jaws, squint – see Cranial nerves I-XII and cervical nerves C1-C8 in upper body)

— Assessment of oral cavity for tears to frenulum, bruising to buccal mucosa, petechiae, tongue, uvula midline, symmetrical smile, and other injuries

— Assessment for previous head injury

— Danger Assessment (eg, previous physical assaults, suicidal ideation and attempts, previous strangulation)

— Pulse oximetry reading

— Head-to-toe assessment, including checking and palpating abdomen

— Peripheral vision test and 6 cardinal fields of gaze

Activity 4-4. Evidence Collection

— Use evidence collection kit for *sexual assault and strangulation*, as stated by the patient or implied by history. Kit should include a reference standard of the patient's DNA from the uninjured buccal area (if injury is present, consider drawing blood for DNA). Swab skin over contusions, fingernails, oral cavity, sides of face, neck, and ears. Genital, vaginal, and cervical swabs should also be collected.

— Document the history given by the patient, using quotation marks for patient's exact words.

— Assess and inspect specific anatomic locations for visible injury and pain on palpation.

— Photograph and measure, documenting all injuries, bruises, and areas the patient notes as painful. All photographs should be taken with and without an ABFO ruler.

— Photograph the 9 diagnostic positions of gaze of the eyes, including the inner aspects of the upper and lower lids.

— Take multiple photographs at 90-degree angles, 360 degrees around the neck.

— Inspect and photograph the oral cavity, including the hard palate, soft palate, uvula, and oropharynx, for petechiae or other injury.

— Inspect and photograph the ears, including anterior and posterior. Initial injury, unless it involves dermal capillary injury, may not be visible but over time may surface, allowing for reassessment and documentation.

— For reference (a baseline), measure and mark the neck at present and at follow-up in 72 hours to 14 days.

— Use an ALS light to scan the neck for substances and to identify injury. At this time, research does not support that ALS light identifies bruising; however, invert filters may identify bruises. More research is necessary to determine the usefulness of both methods. An ALS light can be used to identify substances.

— Photograph the hands using the size mat available on the SDFI website, taking note of the fingernails and any injuries. The advantage of using a size mat is to measure the size and angle of the photographs.

Activity 4-5. Treatment and Care

— The results of the physical examination are consistent with the history of the assault provided by the patient.

— Apply ice indirectly to the neck (eg, cloth or towel barrier between ice and skin) to reduce swelling as tolerated.

— Prepare the patient for radiographic studies.

— Discuss safety planning with the patient.

— Recommend medical observation for 12 to 23 hours, with continuous monitoring of pulse oximetry and vital signs as needed.

— Assess if the patient has a safe place to go after examination and discharge, and if not, involve the advocate or social services as necessary.

— The forensic nurse refers the patient to a community partner (eg, advocate, YWCA, other locally identified agencies) for shelter and victim of crime application.

— Victim advocate offers to assist in obtaining or referring for restraining order protection, if needed. The forensic nurse provides information to the patient and supports their decision about the order of protection.

— Provide a Danger Assessment and discuss the results with the patient, being transparent about the evidence-based risk assessment (eg, "The results reflect a population of persons and may not apply to you as an individual. However, these results can inform your decision about your situation.").

— Depending on jurisdictional mandated reporting laws, report to police or notify the agency within the jurisdiction if the patient requests law enforcement involvement. (Failure to report when mandatory may result in legal action against the nurse and/or health care provider.)

— Discuss findings with the patient and provide patient-specific strangulation discharge information, such as detailed instructions to return to the ED if neurologic signs or symptoms, dyspnea, dysphonia, odynophagia, or seizures develop or worsen. Discuss the possibility of a lifetime increased risk of neurologic consequences.

— Schedule follow-up forensic examination for 72 hours to 14 days after assault for additional medical forensic evaluation if possible within the framework of your program.

— Assess patient access to primary provider care or clinic care for follow-up in 14 days.

Chapter 5: 26-Year-Old Female Patient Assaulted by a Former Intimate Partner

Anatomic Skills 5-1

A. Right jawline or submandibular area

B. Right middle neck

C. Perioral area under the lower lip

D. Under chin

Activity 5-1. Injury Identification

E. 2 cm × 0.5 cm red bruise at right jawline below the ear or submandibular area

F. 2 cm × 1 cm brown bruise at middle neck

G. 2 cm × 2 cm red bruise at right neck

H. No injury noted

Activity 5-2. Assessment

— Use patient-friendly, nonmedical language when evaluating the patient (eg, difficulty breathing, swallowing, or talking).

— What was the method of strangulation (eg, 1 hand, 2 hands, ligature)?

— What were the symptoms of strangulation (eg, loss of consciousness, light-headedness, other neurologic symptoms)?

— Is there any neck pain (now or after strangulation)?

— Is there any difficulty breathing (now or after strangulation)?

— Are there any changes in the patient's voice (now or after strangulation)?

— Are there any changes in vision (now or after strangulation)?

— Does the patient have any difficulty swallowing (now or after strangulation)?

— Does the patient have any pain or bleeding (now or after strangulation)?

— Was there any incontinence of the bowel or bladder? Did the patient change clothes before coming in?

— What are notable characteristics of the patient's behavior and demeanor (eg, flat affect, looking away) and short-term memory?

— How long did the strangulation last (best estimate by patient)? What was the pressure on a scale of 0 to 10?

Activity 5-3. Physical Assessment

— Neurologic checks (eg, full cranial nerve assessment, cervical nerves in upper body, strength)

— Skin assessment for petechial hemorrhages (eg, conjunctiva, retinal hemorrhages, scalp, ears)

— Speech assessment (eg, for clarity, slurring, hoarseness)

— Memory assessment (eg, orientation, sensory memory, recent and remote memory questions)

— Strength assessment and balance (eg, hands, jaws, squint)

— Assessment of oral cavity for tears to frenulum, bruising to buccal mucosa, petechiae, tongue, uvula midline, symmetrical smile, and other injuries

— Assessment for previous head injury

— Danger Assessment (eg, previous physical assaults, suicidal ideation and attempts, previous strangulation)

— Pulse oximetry reading

— Head-to-toe assessment, including checking and palpating abdomen

— Peripheral vision test and 6 cardinal fields of gaze

Activity 5-4. Evidence Collection

— Use evidence collection kit for *sexual assault and strangulation*, as stated by the patient or implied by the history. Kit should include a reference standard of the patient's DNA from the uninjured buccal area (if injury is present, consider drawing blood for DNA). Swab skin over contusions, fingernails, oral cavity, sides of face, and ears.

— Document the history given by the patient, using quotation marks around the patient's exact words.

— Assess and inspect specific anatomic locations for potential injury and pain on palpation.

— Photograph and measure, documenting all injuries, bruises, and areas the patient notes as painful. All photographs should be taken with and without an ABFO ruler.

— Photograph the 9 diagnostic positions of gaze of the eyes, including the inner aspects of the upper and lower lids.

— Take multiple photographs at 90-degree angles, 360 degrees around the neck.

— Inspect and photograph the oral cavity, including the hard palate, soft palate, uvula, and oropharynx, for petechiae or other injury.

— Inspect and photograph the ears, including anterior and posterior. Initial injury, unless it involves dermal capillary injury, may not be visible but over time may surface, allowing for reassessment and documentation.

— For reference (a baseline), measure and mark the neck at present and at follow-up in 72 hours to 14 days.

— Some programs use an ALS light to scan the neck for substances and to highlight injury. At this time, research does not support that ALS light identifies bruising; however, invert filters may identify bruises. More research is necessary to determine the usefulness of both methods. An ALS light can be used to identify substances.

— Photograph the hands using the size mat available on the SDFI website, taking note of the fingernails and any injuries. The advantage of using a size mat is to measure the size and angle of the photographs.

Activity 5-5. Treatment and Care

— Depending on jurisdictional laws, notify child protective services of a child witness present during the crime of domestic violence. In the event charges are filed on behalf of the child, the child may need to provide a report of what was seen and heard. In many jurisdictions, on conviction of domestic violence, additional penalties apply.

— Provide counseling referral for domestic violence and referral for age-specific child counseling for witnessing domestic violence.

— The results of the physical examination are consistent with the history of the assault provided by the patient.

— Apply ice indirectly to the neck (eg, cloth or towel barrier between ice and skin) to reduce swelling as tolerated.

— Prepare the patient for radiographic studies.

— Discuss safety planning with the patient.

— Recommend medical observation for 12 to 23 hours, with continuous monitoring of pulse oximetry and vital signs as needed.

— Assess if the patient has a safe place to go after examination and discharge, and if not, involve the advocate or social services as necessary.

— The forensic nurse refers the patient to a community partner (eg, advocate, YWCA, other locally identified agencies) for shelter and victim of crime application.

— Victim advocate offers to assist in obtaining or referring for restraining order protection, if needed. The forensic nurse provides information to the patient and supports their decision about order of protection.

— Provide a Danger Assessment and discuss the results with the patient, being transparent about the evidence-based risk assessment (eg, "The results reflect a population of persons and may not apply to you as an individual. However, these results can inform your decision about your situation.").

— Depending on jurisdictional mandated reporting laws, report to police or notify the agency within the jurisdiction if the patient requests law enforcement involvement. (Failure to report when mandatory may result in legal action against the nurse or health care provider.)

— Discuss findings with the patient and provide patient-specific strangulation discharge information, such as detailed instructions to return to the ED if neurologic signs and symptoms, dyspnea, dysphonia, odynophagia, or seizures develop or worsen. Provide written instructions if the patient feels comfortable taking them with her. Discuss the possibility of a lifetime increased risk of neurologic consequences.

— Schedule follow-up forensic examination for 72 hours to 14 days after assault for additional medical forensic evaluation if possible within the framework of your program.

— Assess patient access to primary provider care or clinic care for follow-up in 14 days.

Activity 5-6 Lethality Assessment

Indicators of escalating danger include the following:

— Increase in frequency or severity of the assaults

— Increase of new threats of homicide or suicide

— Threats to children present in the home

— Presence of a firearm or deadly weapon in the home

Questions to assess immediate risk of violence include the following. Patients who answer "yes" to at least 3 of the following questions may be at especially high immediate risk of violence.

— Has the physical violence happened more often or gotten worse over the past 6 months?

— Has your partner ever used a weapon or threatened you with a weapon?

— Has your partner ever tried to strangle you?

— Do you believe your partner could kill you?

— Has your partner ever beaten you when you were pregnant?

— Is your partner violently and constantly jealous of you?

— Do you feel unsafe in your home?

Chapter 6: 15-Year-Old Female Patient Assaulted by a Stranger

Anatomic Skills 6-1

A. Left lateral neck

B. Left jawline

C. Mid-left side of the neck

Activity 6-1. Injury Identification

A. Red linear abrasion, about 10 cm, to the left lateral neck

C. 4.5 cm contusion to the left posterior neck

D. Large scleral hemorrhage to the bilateral eyes

E. Petechial hemorrhage on the inside of the lower lip

F. Left to right: 1 cm superficial laceration attached to 2 cm deeper laceration with dried, crusted blood on the forehead above the brow adjacent to hairline

G. 2 cm x 2 cm blue, swollen bruise adjacent to laceration with generalized bruising and swelling, painful when palpated

Activity 6-2. Assessment

— Use patient-friendly, nonmedical language when evaluating the patient (eg, difficulty breathing, swallowing, or talking).

— What was the method of strangulation (eg, 1 hand, 2 hands, ligature)?

— What were the symptoms of strangulation (eg, loss of consciousness, light-headedness, other neurologic symptoms)?

— Is there any neck pain (now or after strangulation)?

— Is there any difficulty breathing (now or after strangulation)?

— Are there any changes in the patient's voice (now or after strangulation)?

— Are there any changes in vision (now or after strangulation)?

— Does the patient have any difficulty swallowing (now or after strangulation)?

— Does the patient have any pain or bleeding (now or after strangulation)?

— Was there any incontinence of the bowel or bladder? Did the patient change clothes before coming in?

— What are notable characteristics of the patient's behavior and demeanor (eg, flat affect, looking away) and short-term memory?

— How long did the strangulation last (best estimate by patient)? What was the pressure on a scale of 0 to 10?

Activity 6-3. Physical Assessment

— Neurologic checks (eg, full cranial nerve assessment, cervical nerves in upper body, strength)

— Skin assessment for petechial hemorrhages (eg, conjunctiva, retinal hemorrhages, scalp, ears)

— Speech assessment (eg, for clarity, slurring, hoarseness)

— Memory assessment (eg, orientation, sensory memory, recent and remote memory questions)

— Strength assessment and balance (eg, hands, jaws, squint)

— Assessment of oral cavity for tears to frenulum, bruising to buccal mucosa, petechiae, tongue, uvula midline, symmetrical smile, and other injuries

— Assessment for previous head injury

— Danger Assessment (eg, previous physical assaults, suicidal ideation and attempts, previous strangulation)

— Pulse oximetry reading

— Head-to-toe assessment, including checking and palpating abdomen

— Peripheral vision test and 6 cardinal fields of gaze

Activity 6-4. Evidence Collection

— Use an evidence collection kit for *sexual assault and strangulation,* as stated by the patient or implied by the history. Kit should include a reference standard of the patient's DNA from the uninjured buccal area (if injury is present, consider drawing blood for DNA). Swab skin over contusions, fingernails, oral cavity, sides of face, and ears.

— Document the history given by the patient, using quotation marks for the patient's exact words.

— Assess and inspect specific anatomic locations for visible injury and pain on palpation.

— Photograph and measure, documenting all injuries, bruises, and areas the patient notes as painful. All photographs should be taken with and without an ABFO ruler.

— Photograph the 9 diagnostic positions of gaze of the eyes, including the inner aspects of the upper and lower lids.

— Take multiple photographs at 90-degree angles, 360 degrees around the neck.

— Inspect and photograph the oral cavity, including the hard palate, soft palate, uvula, and oropharynx, for petechiae or other injury.

— Inspect and photograph the ears, including anterior and posterior. Initial injury, unless it involves dermal capillary injury, may not be visible but over time may surface, allowing for reassessment and documentation.

— For reference (a baseline), measure and mark the neck at present and at follow-up in 72 hours to 14 days.

— Some programs use an ALS light to scan the neck for substances and to highlight injury. At this time, research does not support that ALS light identifies bruising; however, invert filters may identify bruises. More research is necessary to determine the usefulness of both methods. An ALS light can be used to identify substances.

— Photograph the hands using the size mat available on the SDFI website, taking note of the fingernails and any injuries. The advantage of using a size mat is to measure the size and angle of the photographs.

Activity 6-5. Treatment and Care

— The results of the physical examination are consistent with the history of the assault provided by the patient.

— Apply ice indirectly to the neck (eg, cloth or towel barrier between ice and skin) to reduce swelling as tolerated.

— Clean laceration with sterile saline, and assess for primary intention (stitches); refer if stitches are necessary.

— Review diphtheria, pertussis, and tetanus immunization.

— Prepare the patient for radiographic studies.

— Discuss safety planning with the patient.

— Recommend medical observation for 12 to 23 hours, with continuous monitoring of pulse oximetry and vital signs as needed.

— Assess if the patient has a safe place to go after examination and discharge, and if not, involve the advocate or social services as necessary.

— The forensic nurse refers the patient to a community partner (eg, advocate, YWCA, other locally identified agencies) for shelter and victim of crime application.

— Victim advocate offers to assist in obtaining or referring patient for restraining order protection, if needed. The forensic nurse provides information to the patient and supports their decision about order of protection.

— Provide a Danger Assessment and discuss the results with the patient, being transparent about the evidence-based risk assessment (eg, "The results reflect a population of persons and may not apply to you as an individual. However, these results can inform your decision about your situation.").

— Depending on jurisdictional mandated reporting laws, report to police or notify the agency within the jurisdiction if the patient requests law enforcement involvement. (Failure to report when mandatory may result in legal action against the nurse and/or health care provider.)

— Discuss findings with the patient and provide patient-specific strangulation discharge information, such as detailed instructions to return to the ED if neurologic signs or symptoms, dyspnea, dysphonia, odynophagia, or seizures develop or worsen. Discuss the possibility of a lifetime increased risk of neurologic consequences.

— Schedule follow-up forensic examination for 72 hours to 14 days after assault for additional medical forensic evaluation if possible within the framework of your program.

— Assess patient access to primary provider care or clinic care for follow-up in 14 days.

Chapter 7: 24-Year-Old Female Patient Assaulted by a Former Intimate Partner

Anatomic Skills 7-1

A. Chin

B. Left jawline or submandibular area

C. Left middle neck

D. Anterior mid-neck

Anatomic Skills 7-2

E. Right jawline or submandibular area

F. Left jawline or submandibular area

G. Chin

H. Right middle neck

Activity 7-1. Injury Identification

I. Generalized petechiae and erythema noted to entirety of face

J. Multiple linear purple ecchymosis noted to left neck

K. Multiple linear purple ecchymosis noted to left neck

L. Multiple linear purple ecchymosis noted to center of neck

M. Generalized petechiae and erythema noted to entirety of face

N. Purple/red colored ecchymosis noted to right jawline

O. Oval, red/purple ecchymosis noted to right neck

P. Multiple linear purple ecchymosis noted to center neck

Q. Subconjunctival hemorrhage noted to right eye

R. Subconjunctival hemorrhage noted to left eye

Activity 7-2. Assessment

— Use patient-friendly, nonmedical language when evaluating the patient (eg, difficulty breathing, swallowing, or talking).

— What was the method of strangulation (eg, 1 hand, 2 hands, ligature)?

— What were the symptoms of strangulation (eg, loss of consciousness, light-headedness, other neurologic symptoms)?

— Is there any neck pain (now or after strangulation)?

— Is there any difficulty breathing (now or after strangulation)?

— Are there any changes in the patient's voice (now or after strangulation)?

— Are there any changes in vision (now or after strangulation)?

— Does the patient have any difficulty swallowing (now or after strangulation)?

— Does the patient have any pain or bleeding (now or after strangulation)?

— Was there any incontinence of the bowel or bladder? Did the patient change clothes before coming in?

— What are notable characteristics of the patient's behavior and demeanor (eg, flat affect, looking away) and short-term memory?

— How long did the strangulation last (best estimate by patient)? What was the pressure on a scale of 0 to 10?

Activity 7-3. Physical Assessment

— Neurologic checks (eg, full cranial nerve assessment, cervical nerves in upper body, strength)

— Skin assessment for petechial hemorrhages (eg, conjunctiva, retinal splinter hemorrhages, scalp, ears)

— Speech assessment (eg, for clarity, slurring, hoarseness)

— Memory assessment (eg, orientation, sensory memory, recent and remote memory questions)

— Strength assessment and balance (eg, hands, jaws, squint)

— Assessment of oral cavity for tears to frenulum, bruising to buccal mucosa, petechiae, tongue, uvula midline, symmetrical smile, and other injuries

— Assessment for previous head injury

— Danger Assessment (eg, previous physical assaults, suicidal ideation and attempts, previous strangulation)

— Pulse oximetry reading

— Head-to-toe assessment, including checking and palpating abdomen

— Peripheral vision test and 6 cardinal fields of gaze

Activity 7-4. Evidence Collection

— Use evidence collection kit for *sexual assault and strangulation*, as stated by the patient or implied by the history. Kit should include a reference standard of the patient's DNA from the uninjured buccal area (if injury is present, consider drawing blood for DNA). Swab skin over contusions, fingernails, oral cavity, sides of face, and ears.

— Document the history given by the patient, using quotation marks for the patient's exact words.

— Assess and inspect specific anatomic locations for visible injury and pain on palpation.

— Photograph and measure, documenting all injuries, bruises, and areas the patient notes as painful. All photographs should be taken with and without an ABFO ruler.

— Photograph the 9 diagnostic positions of gaze of the eyes, including the inner aspects of the upper and lower lids.

— Take multiple photographs at 90-degree angles, 360 degrees around the neck.

— Inspect and photograph the oral cavity, including the hard palate, soft palate, uvula, and oropharynx, for petechiae or other injury.

— Inspect and photograph the ears, including anterior and posterior. Initial injury, unless it involves dermal capillary injury, may not be visible but over time may surface, allowing for reassessment and documentation.

— For reference (a baseline), measure and mark the neck at present and at follow-up in 72 hours to 14 days.

— Some programs use an ALS light to scan the neck for substances and to highlight injury. At this time, research does not support that ALS light identifies bruising; however, invert filters may identify bruises. More research is necessary to determine the usefulness of both methods. An ALS light can be used to identify substances.

— Photograph the hands using the size mat available on the SDFI website, taking note of the fingernails and any injuries. The advantage of using a size mat is to measure the size and angle of the photographs.

Activity 7-5. Treatment and Care

— The results of the physical examination are consistent with the history of the assault provided by the patient.

— Apply ice indirectly to the neck (eg, cloth or towel barrier between ice and skin) to reduce swelling as tolerated.

— Prepare the patient for radiographic studies.

— Discuss safety planning with the patient.

— Recommend medical observation for 12 to 23 hours, with continuous monitoring of pulse oximetry and vital signs as needed.

— Assess if the patient has a safe place to go after examination and discharge, and if not, involve the advocate or social services as necessary.

— The forensic nurse refers the patient to a community partner (eg, advocate, YWCA, other locally identified agencies) for shelter and victim of crime application.

— Victim advocate offers to assist in obtaining or referring for restraining order protection, if needed. The forensic nurse provides information to the patient and supports their decision about the order of protection.

— Provide a Danger Assessment and discuss the results with the patient, being transparent about the evidence-based risk assessment (eg, "The results reflect a population of persons and may not apply to you as an individual. However, these results can inform your decision about your situation.").

— Depending on jurisdictional mandated reporting laws, report to police or notify the agency within the jurisdiction if the patient requests law enforcement involvement. (Failure to report when mandatory may result in legal action against the nurse and/or health care provider.)

— Discuss findings with the patient and provide patient-specific strangulation discharge information, such as detailed instructions to return to the ED if neurologic signs or symptoms, dyspnea, dysphonia, odynophagia, or seizures develop or worsen. Discuss the possibility of a lifetime increased risk of neurologic consequences.

— Schedule follow-up forensic examination for 72 hours to 14 days after assault for additional medical forensic evaluation if possible within the framework of your program.

— Assess patient access to primary provider care or clinic care for follow-up in 14 days.

Chapter 8: 65-Year-Old Female Patient Assaulted by a Former Intimate Partner

Anatomic Skills 8-1

A. Right neck

B. Left neck

C. Anterior mid-neck

D. Anterior chest

Anatomic Skills 8-2

E. Right submandibular area

F. Chin

G. Left submandibular area

H. Anterior mid-neck

Activity 8-1. Injury Identification

I. Petechiae to right cheek

J. Petechiae to left cheek

K. Linear abrasions to right neck

L. 3 cm red bruise to anterior mid-neck with 0.5 cm abrasion

Activity 8-2. Assessment

— Use patient-friendly, nonmedical language when evaluating the patient (eg, difficulty breathing, swallowing, or talking).

— What was the method of strangulation (eg, 1 hand, 2 hands, ligature)?

— What were the symptoms of strangulation (eg, loss of consciousness, light-headedness, other neurologic symptoms)?

— Is there any neck pain (now or after strangulation)?

— Is there any difficulty breathing (now or after strangulation)?

— Are there any changes in the patient's voice (now or after strangulation)?

— Are there any changes in vision (now or after strangulation)?

— Does the patient have any difficulty swallowing (now or after strangulation)?

— Does the patient have any pain or bleeding (now or after strangulation)?

— Was there any incontinence of the bowel or bladder? Did the patient change clothes before coming in?

— What are notable characteristics of the patient's behavior and demeanor (eg, flat affect, looking away) and short-term memory?

— How long did the strangulation last (best estimate by patient)? What was the pressure on a scale of 0 to 10?

Activity 8-3. Physical Assessment

— Neurologic checks (eg, full cranial nerve assessment, cervical nerves in upper body, strength)

— Skin assessment for petechial hemorrhages (eg, conjunctiva, retinal splinter hemorrhages, scalp, ears)

— Speech assessment (eg, for clarity, slurring, hoarseness)

— Memory assessment (eg, orientation, sensory memory, recent and remote memory questions)

— Strength assessment and balance (eg, hands, jaws, squint)

— Assessment of oral cavity for tears to frenulum, bruising to buccal mucosa, petechiae, tongue, uvula midline, symmetrical smile, and other injuries

— Assessment for previous head injury

— Danger Assessment (eg, previous physical assaults, suicidal ideation and attempts, previous strangulation)

— Pulse oximetry reading

— Head-to-toe assessment, including checking and palpating abdomen

— Peripheral vision test and 6 cardinal fields of gaze

Activity 8-4. Evidence Collection

— Use evidence collection kit for *sexual assault and strangulation*, as stated by the patient or implied by the history. Kit should include a reference standard of the patient's DNA from the uninjured buccal area (if injury is present, consider drawing blood for DNA). Swab skin over contusions, fingernails, oral cavity, sides of face, and ears.

— Document the history given by the patient, using quotation marks around the patient's exact words.

— Assess and inspect specific anatomic locations for visible injury and pain on palpation.

— Photograph and measure, documenting all injuries, bruises, and areas the patient notes as painful. All photographs should be taken with and without an ABFO ruler.

— Photograph the 9 diagnostic positions of gaze of the eyes, including the inner aspects of the upper and lower lids.

— Take multiple photographs at 90-degree angles, 360 degrees around the neck.

— Inspect and photograph the oral cavity, including the hard palate, soft palate, uvula, and oropharynx, for petechiae or other injury.

— Inspect and photograph the ears, including anterior and posterior. Initial injury, unless it involves dermal capillary injury, may not be visible but over time may surface, allowing for reassessment and documentation.

— For reference (a baseline), measure and mark the neck at present and at follow-up in 72 hours to 14 days.

— Some programs use ALS to scan the neck for substances and to highlight injury. At this time, research does not support that ALS light identifies bruising; however, invert filters may identify bruises. More research is necessary to determine the usefulness of both methods. An ALS light can be used to identify substances.

— Photograph the hands using the size mat available on the SDFI website, taking note of the fingernails and any injuries. The advantage of using a size mat is to measure the size and angle of the photographs.

Activity 8-5. Treatment and Care

— The results of the physical examination are consistent with the history of the assault provided by the patient.

— Apply ice indirectly to the neck (eg, cloth or towel barrier between ice and skin) to reduce swelling as tolerated.

— Prepare the patient for radiographic studies.

— Discuss safety planning with the patient.

— Recommend medical observation for 12 to 23 hours, with continuous monitoring of pulse oximetry and vital signs, as needed.

— Assess if the patient has a safe place to go after examination and discharge, and if not, involve the advocate or social services as necessary.

— The forensic nurse refers the patient to a community partner (eg, advocate, YWCA, other locally identified agencies) for shelter and victim of crime application.

— Victim advocate offers to assist in obtaining or referring for restraining order protection, if needed. The forensic nurse provides information to the patient and supports their decision about order of protection.

— Provide a Danger Assessment and discuss the results with the patient, being transparent about the evidence-based risk assessment (eg, "The results reflect a population of persons and may not apply to you as an individual. However, these results can inform your decision about your situation.").

— Depending on jurisdictional mandated reporting laws, report to police or notify the agency within the jurisdiction if the patient requests law enforcement involvement. (Failure to report when mandatory may result in legal action against the nurse or health care provider.)

— Discuss findings with the patient and provide patient-specific strangulation discharge information, such as detailed instructions to return to the ED if neurological signs or symptoms, dyspnea, dysphonia, odynophagia, or seizures develop or worsen. Provide written instructions if the patient feels comfortable taking them with her. Discuss the possibility of a lifetime increased risk of neurologic consequences.

— Schedule follow-up forensic examination for 72 hours to 14 days after assault for additional medical forensic evaluation if possible within the framework of your program.

— Assess patient access to primary provider care or clinic care for follow-up in 14 days.

Activity 8-6 Lethality Assessment

Indicators of escalating danger include the following:

— Increase in frequency or severity of the assaults

— Increase of new threats of homicide or suicide

— Threats to children present in the home

— Presence of a firearm or deadly weapon in the home

Questions to assess immediate risk of violence include the following. Patients who answer "yes" to at least 3 of the following questions may be at especially high immediate risk of violence.

— Has the physical violence happened more often or gotten worse over the past 6 months?

— Has your partner ever used a weapon or threatened you with a weapon?

— Has your partner ever tried to strangle you?

— Do you believe your partner could kill you?

— Has your partner ever beaten you when you were pregnant?

— Is your partner violently and constantly jealous of you?

— Do you feel unsafe in your home?

Chapter 9: 31-Year-Old Female Patient Assaulted by a Former Intimate Partner

Anatomic Skills 9-1

A. Middle front neck

B. Left eye

C. Left inner wrist

Activity 9-1. Injury Identification

B. Scleral hemorrhage at 3 o'clock to the left eye

C. Bruise on left inner wrist

Activity 9-2. Assessment

— Use patient-friendly, nonmedical language when evaluating the patient (eg, difficulty breathing, swallowing, or talking).

— What was the method of strangulation (eg, 1 hand, 2 hands, ligature)?

— What were the symptoms of strangulation (eg, loss of consciousness, light-headedness, other neurologic symptoms)?

— Is there any neck pain (now or after strangulation)?

— Is there any difficulty breathing (now or after strangulation)?

— Are there any changes in the patient's voice (now or after strangulation)?

— Are there any changes in vision (now or after strangulation)?

— Does the patient have any difficulty swallowing (now or after strangulation)?

— Does the patient have any pain or bleeding (now or after strangulation)?

— Was there any incontinence of the bowel or bladder? Did the patient change clothes before coming in?

— What are notable characteristics of the patient's behavior and demeanor (eg, flat affect, looking away) and short-term memory?

— How long did the strangulation last (best estimate by patient)? What was the pressure on a scale of 0 to 10?

Activity 9-3. Physical Assessment

— Neurologic checks (eg, full cranial nerve assessment, cervical nerves in upper body, strength)

— Skin assessment for petechial hemorrhages (eg, conjunctiva, retinal hemorrhages, scalp, ears)

— Speech assessment (eg, for clarity, slurring, hoarseness)

— Memory assessment (eg, orientation, sensory memory, recent and remote memory questions)

— Strength assessment and balance (eg, hands, jaws, squint)

— Assessment of oral cavity for tears to frenulum, bruising to buccal mucosa, petechiae, tongue, uvula midline, symmetrical smile, and other injuries

— Assessment for previous head injury

— Danger Assessment (eg, previous physical assaults, suicide ideation and attempts, previous strangulation)

— Pulse oximetry reading

— Head-to-toe assessment, including checking and palpating abdomen

— Peripheral vision test and 6 cardinal fields of gaze

Activity 9-4. Evidence Collection

— Use evidence collection kit for *sexual assault and strangulation*, as stated by the patient or implied by the history. Kit should include a reference standard of the patient's DNA from the uninjured buccal area (if injury is present, consider drawing blood for the DNA). Swab skin over contusions, fingernails, oral cavity, sides of face, and ears.

— Document the history given by the patient, using quotation marks around the patient's exact words.

— Assess and inspect specific anatomic locations for visible injury and pain on palpation.

— Photograph and measure, documenting all injuries, bruises, and areas the patient notes as painful. All photographs should be taken with and without an ABFO ruler.

— Photograph the 9 diagnostic positions of gaze of the eyes, including the inner aspects of the upper and lower lids.

— Take multiple photographs at 90-degree angles, 360 degrees around the neck.

— Inspect and photograph the oral cavity, including the hard palate, soft palate, uvula, and oropharynx, for petechiae or other injury.

— Inspect and photograph the ears, including anterior and posterior. Initial injury, unless it involves dermal capillary injury, may not be visible but over time may surface, allowing for reassessment and documentation.

— For reference (a baseline), measure and mark the neck at present and at follow-up in 72 hours to 14 days.

— Some programs use an ALS light to scan the neck for substances and to assist in visualizing possible injuries under the skin. At this time, research does not support that ALS light identifies bruising; however, invert filters may identify bruises. More research is necessary to determine the usefulness of both methods. An ALS light can be used to identify substances.

— Photograph the hands using the size mat available on the SDFI website, taking note of the fingernails and any injuries. The advantage of using a size mat is to measure the size and angle of the photographs.

Activity 9-5. Treatment and Care

— The results of the physical examination are consistent with the history of the assault provided by the patient.

— Apply ice indirectly to the neck (eg, cloth or towel barrier between ice and skin) to reduce swelling as tolerated.

— Prepare the patient for radiographic studies.

— Discuss safety planning with the patient.

— Recommend medical observation for 12 to 23 hours, with continuous monitoring of pulse oximetry and vital signs as needed.

— Assess if the patient has a safe place to go after examination and discharge, and if not, involve the advocate or social services as necessary.

— The forensic nurse refers the patient to a community partner (eg, advocate, YWCA, other locally identified agencies) for shelter and victim of crime application.

— Victim advocate offers to assist in obtaining or referring for restraining order protection, if needed. The forensic nurse provides information to the patient and supports their decision about order of protection.

— Provide a Danger Assessment and discuss the results with the patient, being transparent about the evidence-based risk assessment (eg, "The results reflect a population of persons and may not apply to you as an individual. However, these results can inform your decision about your situation.").

— Depending on jurisdictional mandated reporting laws, report to police or notify the agency within the jurisdiction if the patient requests law enforcement involvement. (Failure to report when mandatory may result in legal action against the nurse or health care provider.)

— Discuss findings with the patient and provide patient-specific strangulation discharge information, such as detailed instructions to return to the ED if neurologic signs or symptoms, dyspnea, dysphonia, odynophagia, or seizures develop or worsen. Provide written instructions if the patient feels comfortable taking them with her. Discuss the possibility of a lifetime increased risk of neurologic consequences.

— Schedule follow-up forensic examination for 72 hours to 14 days after assault for additional medical forensic evaluation if possible within the framework of your program.

— Assess patient access to primary provider care or clinic care for follow-up in 14 days.

Activity 9-6 Lethality Assessment

Indicators of escalating danger include the following:

— Increase in frequency or severity of the assaults

— Increase of new threats of homicide or suicide

— Threats to children present in the home

— Presence of a firearm or deadly weapon in the home

Questions to assess immediate risk of violence include the following. Patients who answer "yes" to at least 3 of the following questions may be at especially high risk of immediate violence.

— Has the physical violence happened more often or gotten worse over the past 6 months?

— Has your partner ever used a weapon or threatened you with a weapon?

— Has your partner ever tried to strangle you?

— Do you believe your partner could kill you?

— Has your partner ever beaten you when you were pregnant?

— Is your partner violently and constantly jealous of you?

— Do you feel unsafe in your home?

Chapter 10: 22-Year-Old Female Patient Assaulted by a Former Intimate Partner

Anatomic Skills 10-1

A. Right submandibular area

B. Chin

C. Right mid-neck area

D. Right lower neck

Anatomic Skills 10-2

E. Chin

F. Right neck

G. Anterior mid-neck

H. Left neck

Activity 10-1. Injury Identification

I. ~1.25 cm × 1 cm area of red/purple bruising, right neck

J. Multiple ~1.5 cm linear abrasions, right neck

K. Swelling and tenderness, right superior carotid triangle

L. 1 cm × 0.5 cm red/purple bruise, left neck

M. Subconjunctival hemorrhage 6 to 7 o'clock, right eye

N. ~1 cm × 0.5 cm red/purple bruise, upper helix of left ear

O. 2 cm × 1 cm gray bruise, posterior left ear with petechiae

P. Red/purple bruising with swelling, left top and bottom lips on labial side

Q. ~4 cm × 4 cm double-arch crescent abrasions with scabbing

Activity 10-2. Assessment

— Use patient-friendly, nonmedical language when evaluating the patient (eg, difficulty breathing, swallowing, or talking).

— What was the method of strangulation (eg, 1 hand, 2 hands, ligature)?

— What were the symptoms of strangulation (eg, loss of consciousness, light-headedness, other neurologic symptoms)?

— Is there any neck pain (now or after strangulation)?

— Is there any difficulty breathing (now or after strangulation)?

— Are there any changes in the patient's voice (now or after strangulation)?

— Are there any changes in vision (now or after strangulation)?

— Does the patient have any difficulty swallowing (now or after strangulation)?

— Does the patient have any pain or bleeding (now or after strangulation)?

— Was there any incontinence of the bowel or bladder? Did the patient change clothes before coming in?

— What are notable characteristics of the patient's behavior and demeanor (eg, flat affect, looking away) and short-term memory?

— How long did the strangulation last (best estimate by patient)? What was the pressure on a scale of 0 to 10?

Activity 10-3. Physical Assessment

— Neurologic checks (eg, full cranial nerve assessment, cervical nerves in upper body, strength)

— Skin assessment for petechial hemorrhages (eg, conjunctiva, retinal splinter hemorrhages, scalp, ears)

— Speech assessment (eg, for clarity, slurring, hoarseness)

— Memory assessment (eg, orientation, sensory memory, recent and remote memory questions)

— Strength assessment and balance (eg, hands, jaws, squint)

— Assessment of oral cavity for tears to frenulum, bruising to buccal mucosa, petechiae, tongue, uvula midline, symmetrical smile, and other injuries

— Assessment for previous head injury

— Danger Assessment (eg, previous physical assaults, suicidal ideation and attempts, previous strangulation)

— Pulse oximetry reading

— Head-to-toe assessment, including checking and palpating abdomen

— Peripheral vision test and 6 cardinal fields of gaze

Activity 10-4. Evidence Collection

— Use evidence collection kit for *strangulation*, as stated by the patient or implied by the history. Kit should include a reference standard of the patient's DNA from the uninjured buccal area (if injury is present, consider drawing blood for DNA). Swab skin over contusions, fingernails, oral cavity, sides of face, and ears.

— Document the history given by the patient, using quotation marks around the patient's exact words.

— Assess and inspect specific anatomic locations for visible injury and pain on palpation.

— Photograph and measure, documenting all injuries, bruises, and areas the patient notes as painful. All photographs should be taken with and without an ABFO ruler.

— Photograph the 9 diagnostic positions of gaze of the eyes, including the inner aspects of the upper and lower lids.

— Take multiple photographs at 90-degree angles, 360 degrees around the neck.

— Inspect and photograph the oral cavity, including the hard palate, soft palate, uvula, and oropharynx, for petechiae or other injury.

— Inspect and photograph the ears, including anterior and posterior. Initial injury, unless it involves dermal capillary injury, may not be visible but over time may surface, allowing for reassessment and documentation.

— For reference (a baseline), measure and mark the neck at present and at follow-up in 72 hours to 14 days.

— Some programs use an ALS light to scan the neck for substances and to highlight injury. At this time, research does not support that ALS light identifies bruising; however, invert filters may identify bruises. More research is necessary to determine the usefulness of both methods. An ALS light can be used to identify substances.

— Photograph the hands using the size mat available on the SDFI website, taking note of the fingernails and any injuries. The advantage of using a size mat is to measure the size and angle of the photographs.

Activity 10-5. Treatment and Care

— The results of the physical examination are consistent with the history of the assault provided by the patient.

— Apply ice indirectly to the neck (eg, cloth or towel barrier between ice and skin) to reduce swelling as tolerated.

— Prepare the patient for radiographic studies.

— Discuss safety planning with the patient.

— Recommend medical observation for 12 to 23 hours, with continuous monitoring of pulse oximetry and vital signs as needed.

— Assess if the patient has a safe place to go after examination and discharge, and if not, involve the advocate or social services as necessary.

— The forensic nurse refers the patient to a community partner (eg, advocate, YWCA, other locally identified agencies) for shelter and victim of crime application.

— Victim advocate offers to assist in obtaining or referring for restraining order protection if needed. The forensic nurse provides information to the patient and supports their decision about the order of protection.

— Provide a Danger Assessment and discuss the results with the patient, being transparent about the evidence-based risk assessment (eg, "The results reflect a population of persons and may not apply to you as an individual. However, these results can inform your decision about your situation.").

— Depending on jurisdictional mandated reporting laws, report to police or notify the agency within the jurisdiction if the patient requests law enforcement involvement. (Failure to report when mandatory may result in legal action against the nurse and/or health care provider.)

— Discuss findings with the patient and provide patient-specific strangulation discharge information, such as detailed instructions to return to the ED if neurologic signs or symptoms, dyspnea, dysphonia, odynophagia, or seizures develop or worsen. Provide written instructions if the patient feels comfortable taking them with her. Discuss the possibility of a lifetime increased risk of neurologic consequences.

— Schedule follow-up forensic examination for 72 hours to 14 days after the assault for additional medical forensic evaluation if possible within the framework of your program.

— Assess patient access to primary provider care or clinic care for follow-up in 14 days.

Activity 10-6 Lethality Assessment

Indicators of escalating danger include the following:

— An increase in frequency or severity of the assaults

— Increasing of new threats of homicide or suicide

— Threats to children present in the home

— Presence of a firearm or deadly weapon in the home

Questions to assess immediate risk of violence include the following. Patients who answer "yes" to at least 3 of the following questions may be at especially high immediate risk of violence.

— Has the physical violence happened more often or gotten worse over the past 6 months?

— Has your partner ever used a weapon or threatened you with a weapon?

— Has your partner ever tried to strangle you?

— Do you believe your partner could kill you?

— Has your partner ever beaten you when you were pregnant?

— Is your partner violently and constantly jealous of you?

— Do you feel unsafe in your home?

Chapter 11: 70-year-old Male Patient Assaulted by an Employee

Anatomic Skills 11-1

A. Chin

B. Right neck

C. Left neck

D. Anterior mid-neck

Anatomic Skills 11-2

E. Right submandibular area

F. Chin

G. Right mid-neck

H. Right lower neck

Activity 11-1. Injury Identification

I. 75 cm × 0.25 cm red/purple bruise, left mid-buccal

J. 1 cm × 3.5 cm purple/gray bruise, right mid-neck (with sparring caused by skin wrinkling)

K. 5 cm × 5 cm double-arched abrasion (history of bite) with scabbing on follow-up examination

L. Subconjunctival hematoma 12 to 5 o'clock, left eye

M. 7 cm × 7 cm dark gray bruising (sparing caused by skin wrinkling)

N. 25 cm × 3 cm yellow/gray bruising

Activity 11-2. Assessment

— Use patient-friendly, nonmedical language when evaluating the patient (eg, difficulty breathing, swallowing, or talking).

— What was the method of strangulation (eg, 1 hand, 2 hands, ligature)?

— What were the symptoms of strangulation (eg, loss of consciousness, light-headedness, other neurologic symptoms)?

— Is there any neck pain (now or after strangulation)?

— Is there any difficulty breathing (now or after strangulation)?

— Are there any changes in the patient's voice (now or after strangulation)?

— Are there any changes in vision (now or after strangulation)?

— Does the patient have any difficulty swallowing (now or after strangulation)?

— Does the patient have any pain or bleeding (now or after strangulation)?

— Was there any incontinence of the bowel or bladder? Did the patient change clothes before coming in?

— What are notable characteristics of the patient's behavior and demeanor (eg, flat affect, looking away) and short-term memory?

— How long did the strangulation last (best estimate by patient)? What was the pressure on a scale of 0 to 10?

Activity 11-3. Physical Assessment

— Neurologic checks (eg, full cranial nerve assessment, cervical nerves in upper body, strength)

— Skin assessment for petechial hemorrhages (eg, conjunctiva, retinal splinter hemorrhages, scalp, ears)

— Speech assessment (eg, for clarity, slurring, hoarseness)

— Memory assessment (eg, orientation, sensory memory, recent and remote memory questions)

— Strength assessment and balance (eg, hands, jaws, squint)

— Assessment of oral cavity for tears to frenulum, bruising to buccal mucosa, petechiae, tongue, uvula midline, symmetrical smile, and other injuries

— Assessment for previous head injury

— Danger Assessment (eg, previous physical assaults, suicidal ideation and attempts, previous strangulation)

— Pulse oximetry reading

— Head-to-toe assessment, including checking and palpating abdomen

— Peripheral vision test and 6 cardinal fields of gaze

Activity 11-4. Evidence Collection

— Use evidence collection kit for *strangulation*, as stated by the patient or implied by the history. Kit should include a reference standard of the patient's DNA from the uninjured buccal area (if injury is present, consider drawing blood for DNA). Swab skin over contusions, fingernails, oral cavity, sides of face, and ears.

— Document the history given by the patient, using quotation marks around the patient's exact words.

— Assess and inspect specific anatomic locations for visible injury and pain on palpation.

— Photograph and measure, documenting all injuries, bruises, and areas the patient notes as painful. All photographs should be taken with and without an ABFO ruler.

— Photograph the 9 diagnostic positions of gaze of the eyes, including the inner aspects of the upper and lower lids.

— Take multiple photographs at 90-degree angles, 360 degrees around the neck.

— Inspect and photograph the oral cavity, including the hard palate, soft palate, uvula, and oropharynx, for petechiae or other injury.

— Inspect and photograph the ears, including anterior and posterior. Initial injury, unless it involves dermal capillary injury, may not be visible but over time may surface, allowing for reassessment and documentation.

— For reference (a baseline), measure and mark the neck at present and at follow-up in 72 hours to 14 days.

— Some programs use an ALS light to scan the neck for substances and to highlight injury. At this time, research does not support that ALS light identifies bruising; however, invert filters may identify bruises. More research is necessary to determine the usefulness of both methods. An ALS light can be used to identify substances.

— Photograph the hands using the size mat available on the SDFI website, taking note of the fingernails and any injuries. The advantage of using a size mat is to measure the size and angle of the photographs.

Activity 11-5. Treatment and Care

— The results of the physical examination are consistent with the history of the assault provided by the patient.

— Apply ice indirectly to the neck (eg, cloth or towel barrier between ice and skin) to reduce swelling as tolerated.

— Prepare the patient for radiographic studies.

— Discuss safety planning with the patient.

— Recommend medical observation for 12 to 23 hours, with continuous monitoring of pulse oximetry and vital signs as needed.

— Assess if the patient has a safe place to go after examination and discharge, and if not, involve the advocate or social services as necessary.

— The forensic nurse refers the patient to a community partner (eg, advocate, YWCA, other locally identified agencies) for shelter and victim of crime application.

— Victim advocate offers to assist in obtaining or referring for restraining order protection if needed. The forensic nurse provides information to the patient and supports their decision about the order of protection.

— Provide a Danger Assessment and discuss the results with the patient, being transparent about the evidence-based risk assessment (eg, "The results reflect a population of persons and may not apply to you as an individual. However, these results can inform your decision about your situation.").

— Depending on jurisdictional mandated reporting laws, report to police or notify the agency within the jurisdiction if the patient requests law enforcement involvement. (Failure to report when mandatory may result in legal action against the nurse and/or health care provider.)

— Discuss findings with the patient and provide patient-specific strangulation discharge information, such as detailed instructions to return to the ED if neurologic signs or symptoms, dyspnea, dysphonia, odynophagia, or seizures develop or worsen. Discuss the possibility of a lifetime increased risk of neurologic consequences.

— Schedule follow-up forensic examination for 72 hours to 14 days after assault for additional medical forensic evaluation if possible within the framework of your program.

— Assess patient access to primary provider care/clinic care for follow-up in 14 days.

Chapter 12: 56-Year-Old Female Patient Assaulted by an Ex-Husband

Anatomic Skills 12-1

A. Chin

B. Anterior mid-neck

Anatomic Skills 12-2

C. Upper lip

D. Tongue

Activity 12-1. Injury Identification

E. 6 cm x 1.5 cm red/purple irregularly shaped bruise, left lateral mid-neck

F. Multiple red linear abrasions, 1 cm to 1.5 cm long, right lateral mid-neck and under jawline

G. Red linear abrasion, 2 cm long, anterior midline neck

H. Dark red pattern bruising with abrasions, left lateral tongue (possible self-inflicted bite per history)

Activity 12-2. Assessment

— What was the method of strangulation (eg, 1 hand, 2 hands, ligature)?

— What were the symptoms of strangulation (eg, loss of consciousness, light-headedness, other neurologic symptoms)?

— Is there any neck pain (now or after strangulation)?

— Is there any difficulty breathing (now or after strangulation)?

— Are there any changes in the patient's voice (now or after strangulation)?

— Are there any changes in vision (now or after strangulation)?

— Does the patient have any difficulty swallowing (now or after strangulation)?

— Does the patient have any pain or bleeding (now or after strangulation)?

— Was there any incontinence of the bowel or bladder? Did the patient change clothes before coming in?

— What are notable characteristics of the patient's behavior and demeanor (eg, flat affect, looking away) and short-term memory?

— How long did the strangulation last (best estimate by patient)? What was the pressure on a scale of 0 to 10?

Activity 12-3. Physical Assessment

— Use patient-friendly, nonmedical language when evaluating the patient (eg, difficulty breathing, swallowing, or talking).

— Neurologic checks (eg, full cranial nerve assessment, cervical nerves in upper body, strength)

— Skin assessment for petechial hemorrhages (eg, conjunctiva, retinal splinter hemorrhages, scalp, ears)

— Speech assessment (eg, for clarity, slurring, hoarseness)

— Memory assessment (eg, orientation, sensory memory, recent and remote memory questions)

— Strength assessment and balance (eg, hands, jaws, squint)

— Assessment of oral cavity for tears to frenulum, bruising to buccal mucosa, petechiae, tongue, uvula midline, symmetrical smile, and other injuries

— Assessment for previous head injury

— Danger Assessment (eg, previous physical assaults, suicide ideation and attempts, previous strangulation)

— Pulse oximetry reading

— Head-to-toe assessment, including checking and palpating abdomen

— Peripheral vision test and 6 cardinal fields of gaze

Activity 12-4. Evidence Collection

— Use evidence collection kit for *strangulation*, as stated by the patient or implied by the history. Kit should include a reference standard of the patient's DNA from the uninjured buccal area (if injury is present, consider drawing blood for DNA). Swab skin over contusions, fingernails, oral cavity, sides of face, and ears.

— Document the history given by the patient, using quotation marks around the patient's exact words.

— Assess and inspect specific anatomic locations for visible injury and pain on palpation.

— Photograph and measure, documenting all injuries, bruises, and areas the patient notes as painful. All photographs should be taken with and without an ABFO ruler.

— Photograph the 9 diagnostic positions of gaze of the eyes, including the inner aspects of the upper and lower lids.

— Take multiple photographs at 90-degree angles, 360 degrees around the neck.

— Inspect and photograph the oral cavity, including the hard palate, soft palate, uvula, and oropharynx, for petechiae or other injury.

— Inspect and photograph the ears, including anterior and posterior. Initial injury, unless it involves dermal capillary injury, may not be visible but over time may surface, allowing for reassessment and documentation.

— For reference (a baseline), measure and mark the neck at present and at follow-up in 72 hours to 14 days.

— Some programs use an ALS light to scan the neck for substances and to highlight injury. At this time, research does not support that ALS light identifies bruising; however, invert filters may identify bruises. More research is necessary to determine the usefulness of both methods. An ALS light can be used to identify substances.

— Photograph the hands using the size mat available on the SDFI website, taking note of the fingernails and any injuries. The advantage of using a size mat is to measure the size and angle of the photographs.

Activity 12-5. Treatment and Care

— The results of the physical examination are consistent with the history of the assault provided by the patient.

— Apply ice indirectly to the neck (eg, cloth or towel barrier between ice and skin) to reduce swelling as tolerated.

— Prepare the patient for radiographic studies.

— Discuss safety planning with the patient.

— Recommend medical observation for 12 to 23 hours, with continuous monitoring of pulse oximetry and vital signs as needed.

— Assess if the patient has a safe place to go after examination and discharge, and if not, involve the advocate or social services as necessary.

— The forensic nurse refers the patient to a community partner (eg, advocate, YWCA, other locally identified agencies) for shelter and victim of crime application.

— Victim advocate offers to assist in obtaining or referring for restraining order protection if needed. The forensic nurse provides information to the patient and supports their decision about the order of protection.

— Provide a Danger Assessment and discuss the results with the patient, being transparent about the evidence-based risk assessment (eg, "The results reflect a population of persons and may not apply to you as an individual. However, these results can inform your decision about your situation.").

— Depending on jurisdictional mandated reporting laws, report to police or notify the agency within the jurisdiction if the patient requests law enforcement involvement. (Failure to report when mandatory may result in legal action against the nurse and/or health care provider.)

— Discuss findings with the patient and provide patient-specific strangulation discharge information, such as detailed instructions to return to the ED if neurologic signs or symptoms, dyspnea, dysphonia, odynophagia, or seizures develop or worsen. Provide written instructions if the patient feels comfortable taking them with her. Discuss the possibility of a lifetime increased risk of neurologic consequences.

— Schedule follow-up forensic examination for 72 hours to 14 days after assault for additional medical forensic evaluation if possible within the framework of your program.

— Assess patient access to primary provider care or clinic care for follow-up in 14 days.

Activity 12-6 Lethality Assessment

Indicators of escalating danger include the following:

— Increase in frequency or severity of the assaults

— Increase of new threats of homicide or suicide

— Threats to children present in the home

— Presence of a firearm or deadly weapon in the home

Questions to assess immediate risk of violence include the following. Patients who answer "yes" to at least 3 of the following questions may be at especially high immediate risk of violence.

— Has the physical violence happened more often or gotten worse over the past 6 months?

— Has your partner ever used a weapon or threatened you with a weapon?

— Has your partner ever tried to strangle you?

— Do you believe your partner could kill you?

— Has your partner ever beaten you when you were pregnant?

— Is your partner violently and constantly jealous of you?

— Do you feel unsafe in your home?

Chapter 13: 30-year-old Female Patient Assaulted and Strangled by an Intimate Partner

Anatomic Skills 13-1

A. Right clavicle

B. Suprasternal notch

C. Left lateral neck

Activity 13-1. Injury Identification

D. Florid petechial hemorrhage of the face

E. Fingernail abrasions

F. Scleral hemorrhages

G. Petechial hemorrhage

H. Pattern contusions to the anterior neck (necklace)

I. Intraoral contusion

J. Florid petechial hemorrhages

K. Forehead abrasion (fall to floor)

L. Tongue laceration (may be associated with an anoxic seizure)

Activity 13-2. Petechial Hemorrhages

Florid petechial hemorrhage of the face indicates a relatively long period of venous obstruction. In the experience of the author, florid facial petechial hemorrhage is always associated with either unconsciousness or fatal strangulation.

Activity 13-3. Assessment

— Use patient-friendly, nonmedical language when evaluating the patient (eg, difficulty breathing, swallowing, or talking).

— What was the method of strangulation (eg, 1 hand, 2 hands, ligature)?

— What were the symptoms of strangulation (eg, loss of consciousness, light-headedness, or other neurologic symptoms?

— Is there any neck pain (now or after strangulation)?

— Is there any difficulty breathing (now or after strangulation)?

— Are there any changes in the patient's voice (now or after strangulation)?

— Are there any changes in vision (now or after strangulation)?

— Does the patient have any difficulty swallowing (now or after strangulation)?

— Does the patient have any pain or bleeding (now or after strangulation)?

— Was there any incontinence of the bowel or bladder? Did the patient change clothes before coming in?

— What are notable characteristics of the patient's behavior and demeanor (eg, flat affect, looking away) and short-term memory?

— How long did the strangulation last (best estimate by patient)? What was the pressure on a scale of 0 to 10?

Activity 13-4. Physical Assessment

— Neurologic checks (eg, full cranial nerve assessment, cervical nerves in upper body, strength)

— Skin assessment for petechial hemorrhages (eg, conjunctiva, retinal splinter hemorrhages, scalp, ears)

— Speech assessment (eg, for clarity, slurring, hoarseness)

— Memory assessment (eg, orientation, sensory memory, recent and remote memory questions)

— Strength assessment and balance (eg, hands, jaws, squint)

— Assessment of oral cavity for tears to frenulum, bruising to buccal mucosa, petechiae, tongue, uvula midline, symmetrical smile, and other injuries

— Assessment for previous head injury

— Danger Assessment (eg, previous physical assaults, suicidal ideation and attempts, previous strangulation)

— Pulse oximetry reading

— Head-to-toe assessment, including checking and palpating abdomen

— Peripheral vision test and 6 cardinal fields of gaze

Activity 13-5. Evidence Collection

— Use evidence collection kit for *sexual assault and strangulation*, as stated by the patient or implied by the history. Kit should include a reference standard of the patient's DNA from the uninjured buccal area (if injury is present, consider drawing blood for DNA). Swab skin over contusions, fingernails, oral cavity, sides of face, and ears.

— Document the history given by the patient, using quotation marks for the patient's exact words.

— Assess and inspect specific anatomic locations for visible injury and pain on palpation.

— Photograph and measure, documenting all injuries, bruises, and areas the patient notes as painful. All photographs should be taken with and without an ABFO ruler.

— Photograph the 9 diagnostic positions of gaze of the eyes, including the inner aspects of the upper and lower lids.

— Take multiple photographs at 90-degree angles, 360 degrees around the neck.

— Inspect and photograph the oral cavity, including the hard palate, soft palate, uvula, and oropharynx, for petechiae or other injury.

— Inspect and photograph the ears, including anterior and posterior. Initial injury, unless it involves dermal capillary injury, may not be visible but over time may surface, allowing for reassessment and documentation.

— For reference (a baseline), measure and mark the neck at present and at follow-up in 72 hours to 14 days.

— Some programs use an ALS light to scan the neck for substances and to highlight injury. At this time, research does not support that ALS light identifies bruising; however, invert filters may identify bruises. More research is necessary to determine the usefulness of both methods. An ALS light can be used to identify substances.

— Photograph the hands using the size mat available on the SDFI website, taking note of the fingernails and any injuries. The advantage of using a size mat is to measure the size and angle of the photographs.

Activity 13-6. Treatment and Care

— Computed tomography angiography (CTA) of the neck to rule out internal injuries and carotid or vertebral dissections is medically indicated. The history of being lifted up by the neck can result in stretching of the internal carotid artery and cause a carotid dissection.

— The results of the physical examination are consistent with the history of the assault provided by the patient.

— Apply ice indirectly to the neck (eg, cloth or towel barrier between ice and skin) to reduce swelling as tolerated.

— Prepare the patient for the CTA and other radiographic studies.

— Discuss safety planning with the patient.

— Recommend medical observation for 12 to 23 hours, with continuous monitoring of pulse oximetry and vital signs, as needed.

— Discharge is safe after a negative CTA unless there are positive toxicology results or progression of symptoms.

— Assess if the patient has a safe place to go after examination and discharge, and if not, involve the advocate or social services as necessary.

— The forensic nurse refers the patient to a community partner (eg, advocate, YWCA, other locally identified agencies) for shelter and victim of crime application.

— Victim advocate offers to assist in obtaining or referring for restraining order protection, if needed. The forensic nurse provides information to the patient and supports their decision about the order of protection.

— Provide a Danger Assessment and discuss the results with the patient, being transparent about the evidence-based risk assessment (eg, "The results reflect a population of persons and may not apply to you as an individual. However, these results can inform your decision about your situation.").

— Depending on jurisdictional mandated reporting laws, report to police or notify the agency within the jurisdiction if the patient requests law enforcement involvement. (Failure to report when mandatory may result in legal action against the nurse and/or health care provider.)

— Discuss findings with the patient and provide patient-specific strangulation discharge information, such as detailed instructions to return to the ED if neurologic signs or symptoms, dyspnea, dysphonia, odynophagia, or seizures develop or worsen. Provide written instructions if the patient feels comfortable taking them with her. Discuss the possibility of a lifetime increased risk of neurologic consequences.

— Schedule follow-up forensic examination for 72 hours to 14 days after assault for additional medical forensic evaluation if possible within the framework of your program.

— Assess patient access to primary provider care or clinic care for follow-up in 14 days.

Activity 13-7. Lethality Assessment

Indicators of escalating danger include the following:

— Increase in frequency or severity of the assaults

— Increase of new threats of homicide or suicide

— Threats to children present in the home

— Presence of a firearm or deadly weapon in the home

Questions to assess immediate risk of violence include the following. Patients who answer "yes" to at least 3 of the following questions may be at especially high immediate risk of violence.

— Has the physical violence happened more often or gotten worse over the past 6 months?

— Has your partner ever used a weapon or threatened you with a weapon?

— Has your partner ever tried to strangle you?

— Do you believe your partner could kill you?

— Has your partner ever beaten you when you were pregnant?

— Is your partner violently and constantly jealous of you?

— Do you feel unsafe in your home?

Chapter 14: 25-Year-Old Female Patient Assaulted by a Stranger

Anatomic Skills 14-1

A. Midline chest

B. Neck

Anatomic Skills 14-2

C. 5 cm x 7 cm black-blue bruise, middle left chest

Activity 14-1. Injury Identification

D. Multiple blue-black bruises, mastoid area of the head

E. Multiple blue-black bruises, posterior right ear

Activity 14-2. Injury Identification

Multiple scattered bruises and abrasions to the right lateral neck

Activity 14-3. Assessment

— Use patient-friendly, nonmedical language when evaluating the patient (eg, difficulty breathing, swallowing, or talking).

— What was the method of strangulation (eg, 1 hand, 2 hands, ligature)?

— What were the symptoms of strangulation (eg, loss of consciousness, light-headedness, other neurologic symptoms)?

— Is there any neck pain (now or after strangulation)?

— Is there any difficulty breathing (now or after strangulation)?

— Are there any changes in the patient's voice (now or after strangulation)?

— Are there any changes in vision (now or after strangulation)?

— Does the patient have any difficulty swallowing (now or after strangulation)?

— Does the patient have any pain or bleeding (now or after strangulation)?

— Was there any incontinence of the bowel or bladder? Did the patient change clothes before coming in?

— What are notable characteristics of the patient's behavior and demeanor (eg, flat affect, looking away) and short-term memory?

— How long did the strangulation last (best estimate by patient)? What was the pressure on a scale of 0 to 10?

Activity 14-4. Physical Assessment

— Neurologic checks (eg, full cranial nerve assessment, cervical nerves in upper body, strength)

— Skin assessment for petechial hemorrhages (eg, conjunctiva, retinal splinter hemorrhages, scalp, ears)

— Speech assessment (eg, for clarity, slurring, hoarseness)

— Memory assessment (eg, orientation, sensory memory, recent and remote memory questions)

— Strength assessment and balance (eg, hands, jaws, squint)

— Assessment of oral cavity for tears to frenulum, bruising to buccal mucosa, petechiae, tongue, uvula midline, symmetrical smile, and other injuries

— Assessment for previous head injury

— Danger Assessment (eg, previous physical assaults, suicidal ideation and attempts, previous strangulation)

— Pulse oximetry reading

— Head-to-toe assessment, including checking and palpating abdomen

— Peripheral vision test and 6 cardinal fields of gaze

Activity 14-5. Evidence Collection

— Use evidence collection kit for *sexual assault and nonfatal strangulation*, as stated by the patient or implied by the history. Kit should include a reference standard of the patient's DNA from the uninjured buccal area (if injury is present, consider drawing blood for DNA). Swab skin over contusions, fingernails, oral cavity, sides of face, and ears.

— Document the history given by the patient, using quotation marks around the patient's exact words.

— Assess and inspect specific anatomic locations for visible injury and pain on palpation.

— Photograph and measure, documenting all injuries, bruises, and areas the patient notes as painful. All photographs should be taken with and without an ABFO ruler.

— Photograph the 9 diagnostic positions of gaze of the eyes, including the inner aspects of the upper and lower lids.

— Take multiple photographs at 90-degree angles, 360 degrees around the neck.

— Inspect and photograph the oral cavity, including the hard palate, soft palate, uvula, and oropharynx, for petechiae or other injury.

— Inspect and photograph the ear, including posterior and anterior. Initial injury, unless it involves dermal capillary injury, may not be visible but over time may surface, allowing for reassessment and documentation.

— For reference (a baseline), measure and mark the neck at present and at follow-up in 72 hours to 14 days.

— Some programs use an ALS light to scan the neck for substances and to highlight injury. At this time, research does not support that ALS light identifies bruising; however, invert filters may identify bruises. More research is necessary to determine the usefulness of both methods. An ALS light can be used to identify substances.

— Photograph the hands using the size mat available on the SDFI website, taking note of the fingernails and any injuries. The advantage of using a size mat is to measure the size and angle of the photographs.

Activity 14-6. Treatment and Care

— The results of the physical examination are consistent with the history of the assault provided by the patient.

— Apply ice indirectly to the neck (eg, cloth or towel barrier between ice and skin) to reduce swelling, as tolerated.

— Prepare the patient for radiographic studies.

— Discuss safety planning with the patient.

— Recommend medical observation for 12 to 23 hours, with continuous monitoring of pulse oximetry and vital signs, as needed.

— Assess if the patient has a safe place to go after examination and discharge, and if not, involve the advocate or social services as necessary.

— The forensic nurse refers the patient to a community partner (eg, advocate, YWCA, other locally identified agencies) for shelter and victim of crime application.

— Victim advocate offers to assist in obtaining or referring for restraining order protection, if needed. The forensic nurse provides information to the patient and supports their decision about the order of protection.

— Provide a Danger Assessment and discuss the results with the patient, being transparent about the evidence-based risk assessment (eg, "The results reflect a population of persons and may not apply to you as an individual. However, these results can inform your decision about your situation.").

— Depending on jurisdictional mandated reporting laws, report to police or notify the agency within the jurisdiction if the patient requests law enforcement involvement. (Failure to report when mandatory may result in legal action against the nurse and/or health care provider.)

— Discuss findings with the patient and provide patient-specific strangulation discharge information, such as detailed instructions to return to the ED if neurologic signs or symptoms, dyspnea, dysphonia, odynophagia, or seizures develop or worsen. Discuss the possibility of a lifetime increased risk of neurologic consequences.

— Schedule follow-up forensic examination for 72 hours to 14 days after assault for additional medical forensic evaluation if possible within the framework of your program.

— Assess patient access to primary provider care or clinic care for follow-up in 14 days.

Chapter 15: 46-Year-old Female Patient Assaulted and Strangled by Her Husband

Anatomic Skills 15-1

A. Right pre-auricular area

B. Right infraorbital area

Activity 15-1. Injury Identification

C. Right periorbital ecchymosis

D. Laceration over infraorbital notch (associated with the injury to infraorbital nerve, causing numbness over the right cheek)

E. Ligature mark (from collar of shirt)

F. Nondisplaced nasal fracture

G. Soft tissue swelling, right cheek

H. Right orbital floor "blowout" fracture

I. Blood in right maxillary sinus

J. Contusion, right ear

K. 1 cm x 1 cm contusions, likely caused by fingertips

L. Ecchymosis associated with ulnar styloid fracture

Activity 15-2. Assessment

— Use patient-friendly, nonmedical language when evaluating the patient (eg, difficulty breathing, swallowing, or talking).

— What was the method of strangulation (eg, 1 hand, 2 hands, ligature)?

— What were the symptoms of strangulation (eg, loss of consciousness, light-headedness, other neurologic symptoms)?

— Is there any neck pain (now or after strangulation)?

— Is there any difficulty breathing (now or after strangulation)?

— Are there any changes in the patient's voice (now or after strangulation)?

— Are there any changes in vision (now or after strangulation)?

— Does the patient have any difficulty swallowing (now or after strangulation)?

— Does the patient have any pain or bleeding (now or after strangulation)?

— Was there any incontinence of the bowel or bladder? Did the patient change clothes before coming in?

— What are notable characteristics of the patient's behavior and demeanor (eg, flat affect, looking away) and short-term memory?

— How long did the strangulation last (best estimate by patient)? What was the pressure on a scale of 0 to 10?

Activity 15-3. Physical Assessment

— Neurologic checks (eg, full cranial nerve assessment, cervical nerves in upper body, strength)

— Skin assessment for petechial hemorrhages (eg, conjunctiva, retinal splinter hemorrhages, scalp, ears)

— Speech assessment (eg, for clarity, slurring, hoarseness)

— Memory assessment (eg, orientation, sensory memory, recent and remote memory questions)

— Strength assessment and balance (eg, hands, jaws, squint)

— Assessment of oral cavity for tears to frenulum, bruising to buccal mucosa, petechiae, tongue, uvula midline, symmetrical smile, and other injuries

— Assessment for previous head injury

— Danger Assessment (eg, previous physical assaults, suicidal ideation and attempts, previous strangulation)

— Pulse oximetry reading

— Head-to-toe assessment, including checking and palpating abdomen

— Peripheral vision test and 6 cardinal fields of gaze

Activity 15-4. Evidence Collection

— Use evidence collection kit for *nonfatal strangulation*, as stated by the patient or implied by the history. Kit should include a reference standard of the patient's DNA from the uninjured buccal area (if injury is present, consider drawing blood for DNA). Swab skin over contusions, fingernails, sides of face, and ears.

— Document the history given by the patient, using quotation marks for the patient's exact words.

— Assess and inspect specific anatomic locations for visible injury and pain on palpation.

— Photograph and measure, documenting all injuries, bruises, and areas the patient notes as painful. All photographs should be taken with and without an ABFO ruler.

— Photograph the 9 diagnostic positions of gaze of the eyes, including the inner aspects of the upper and lower lids.

— Take multiple photographs at 90-degree angles, 360 degrees around the neck.

— Inspect and photograph the oral cavity, including the inner cheeks, hard palate, soft palate, uvula, and oropharynx, for petechiae or other injury.

— Inspect and photograph the ears, including anterior and posterior. Initial injury, unless it involves dermal capillary injury, may not be visible but over time may surface, allowing for reassessment and documentation.

— For reference (a baseline), measure and mark the neck's circumference at present and at follow-up in 72 hours to 14 days.

— Some programs use an ALS light to scan the neck for substances and to highlight injury. At this time, research does not support that ALS light identifies bruising; however, invert filters may identify bruises. More research is necessary to determine the usefulness of both methods. An ALS light can be used to identify substances.

— Photograph the hands using the size mat available on the SDFI website, taking note of the fingernails and any injuries. The advantage of using a size mat is to measure the size and angle of the photographs.

Activity 15-5. Treatment and Care

— The results of the physical examination are consistent with the history of the assault provided by the patient.

— Apply ice indirectly to the neck (eg, cloth or towel barrier between ice and skin) to reduce swelling as tolerated.

— Prepare the patient for radiographic studies.

— Discuss safety planning with the patient.

— Recommend medical observation for 12 to 23 hours, with continuous monitoring of pulse oximetry and vital signs as needed.

— Assess if the patient has a safe place to go after examination and discharge, and if not, involve the advocate or social services as necessary.

— The forensic nurse refers the patient to a community partner (eg, advocate, YWCA, other locally identified agencies) for shelter and victim of crime application.

— Victim advocate offers to assist in obtaining or referring for restraining order protection, if needed. The forensic nurse provides information to the patient and supports their decision about the order of protection.

— Provide a Danger Assessment and discuss the results with the patient, being transparent about the evidence-based risk assessment (eg, "The results reflect a population of persons and may not apply to you as an individual. However, these results can inform your decision about your situation.").

— Depending on jurisdictional mandated reporting laws, report to police or notify the agency within the jurisdiction if the patient requests law enforcement involvement. (Failure to report when mandatory may result in legal action against the nurse and/or health care provider.)

— Discuss findings with the patient and provide patient-specific strangulation discharge information, such as detailed instructions to return to the ED if neurologic signs or symptoms, dyspnea, dysphonia, odynophagia, or seizures develop or worsen. Provide written instructions if the patient feels comfortable taking them with her. Discuss the possibility of a lifetime increased risk of neurologic consequences.

— Schedule follow-up forensic examination for 72 hours to 14 days after assault for additional medical forensic evaluation if possible within the framework of your program.

— Assess patient access to primary provider care or clinic care for follow-up in 14 days.

Activity 15-6 Lethality Assessment

Indicators of escalating danger include the following:

— Increase in frequency or severity of the assaults

— Increase of new threats of homicide or suicide

— Threats to children present in the home

— Presence of a firearm or deadly weapon in the home

Questions to assess immediate risk of violence include the following. Patients who answer "yes" to at least 3 of the following questions may be at especially high immediate risk of violence.

— Has the physical violence happened more often or gotten worse over the past 6 months?

— Has your partner ever used a weapon or threatened you with a weapon?

— Has your partner ever tried to strangle you?

— Do you believe your partner could kill you?

— Has your partner ever beaten you when you were pregnant?

— Is your partner violently and constantly jealous of you?

— Do you feel unsafe in your home?

www.ingramcontent.com/pod-product-compliance
Lightning Source LLC
LaVergne TN
LVHW070909210926
848482LV00017B/1031